ECG in the Child and Adolescent

NORMAL STANDARDS AND PERCENTILE CHARTS

ECG in the Child and Adolescent

NORMAL STANDARDS AND PERCENTILE CHARTS

Hung-Chi Lue, M.D., Ph.D., F.A.C.C., F.C.C.P.
Attending Pediatric Cardiologist and Physician-in-Chief,
Min-Sheng General Hospital; *and* Emeritus Professor of Pediatrics,
College of Medicine, National Taiwan University

WITH THE COLLABORATION OF

Yung-Chang Lai, M.D.
Mei-Hwan Wu, M.D., Ph.D., F.A.C.C.
Jou-Kou Wang, M.D., Ph.D.
Ming-Lon Young, M.D., M.P.H.
Yung-Ching Chang, M.D.
Shu-Jen Yeh, M.D.
Jiuann-Huey Lin, M.D.

Blackwell
Futura

Blackwell Futura is an imprint of Blackwell Publishing

Blackwell Publishing, Inc., 350 Main Street, Malden, Massachusetts 02148-5020, USA
Blackwell Publishing Ltd, 9600 Garsington Road, Oxford OX4 2DQ, UK
Blackwell Science Asia Pty Ltd, 550 Swanston Street, Carlton, Victoria 3053, Australia

First published 2006

1 2006

ISBN-13: 978-1-4051-5899-2
ISBN-10: 1-4051-5899-9

Library of Congress Cataloguing-in-Publication Data

Lue, Hung-Chi, 1931–
ECG in the child and adolescent : normal standards and percentile charts / Hung-Chi Lue ; with the collaboration of Yung-Chang Lai ... [et al.].
p. ; cm.
Includes bibliographical references.
ISBN-13: 978-1-4051-5899-2 (hardcover : alk. paper)
ISBN-10: 1-4051-5899-9 (hardcover : alk. paper)
1. Pediatric cardiology—Standards—Tables. 2. Electrocardiography—Interpretation—Tables. I. Lai, Yung-Chang. II. Title.
[DNLM: 1. Electrocardiography—standards—Tables. 2. Adolescent. 3. Child. 4. Infant. WS 16 L948e 2007]
RJ423.5.E43L84 2007
618.92'12—dc22

2006014415

A catalogue record for this title is available from the British Library

Acquisitions: Gina Almond
Development: Fiona Pattison
Set in Palatino 9.5pt/12pt by TechBooks

For further information on Blackwell Publishing, visit our website:
www.blackwellfutura.com

The publisher's policy is to use permanent paper from mills that operate a sustainable forestry policy, and which has been manufactured from pulp processed using acid-free and elementary chlorine-free practices. Furthermore, the publisher ensures that the text paper and cover board used have met acceptable environmental accreditation standards.

Contents

Preface

Electrocardiograms (ECGs) are the graphic representation of body surface potential differences generated by the electrical activity of the heart. Bipolar limb leads, augmented unipolar limb leads and precordial leads have been used routinely for recording the ECG, which remains an essential part of the cardiac examination, even after the advent of cardiac catheterization, angiocardiography, echocardiography and many other sophisticated diagnostic modalities.

Fundamental changes in circulation occur immediately after birth, followed by typical and characteristic changes in physiology, position and size of the cardiac chambers relative to the body, throughout infancy, childhood and adolescence. Normal adult values are abnormal in children. Likewise, many of the normal pediatric values are abnormal in the adult. Studies on the developing ECGs reflecting these changes in the healthy pediatric population are of utmost importance, but are still few and limited. Reliable normal standards for P-QRS-T wave intervals and amplitudes are needed as the reference for the diagnosis and evaluation of children with heart disease. Traditionally, normal ECG values in the pediatric population were derived from those published by Ziegler RF (1951) and Davignon *et al.* (1979). We found that the available interpretation packages were inadequate, and not easy to use.

Normal ECG standards for infants, children and adolescents provide not only the reference for physicians in their daily practice of ECG reading, but also provide the database for the study of growing and developing heart and for the computer-assisted electrocardiography analysis. To establish such a set of normal ECG standards and percentile charts in the young in 1995, we started to collect and analyse the electrocardiographic data from healthy newborns, infants, children and adolescents.

Thanks must go to Drs. Y. C. Lai, M. H. Wu, J. K. Wang, M. L. Young, Y. C. Chang, S. J. Yeh, J. H. Lin, and Ms. S. C. Lin together with her team of technicians, who collaborated in this study. Without their efforts collection of the ECGs for analysis of normal standards and percentile charts would not have been possible. The author is grateful to Dr. W. Y. Shau for his advice in the statistical analysis of the normative data, and also to Ms. Renee Shen for her secretarial work.

The author is grateful to the Fukuda Denshi for providing us the FCP-4301 Electrocardiograph with a 500 Hz acquisition program, as recommended by the American Heart Association. Last but not least, the author is grateful to Blackwell Publishing for their efforts in editing and printing.

Hung-Chi Lue

Preface

Foreword

One of the most tedious and often unrewarding tasks in medical investigation is obtaining massive normative data on a general population, so that normal standards can be made available to physicians throughout the world. Dr. Hung-Chi Lue and his colleagues have completed a monumental effort of gathering electrocardiographic data on over 1,800 normal infants, children and adolescents, and they have produced a unique monograph which provides normal standards and percentile charts. These published tables will undoubtedly be the basis for comparing values obtained from all components of electrocardiograms on pediatric cardiac patients to the normal range of measurements. These data also should be the basis for the development of valid computer analyses of pediatric electrocardiograms; the present interpretation packages being woefully inadequate.

Although the morphologic diagnostic aspects of electrocardiography have less impact in the modern era because of the advent of echocardiography, the electrocardiogram is vital for the diagnosis and evaluation of patients with cardiac rhythm disorders. Reliable standards for P-QRS-T wave intervals are required to evaluate children with tachyarrhythmias, bradyarrhythmias, first, second, and third degree heart block, WPW, and long QT syndromes.

The format is an especially attractive feature of this monograph. The authors provide 95th and 5th percentile data for all interval and amplitude measurements for all ages, giving access to the limits of normality, so that data from an individual patient can be quickly interpreted in terms of comparison to the general population. The easy-to-use tables will result in data being accessed more often by clinicians and investigators in the field.

This monograph will be especially helpful to those who teach pediatric electrocardiography to medical students, residents, and pediatric cardiology fellows. Many of the teaching points regarding the diagnosis of left, right, and biventricular hypertrophy at various stages, in terms of what is abnormal amplitude of Q, R and S waves as well as RS ratios in the right and left precordial leads, can now be validated (or invalidated), on the basis of this extensive data base for normals.

Those of us in pediatric cardiology owe a debt of thanks to Dr. Lue and his associates for collecting this data, analyzing the material by age groups, and presenting the results in table form which is so easily accessible. The painstakingly careful methodology and large patient population gives us confidence in the reliability of this database, which I hope will be used for the development of accurate computer analyses of pediatric ECG's. Dr. Hung-Chi Lue has made so many contributions to pediatric cardiology that the success of this endeavor is to be expected. He is an international leader in our field, and the widespread use of this reference manual by his colleagues throughout the world will be another milestone in his outstanding career.

Welton M. Gersony, M.D.
Alexander S. Nadas Professor of Pediatrics
College of Physicians and Surgeons
Columbia University

At the beginning of the twenty-first century, pediatric cardiologists face a uniquely different situation than half a century ago. The diagnostic tools and therapeutic methods available today were almost unimaginable then. Even thinking back only several decades to the days when a combination of the physical examination, the chest roentgenogram, and the electrocardiogram were all that was available to assist in the outpatient clinic and subsequently to the time when physiologic and anatomic data obtained in the catheterization laboratory became more completely understood, the cardiologist today fully appreciates these practical clinical advantages.

Unfortunately, for many present day physicians and students alike, there is a feeling that these valuable diagnostic implements have fully given way to the newer tools such as echocardiography. This is obviously unwarranted.

Important practical clinical information and understanding are made available by the electrocardiographic examination. Of particular importance to both pediatricians and pediatric cardiologists, however, is the fact that the electrocardiogram varies so extensively with the age of the patient. Understanding this has been an issue since the ECG began to be used in pediatric patients and continued later when the difficulties were even more problematic at the time when computerization of pediatric electrocardiography was initially undertaken.

The ECG has stood the test of time and, in contrast to the phonocardiogram, remains important to the cardiologist each and every day. To assist in the implementation of this clinical tool, Professor Hung-Chi Lue has created an impressive and inclusive database showing what is normal and what is not. The careful electrocardiographic examination of almost two-thousand youngsters has provided new and valuable categorized information.

It should not be surprising that Professor Lue has successfully undertaken and completed this gigantic task. As one of the world's leaders in so many aspects of pediatric cardiology, Dr. Lue's continuing contributions – again and again – have been recognized and favorably received not only by the international medical community, but also by his peers in pediatric cardiology. No doubt this book will be equally well received because of the extraordinary detail with which he has displayed these unique data in a clinically usable format.

Professor Hung-Chi Lue is to be congratulated for this effort which will be used by clinicians around the world.

Edward L. Kaplan, M.D.
Professor of Pediatrics
University of Minnesota Medical School

Introduction

The study population consisted of 1884 healthy newborns, infants, children and adolescents enrolled from nurseries, well-baby clinics, kindergartens, and elementary and secondary schools. All children were screened by a specially designed questionnaire, then examined on supine position by a pediatrician, and checked by a pediatric cardiologist. Age was expressed as days, months and years attained at the last birthday. They were divided into twelve age groups: newborns aged less than 1 day, 1–3 days, 3–7 days, and 7–30 days; infants aged 1–3 months, 3–6 months, and 6–12 months; children of 1–3 years, 3–6 years, 6–9 years, 9–13 years and adolescents, 13–18 years.

Appropriate ECG electrodes were placed with no electrical contact between adjacent electrodes to minimize the short-range age-independent ECG variation. ECG was recorded on standardized paper with a stylus, at 10 mm/mV paper speed of 25mm/s, at rest and on supine position. For large amplitude complexes, the half-standard (5 mm/mV) was used. Acquisition of ECG database was performed by an automatic ECG analysis and management program using a Fukuda Denshi FCP-4301 Floppy Utility, Reference MS-DOS/IBM-AT, ECG machine. A 12 lead conventional ECG was taken. Lead V3R was not taken. Analog-to-digital conversion was performed by Fukuda signal acquisition module. The analog potential was digitalized into 5-UV units at a sampling rate of 500 Hz (once every 2 milliseconds). The percentile charts for age were constructed with a variable span smoother (Friedman, 1984).

Morphology measurements were made from the median voltages of the identical P-QRS-T cycles representative of a normal complex selected by the above mentioned analysis program. Amplitude measurements were made using the PR segment as reference for the baseline. The onsets and offsets of the P, QRS, and T were determined by an analysis of the simultaneous slopes in all 12 leads from the earliest onset in any lead to the latest deflection in any lead.

Visual verification using a magnifier and appropriate lighting was systematically performed, by a fellow in pediatric cardiology and an attending cardiologist, on all electrocardiograms in the upper and lower 5th percentile in each age group, with measurements made to the nearest 0.1 mm. In instances of computer wave-recognition errors and of more than 10% differences between visual and computer measurements, the visually determined value was substituted in the data file.

The following ECG parameters were obtained: heart rate, PR interval, QT interval, QTc, QRS duration, RR interval, P-QRS-T axes, P amplitude, Q amplitude, R amplitude, S amplitude, T amplitude and ventricular activation time.

A total of 117 to 125 records, with noises, baseline drifting, bundle branch blocks, WPW, extrasystoles and ECG rhythms other than sinus rhythm detected by computer and verified by one cardiologist and the author were excluded from the data file.

The relation between ECG wave amplitudes and durations, as well as some other ECG indices, (heart rate, age), commonly used in pediatric cardiology were calculated. The normal standards for each age group, including the number of subjects analyzed, the mean and standard deviation and the 95th and 5th percentile values of the variables were listed in tables, and the 5th, 25th, 50th, 75th and 95th values were illustrated in percentile format charts.

How to use this book

The electrocardiogram varies extensively with the age of patients. Easy to use tables and charts of heart rate, duration, interval, axis, amplitude, and calculated values by age provided in this book may help the clinicians and investigators to:

1 Learn the characteristic ECG changes along with the growth and development of infants and children to adolescence. This can be readily recognized at a glance over the percentile charts and the corresponding tables.

2 Find the normal standards of ECG tracings in the young. The mean (± SD) and the limits (5th and 95th percentile) of normality in twelve age groups are provided.

3 Compare the ECG tracings recorded from an individual with the data in this book, thus helping make the assessment and interpretation.

References

Bailey JJ, Berson AS, Garson A Jr, Horan LG, Macfarlane PW, Mortara DW, Zywietz C. (1990) Recommendations for standardization and specifications in automated electrocardigraphy: Band width and digital signal processing. *Circulation* **81**: 730–9.

Davignon A, Rautaharju P, Boisselle E, Soumis F, Megelas M, Choquette A. (1979) Normal ECG standards for infants and children. *Pediatr Cardiol* **1**: 123–52.

Friedman JH. (1984) A Variable Span Smoother. Tech. Rep. No. 5, Laboratory for Computational Statistics, Dept. of Statistics, Stanford Univ., California.

New York Heart Association. (1953) Nomenclature and Criteria for Diagnosis of Diseases of the Heart and Blood Vessels. New York Heart Assoc., New York.

Rijnbeek PR, Witsenburg M. Schrama E, Hess J, Kors JA. (2001) New normal limits for the paediatric electrocardiogram. *Eur Heart J* **22**: 702–11.

Schwartz PJ, Garson A, Jr. Paul T, Stramba-Badiale M, Vetter JL, Villain E, Wren C. (2002) Guidelines for the interpretation of the neonatal electrocardiogram. *Eur Heart J* **23**: 1329–44.

Ziegler RF. (1951) Electrographic Studies in Normal Infants and Children. Charles C Thomas, Springfield, Ill.

PART 1

Heart rate, P-QRS-T interval and duration by age

Heart rate by age

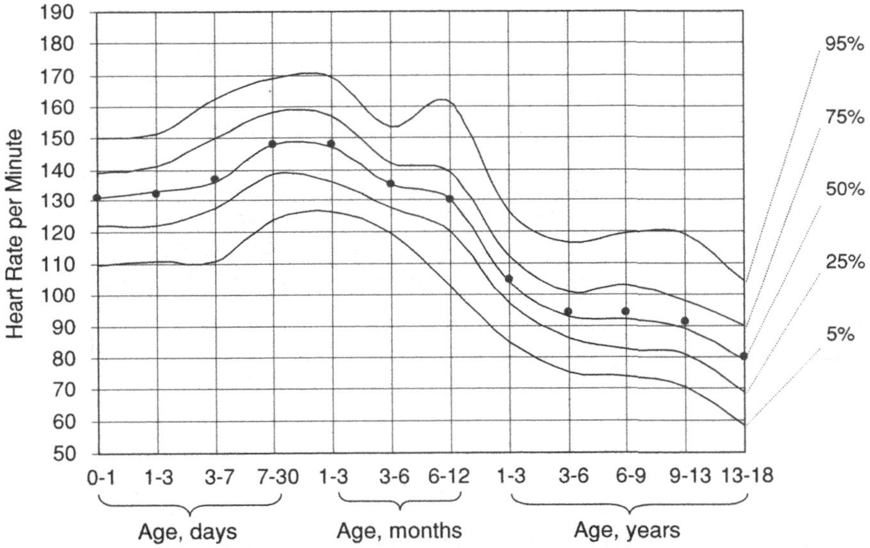

Figure 1.1 Heart rate by age, each curve corresponding to the indicated percentile level (• = mean). Striking changes in heart rate are noted from newborn to adolescence. The heart rate increases from birth to ages 7–30, days and 1–3 months. From that age forward, the heart rate decreases with increasing age, most rapidly from age 6–12 months to 1–3 years.

	Days				*Months*			*Years*				
Age	*0–1*	*1–3*	*3–7*	*7–30*	*1–3*	*3–6*	*6–12*	*1–3*	*3–6*	*6–9*	*9–13*	*13–18*
95%	150	152	163	169	169	154	161	126	117	119	119	105
Mean	**131**	**132**	**137**	**148**	**148**	**135**	**130**	**105**	**94**	**94**	**91**	**80**
(±SD)	**12.86**	**13.07**	**15.91**	**15.58**	**14.66**	**11.70**	**18.67**	**13.09**	**11.96**	**14.68**	**14.08**	**14.50**
5%	109	111	111	124	126	120	103	85	75	74	70	58
(N)	109	128	95	100	113	91	97	113	107	99	289	510

PR interval by age

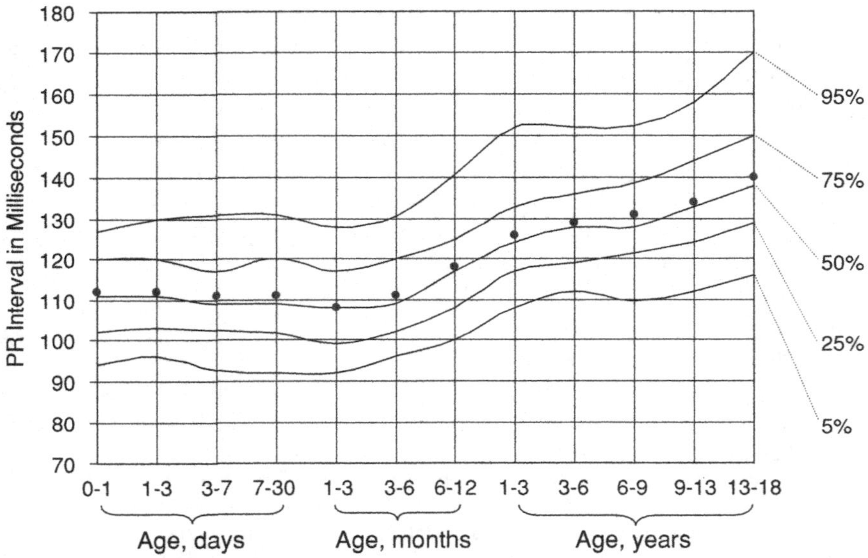

Figure 1.2 PR interval by age, each curve corresponding to the indicated percentile level (• = mean). The PR interval remains little changed after birth and during early infancy. It increases with increasing age, from age 6 months through to adolescence.

	Days				*Months*			*Years*				
Age	*0–1*	*1–3*	*3–7*	*7–30*	*1–3*	*3–6*	*6–12*	*1–3*	*3–6*	*6–9*	*9–13*	*13–18*
95%	127	130	131	131	128	131	140	152	152	152	158	170
Mean	**112**	**112**	**111**	**111**	**108**	**111**	**118**	**126**	**129**	**131**	**134**	**140**
(±SD)	**10.65**	**11.54**	**12.65**	**13.48**	**11.81**	**11.36**	**12.93**	**10.85**	**10.56**	**14.52**	**17.35**	**17.94**
5%	94	96	93	92	92	96	100	108	112	110	112	116
(N)	109	128	95	100	113	91	97	113	107	99	289	510

PR interval by heart rate

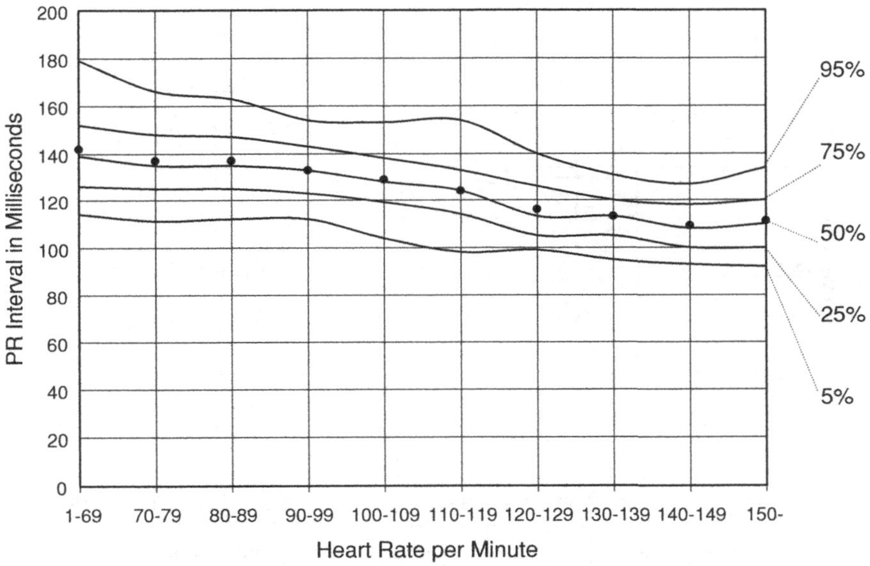

Figure 1.3 PR Interval by heart rate, each curve corresponding to the indicated percentile level (• = mean). The PR interval decreases slightly along with increasing heart rate during the entire pediatric ages.

Heart rate	*1–69*	*70–79*	*80–89*	*90–99*	*100–109*	*110–119*	*120–129*	*130–139*	*140–149*	*150–*
95%	179	166	163	154	153	154	140	131	127	134
Mean	**142**	**137**	**137**	**133**	**129**	**124**	**116**	**113**	**109**	**111**
(±SD)	**21.54**	**18.53**	**15.96**	**13.71**	**14.91**	**17.48**	**14.94**	**0.00**	**0.00**	**0.00**
5%	114	111	112	112	104	98	99	95	93	92
(N)	143	206	274	247	178	127	174	200	158	177

CHAPTER 1.4

QT interval by age

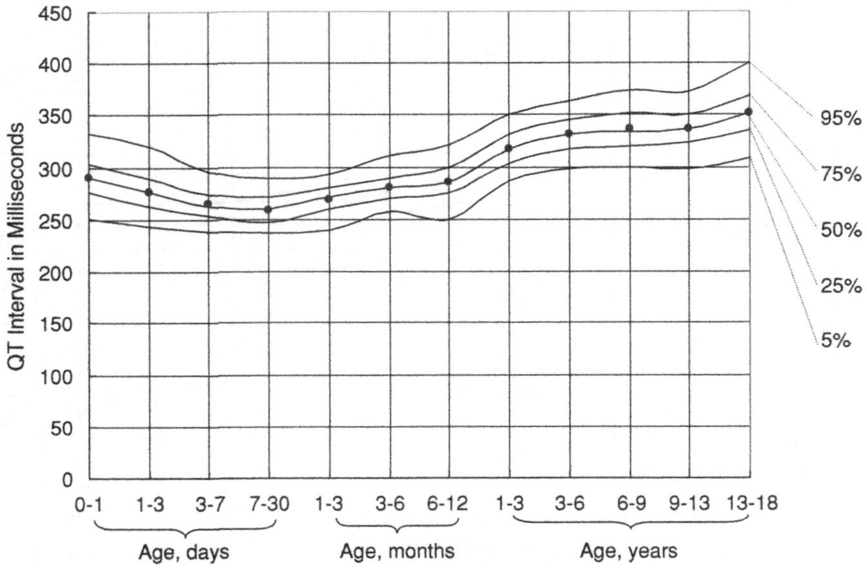

Figure 1.4 QT interval by age, each curve corresponding to the indicated percentile level (• = mean). The QT interval decreases slightly after birth, reaching the lowest at age 7–30 days. From that age forward, the QT interval increases along with increasing age up to adolescence.

	Days				*Months*			*Years*				
Age	*0–1*	*1–3*	*3–7*	*7–30*	*1–3*	*3–6*	*6–12*	*1–3*	*3–6*	*6–9*	*9–13*	*13–18*
95%	333	320	296	289	293	311	321	350	363	373	372	400
Mean	**291**	**277**	**265**	**259**	**269**	**281**	**285**	**318**	**331**	**336**	**337**	**352**
(±SD)	**26.63**	**23.09**	**17.92**	**17.85**	**18.90**	**15.95**	**23.81**	**21.69**	**21.11**	**23.41**	**26.02**	**27.00**
5%	251	244	239	237	240	258	249	287	298	300	298	309
(N)	109	128	95	100	113	91	97	113	107	99	289	510

QT interval by heart rate

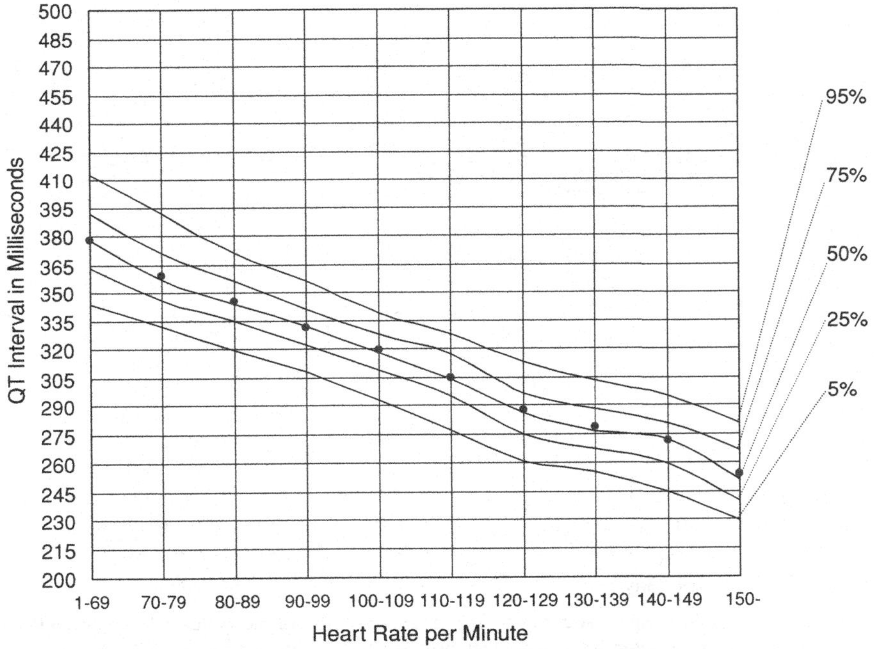

Figure 1.5 QT interval by heart rate, each curve corresponding to the indicated percentile level (• = mean). The QT interval decreases in striking accordance with the increasing heart rate.

Heart rate	*1–69*	*70–79*	*80–89*	*90–99*	*100–109*	*110–119*	*120–129*	*130–139*	*140–149*	*150–*
95%	413	392	371	356	339	328	313	303	295	280
Mean	**378**	**359**	**345**	**331**	**319**	**305**	**287**	**278**	**271**	**254**
(±SD)	**21.54**	**17.50**	**15.46**	**14.51**	**15.18**	**16.39**	**15.61**	**0.00**	**0.00**	**0.00**
5%	344	332	319	308	293	277	261	255	245	229
(N)	143	206	274	247	178	127	174	200	158	177

QTc interval by age

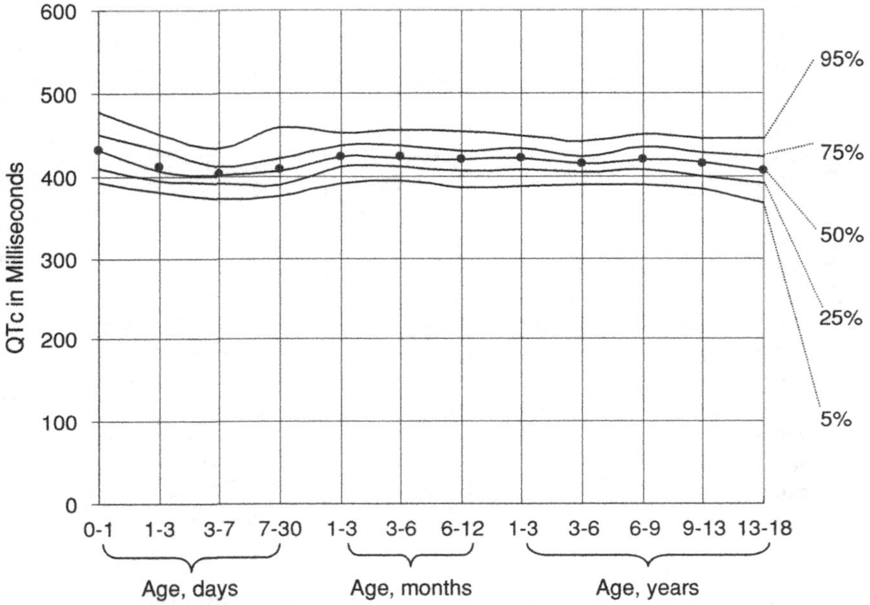

Figure 1.6 QTc interval by age, each curve corresponding to the indicated percentile level (• = mean). The corrected QT interval decreases slightly after birth, and returns to the previous level by age 1–3 months, then remains unchanged until adolescence.

	Days				*Months*			*Years*				
Age	*0–1*	*1–3*	*3–7*	*7–30*	*1–3*	*3–6*	*6–12*	*1–3*	*3–6*	*6–9*	*9–13*	*13–18*
95%	478	451	434	459	452	455	453	449	442	450	445	446
Mean	**431**	**412**	**402**	**408**	**423**	**424**	**419**	**421**	**415**	**420**	**415**	**407**
(±SD)	**26.44**	**23.09**	**19.15**	**25.15**	**20.56**	**17.50**	**20.17**	**16.27**	**15.83**	**18.09**	**17.35**	**23.52**
5%	392	380	372	375	391	395	386	388	389	390	384	367
(N)	109	128	95	100	113	91	97	113	107	99	289	510

QTc interval by heart rate

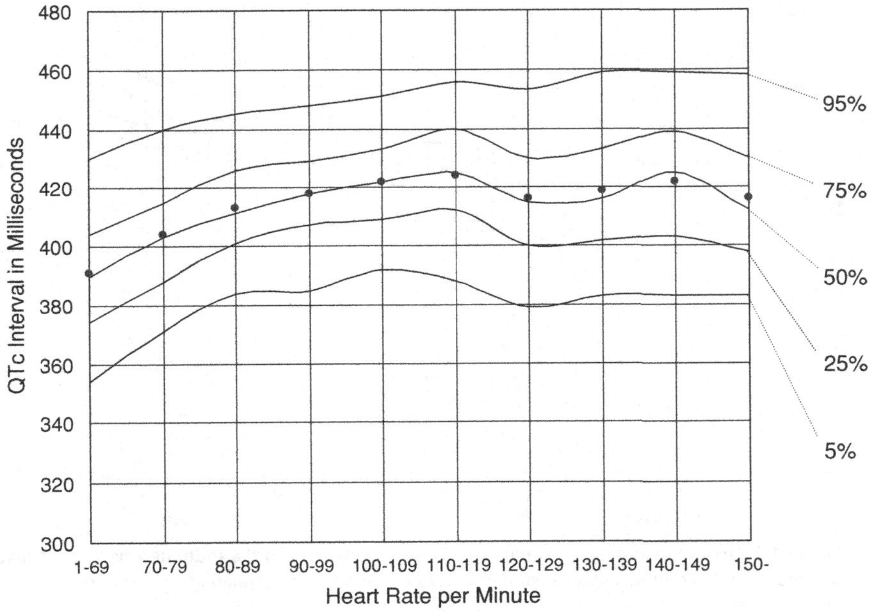

Figure 1.7 QTc interval by heart rate, each curve corresponding to the indicated percentile level (• = mean). The corrected QT interval increases slightly and steadily with increasing heart rate up to a rate of 110–119 per minute, then remains little or unchanged.

Heart rate	*1–69*	*70–79*	*80–89*	*90–99*	*100–109*	*110–119*	*120–129*	*130–139*	*140–149*	*150–*
95%	430	440	445	448	451	456	453	459	459	458
Mean	**391**	**404**	**413**	**418**	**422**	**424**	**416**	**419**	**422**	**416**
(±SD)	**22.76**	**19.70**	**17.90**	**18.44**	**19.74**	**22.19**	**21.81**	**0.00**	**0.00**	**0.00**
5%	354	371	384	385	392	388	379	383	383	383
(N)	143	206	274	247	178	127	174	200	158	177

CHAPTER 1.8

QRS duration by age

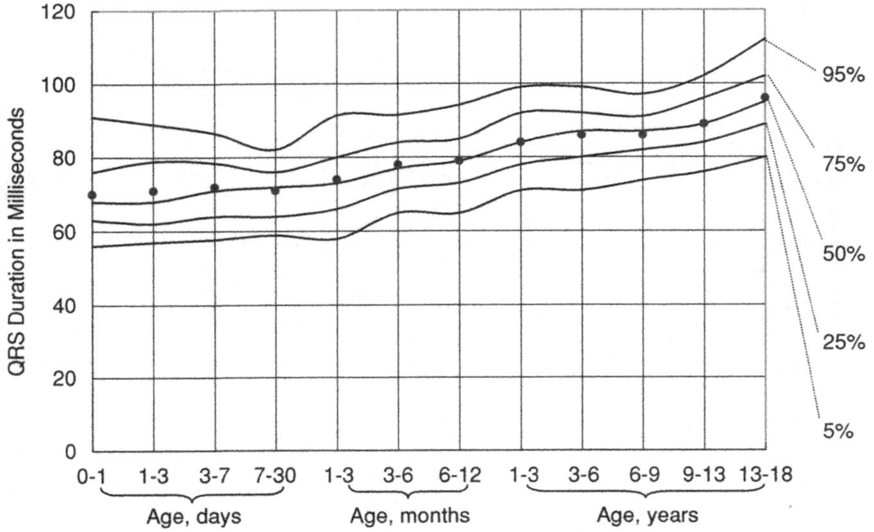

Figure 1.8 QRS duration by age, each curve corresponding to the indicated percentile level (• = mean). QRS duration steadily and gradually increases with increasing age, from birth to adolescence.

	Days				*Months*			*Years*				
Age	*0–1*	*1–3*	*3–7*	*7–30*	*1–3*	*3–6*	*6–12*	*1–3*	*3–6*	*6–9*	*9–13*	*13–18*
95%	91	89	87	82	91	92	94	99	99	97	102	112
Mean	**70**	**71**	**72**	**71**	**74**	**78**	**79**	**84**	**86**	**86**	**89**	**96**
(±SD)	**10.65**	**11.54**	**9.44**	8.06	**10.55**	**8.31**	**9.04**	**10.85**	**10.56**	**7.53**	**8.67**	**9.85**
5%	56	57	58	59	58	65	65	71	71	74	76	80
(N)	109	128	95	100	113	91	97	113	107	99	289	510

RR interval by age

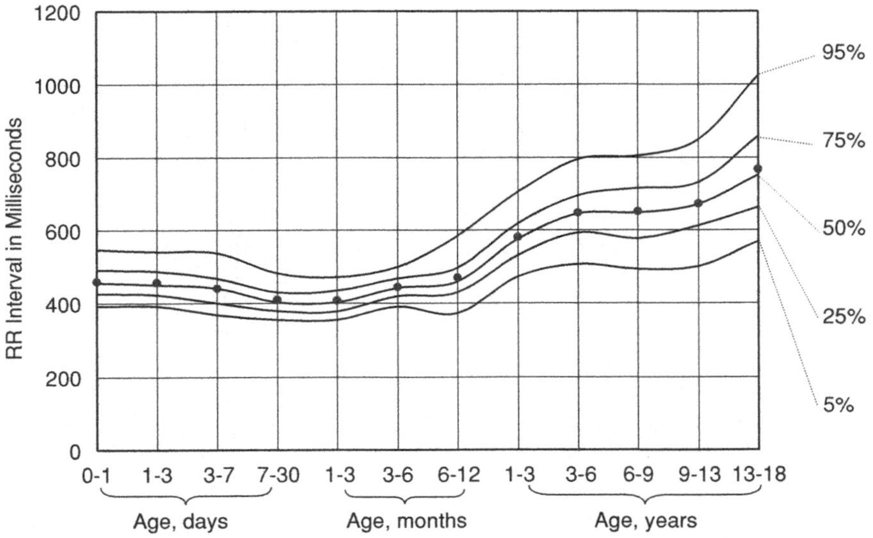

Figure 1.9 RR interval by age, each curve corresponding to the indicated percentile level (• = mean). The RR interval decreases slightly from birth to ages 7–30 days and 1–3 months. From that age forward, the RR interval increases with a wider range along with increasing age until adolescence.

	Days				*Months*			*Years*				
Age	*0–1*	*1–3*	*3–7*	*7–30*	*1–3*	*3–6*	*6–12*	*1–3*	*3–6*	*6–9*	*9–13*	*13–18*
95%	547	541	537	483	472	500	583	705	795	805	849	1023
Mean	**460**	**458**	**441**	**410**	**407**	**445**	**471**	**580**	**646**	**650**	**672**	**767**
(±SD)	**47.94**	**46.18**	**53.46**	**48.33**	**40.57**	**37.92**	**71.09**	**75.93**	**79.16**	**96.94**	**95.41**	**138.81**
5%	391	391	368	354	354	390	372	473	507	494	501	568
(N)	109	128	95	100	120	92	97	113	107	100	289	514

PART 2

Frontal plane P-QRS-T axis by age

CHAPTER 2.1

Frontal plane P axis by age

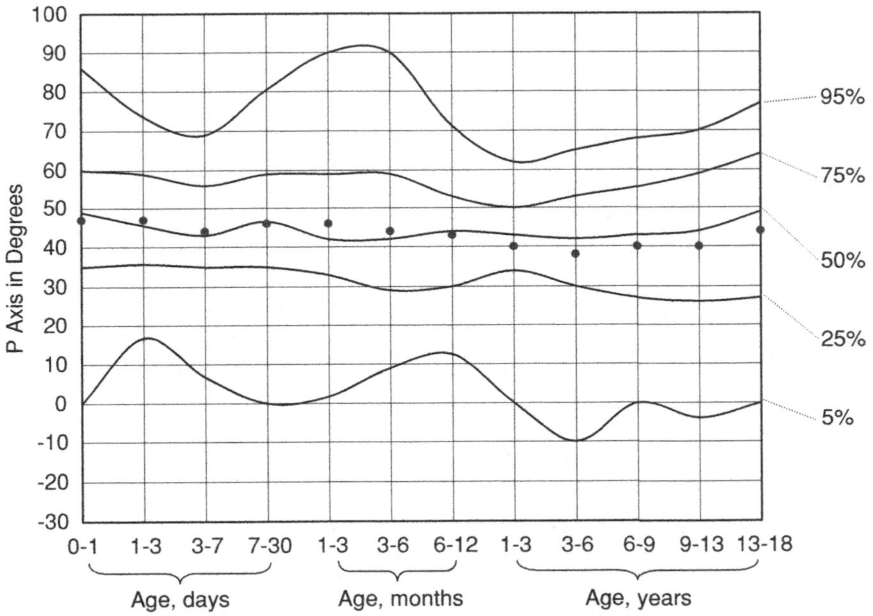

Figure 2.1 Frontal plane P axis by age, each curve corresponding to the indicated percentile level (• = mean). From newborn to adolescence, the frontal plane P axes, as in adults, direct constantly to the left and inferiorly between zero and 90 degrees.

	Days				*Months*			*Years*				
Age	*0–1*	*1–3*	*3–7*	*7–30*	*1–3*	*3–6*	*6–12*	*1–3*	*3–6*	*6–9*	*9–13*	*13–18*
95%	86	74	69	81	90	90	71	62	65	68	70	77
Mean	**47**	**47**	**44**	**46**	**46**	**44**	**43**	**40**	**38**	**40**	**40**	**44**
(±SD)	**22.24**	**17.05**	**18.15**	**24.79**	**25.13**	**27.16**	**18.67**	**16.27**	**21.11**	**21.02**	**26.02**	**26.88**
5%	0	17	7	0	2	9	12	0	−10	0	−4	0
(N)	109	128	95	100	113	91	97	113	107	99	289	510

Frontal plane QRS axis by age

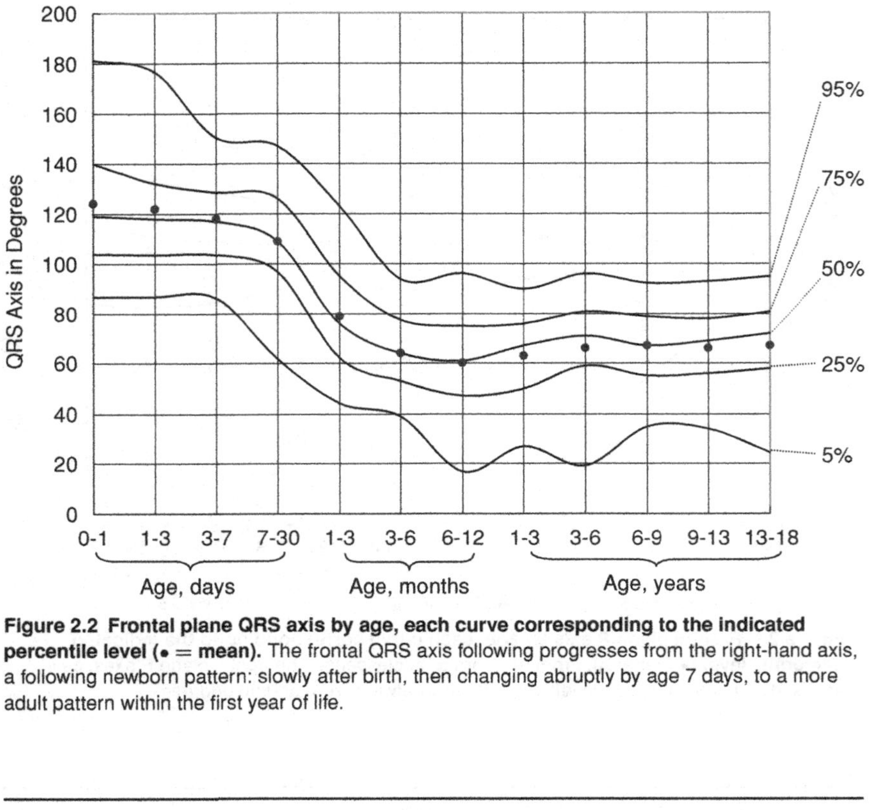

Figure 2.2 Frontal plane QRS axis by age, each curve corresponding to the indicated percentile level (• = mean). The frontal QRS axis following progresses from the right-hand axis, a following newborn pattern: slowly after birth, then changing abruptly by age 7 days, to a more adult pattern within the first year of life.

	Days				*Months*			*Years*				
Age	*0–1*	*1–3*	*3–7*	*7–30*	*1–3*	*3–6*	*6–12*	*1–3*	*3–6*	*6–9*	*9–13*	*13–18*
95%	181	177	150	147	123	94	96	90	96	92	93	95
Mean	**124**	**122**	**118**	**109**	**79**	**64**	**60**	**63**	**66**	**67**	**66**	**67**
(±SD)	**28.56**	**27.59**	**20.62**	**26.35**	**25.80**	**18.53**	**24.49**	**21.69**	**21.11**	**18.60**	**17.35**	**21.48**
5%	87	87	87	62	44	39	17	27	19	35	34	24
(N)	109	128	95	100	113	91	97	113	107	99	289	510

Frontal plane T axis by age

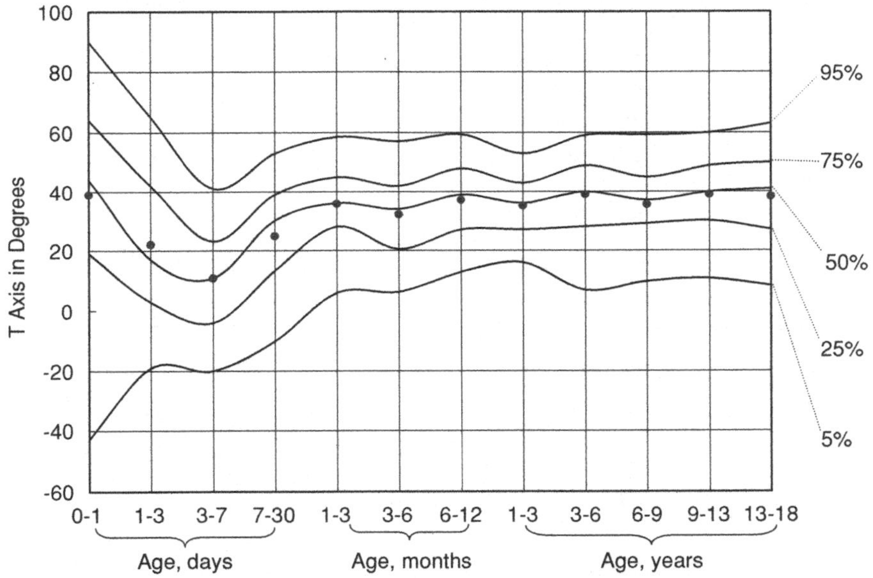

Figure 2.3 Frontal plane T axis by age, each curve corresponding to the indicated percentile level (• = mean). The frontal plane T wave axis abruptly changes from a wide range of T axis after birth, to a narrower range at age 3–7 days. The T axis moves back to the previous levels during the subsequent days, then reaching the adult pattern by age 3–6 years.

	Days				*Months*			*Years*				
Age	*0–1*	*1–3*	*3–7*	*7–30*	*1–3*	*3–6*	*6–12*	*1–3*	*3–6*	*6–9*	*9–13*	*13–18*
95%	90	65	41	53	58	57	59	53	59	59	60	63
Mean	**39**	**22**	**11**	**25**	**36**	**32**	**37**	**35**	**39**	**35**	**39**	**38**
(±SD)	**42.61**	**23.09**	**19.98**	**20.20**	**14.82**	**16.01**	**16.61**	**10.85**	**15.83**	**15.94**	**17.35**	**17.09**
5%	−43	−19	−20	−10	6	7	13	16	7	10	11	8
(N)	109	128	95	100	113	91	97	113	107	99	289	510

PART 3

P-QRS-T amplitude by age

CHAPTER 3.1

P amplitude by age in lead II

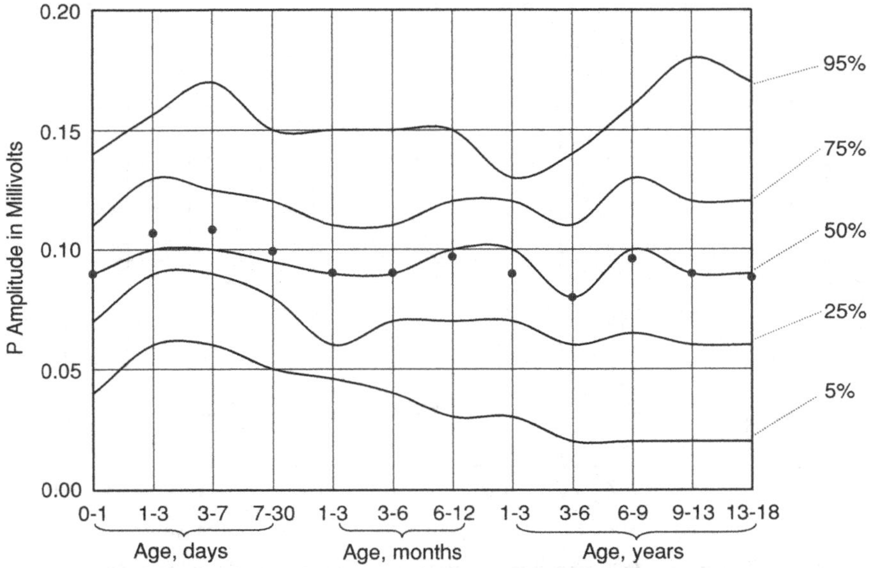

Figure 3.1 P amplitude by age in lead II, each curve corresponding to the indicated percentile level (• = mean). The mean of the P wave amplitudes in lead II of newborns to adolescents stays little changed, but a wider range of amplitudes is noted after the first year of life.

	Days				*Months*			*Years*				
Age	*0–1*	*1–3*	*3–7*	*7–30*	*1–3*	*3–6*	*6–12*	*1–3*	*3–6*	*6–9*	*9–13*	*13–18*
95%	0.14	0.16	0.17	0.15	0.15	0.15	0.15	0.13	0.14	0.16	0.18	0.17
Mean	**0.09**	**0.11**	**0.11**	**0.10**	**0.09**	**0.09**	**0.10**	**0.09**	**0.08**	**0.10**	**0.09**	**0.09**
(±SD)	**0.05**	**0.03**	**0.03**	**0.03**	**0.03**	**0.04**	**0.04**	**0.05**	**0.05**	**0.04**	**0.09**	**0.05**
5%	0.04	0.06	0.06	0.05	0.05	0.04	0.03	0.03	0.02	0.02	0.02	0.02
(N)	109	128	95	100	113	91	97	113	107	99	289	510

Q amplitude by age in lead I

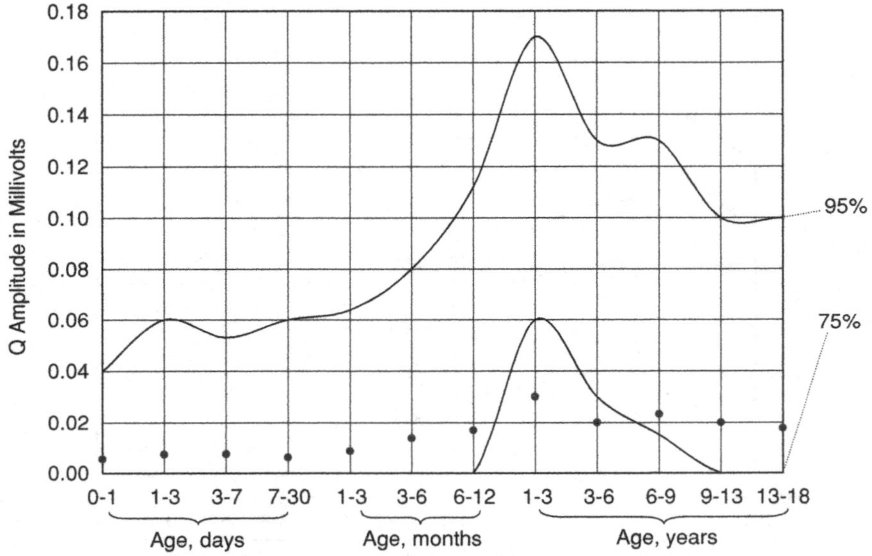

Figure 3.2 Q amplitude by age in lead I, each curve corresponding to the indicated percentile level (• = mean). Q waves in lead I are absent or small during infancy.

	Days				*Months*			*Years*				
Age	*0–1*	*1–3*	*3–7*	*7–30*	*1–3*	*3–6*	*6–12*	*1–3*	*3–6*	*6–9*	*9–13*	*13–18*
95%	0.04	0.06	0.05	0.06	0.06	0.08	0.11	0.17	0.13	0.13	0.10	0.10
Mean	**0.01**	**0.01**	**0.01**	**0.01**	**0.01**	**0.01**	**0.02**	**0.03**	**0.02**	**0.02**	**0.02**	**0.02**
(±SD)	**0.02**	**0.03**	**0.02**	**0.02**	**0.02**	**0.03**	**0.04**	**0.05**	**0.05**	**0.05**	**0.00**	**0.04**
5%	0	0	0	0	0	0	0	0	0	0	0	0
(N)	109	128	95	100	113	91	97	113	107	99	289	510

Q amplitude by age in lead II

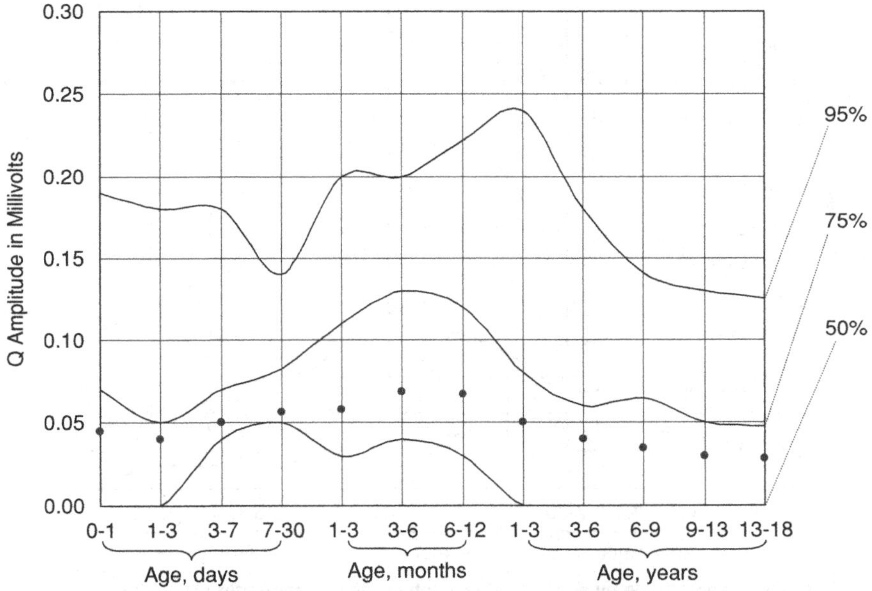

Figure 3.3 Q amplitude by age in lead II, each curve corresponding to the indicated percentile level (• = mean). Q waves in lead II are generally small or absent. The amplitude is relatively larger during ages 1–3 months, 3–6 months, 6–12 months and 1–3 years.

	Days				*Months*			*Years*				
Age	*0–1*	*1–3*	*3–7*	*7–30*	*1–3*	*3–6*	*6–12*	*1–3*	*3–6*	*6–9*	*9–13*	*13–18*
95%	0.19	0.18	0.18	0.14	0.20	0.20	0.22	0.24	0.18	0.14	0.13	0.13
Mean	**0.04**	**0.04**	**0.05**	**0.06**	**0.06**	**0.07**	**0.07**	**0.05**	**0.04**	**0.03**	**0.03**	**0.03**
(±SD)	**0.07**	**0.06**	**0.06**	**0.06**	**0.07**	**0.08**	**0.08**	**0.11**	**0.05**	**0.05**	**0.09**	**0.05**
5%	0	0	0	0	0	0	0	0	0	0	0	0
(N)	109	128	95	100	113	91	97	113	107	99	289	510

Q amplitude by age in lead III

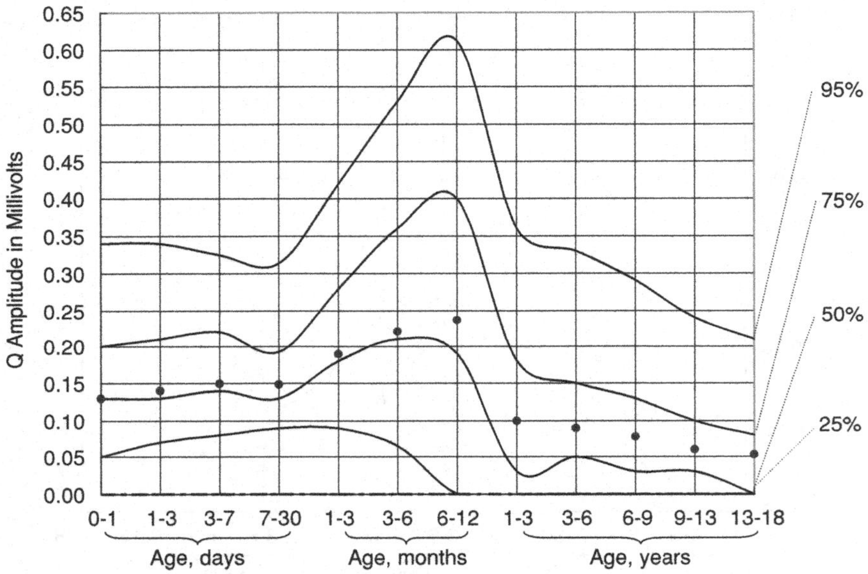

Figure 3.4 Q amplitude by age in lead III, each curve corresponding to the indicated percentile level (• = mean). Q waves in lead III are more prominent at ages 1–3 months, 3–6 months, and 6–12 months, with a deflection up to 6.1 mm.

	Days				*Months*			*Years*				
Age	*0–1*	*1–3*	*3–7*	*7–30*	*1–3*	*3–6*	*6–12*	*1–3*	*3–6*	*6–9*	*9–13*	*13–18*
95%	0.34	0.34	0.33	0.31	0.42	0.53	0.61	0.36	0.33	0.29	0.24	0.21
Mean	**0.13**	**0.14**	**0.15**	**0.15**	**0.19**	**0.22**	**0.24**	**0.1**	**0.09**	**0.08**	**0.06**	**0.05**
(±SD)	**0.11**	**0.12**	**0.10**	**0.10**	**0.14**	**0.17**	**0.22**	**0.11**	**0.11**	**0.11**	**0.09**	**0.07**
5%	0	0	0	0	0	0	0	0	0	0	0	0
(N)	109	128	95	100	113	91	97	113	107	99	289	510

Q amplitude by age in lead aVR

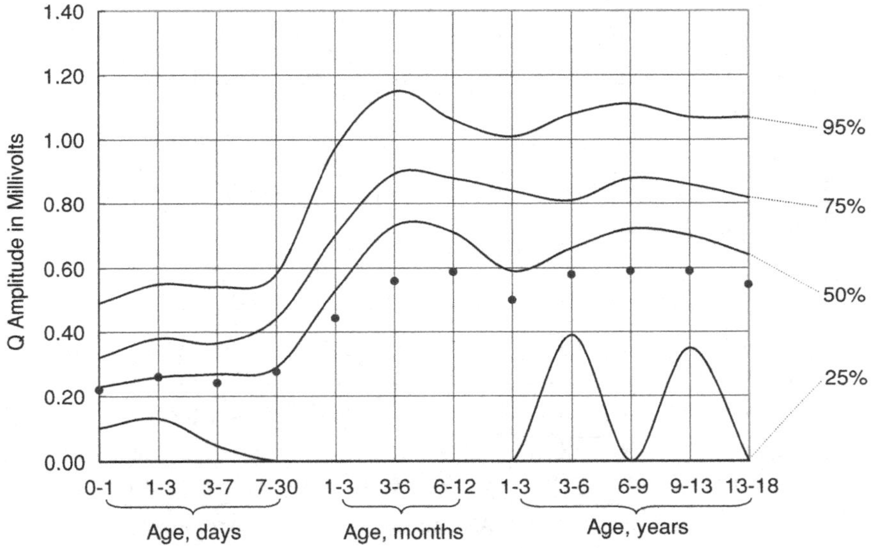

Figure 3.5 Q amplitude by age in lead aVR, each curve corresponding to the indicated percentile level (• = mean). Q waves recorded in aVR are absent, small or prominent. The Q wave amplitude produced becomes larger with a wider range after 1 month of age and thereafter.

	Days				*Months*			*Years*				
Age	*0–1*	*1–3*	*3–7*	*7–30*	*1–3*	*3–6*	*6–12*	*1–3*	*3–6*	*6–9*	*9–13*	*13–18*
95%	0.49	0.55	0.54	0.58	0.97	1.15	1.06	1.01	1.08	1.11	1.07	1.07
Mean	**0.22**	**0.26**	**0.24**	**0.28**	**0.44**	**0.56**	**0.59**	**0.5**	**0.58**	**0.59**	**0.59**	**0.55**
(±SD)	**0.16**	**0.17**	**0.18**	**0.21**	**0.34**	**0.43**	**0.40**	**0.38**	**0.37**	**0.41**	**0.35**	**0.37**
5%	0	0	0	0	0	0	0	0	0	0	0	0
(N)	109	128	95	100	113	91	97	113	107	99	289	510

Q amplitude by age in lead aVL

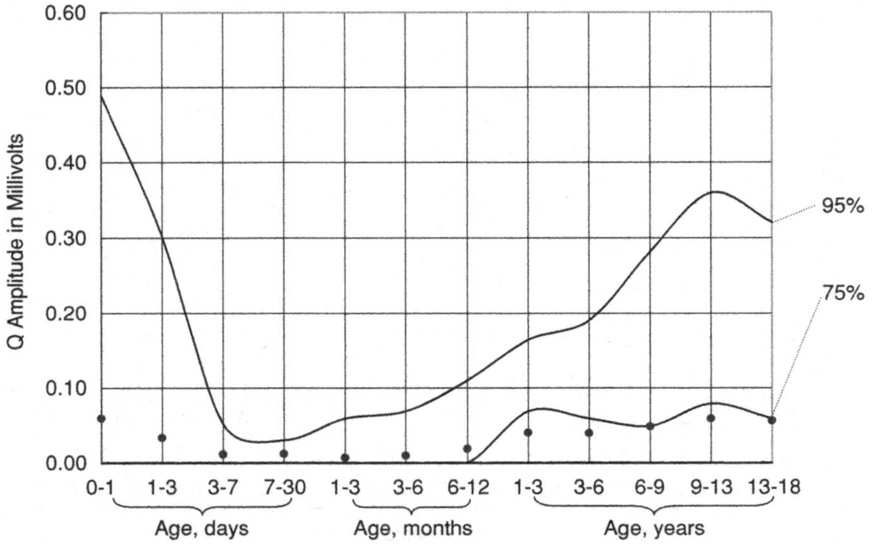

Figure 3.6 Q amplitude by age in lead aVL, each curve corresponding to the indicated percentile level (• = mean). Q waves in lead aVL are absent or small during infancy. The Q wave deflections can be large, up to 4.9 mm, immediately and 1–3 days after birth, and up to 3.6 mm also after age 3–6 years.

	Days				*Months*			*Years*					
Age	*0–1*	*1–3*	*3–7*	*7–30*	*1–3*	*3–6*	*6–12*	*1–3*	*3–6*	*6–9*	*9–13*	*13–18*
95%	0.49	0.30	0.05	0.03	0.06	0.07	0.11	0.16	0.19	0.28	0.36	0.32
Mean	**0.06**	**0.03**	**0.01**	**0.01**	**0.01**	**0.01**	**0.02**	**0.04**	**0.04**	**0.05**	**0.06**	**0.06**
(±SD)	**0.16**	**0.12**	**0.05**	**0.07**	**0.03**	**0.03**	**0.04**	**0.06**	**0.05**	**0.10**	**0.09**	**0.12**
5%	0	0	0	0	0	0	0	0	0	0	0	0
(N)	109	128	95	100	113	91	97	113	107	99	289	510

Q amplitude by age in lead aVF

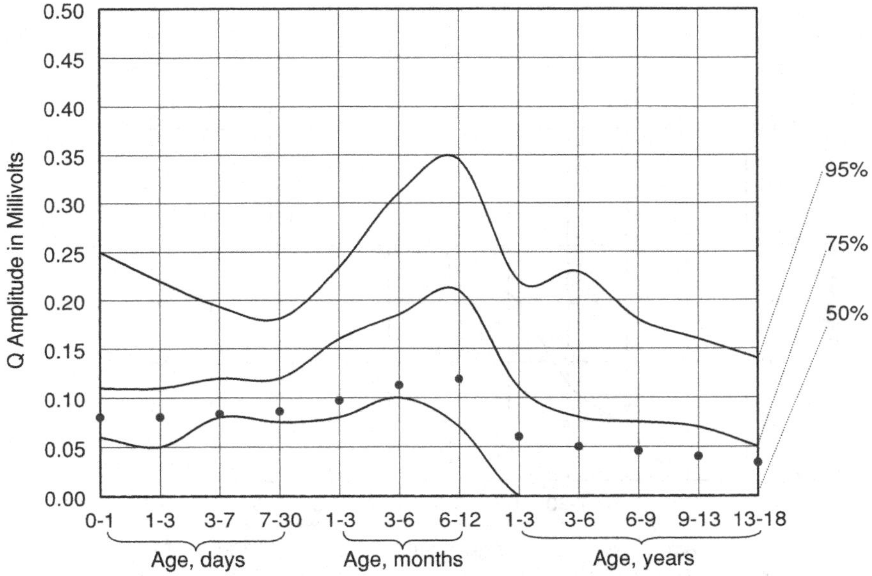

Figure 3.7 Q amplitude by age in lead aVF, each curve corresponding to the indicated percentile level (• = mean). Q waves in aVF are absent of small deflections.

	Days				*Months*			*Years*				
Age	*0–1*	*1–3*	*3–7*	*7–30*	*1–3*	*3–6*	*6–12*	*1–3*	*3–6*	*6–9*	*9–13*	*13–18*
95%	0.25	0.22	0.19	0.18	0.23	0.31	0.35	0.22	0.23	0.18	0.16	0.14
Mean	**0.08**	**0.08**	**0.08**	**0.09**	**0.10**	**0.11**	**0.12**	**0.06**	**0.05**	**0.05**	**0.04**	**0.03**
(±SD)	**0.05**	**0.06**	**0.07**	**0.07**	**0.09**	**0.11**	**0.13**	**0.11**	**0.05**	**0.07**	**0.09**	**0.05**
5%	0	0	0	0	0	0	0	0	0	0	0	0
(N)	109	128	95	100	113	91	97	113	107	99	289	510

Q amplitude by age in lead V4

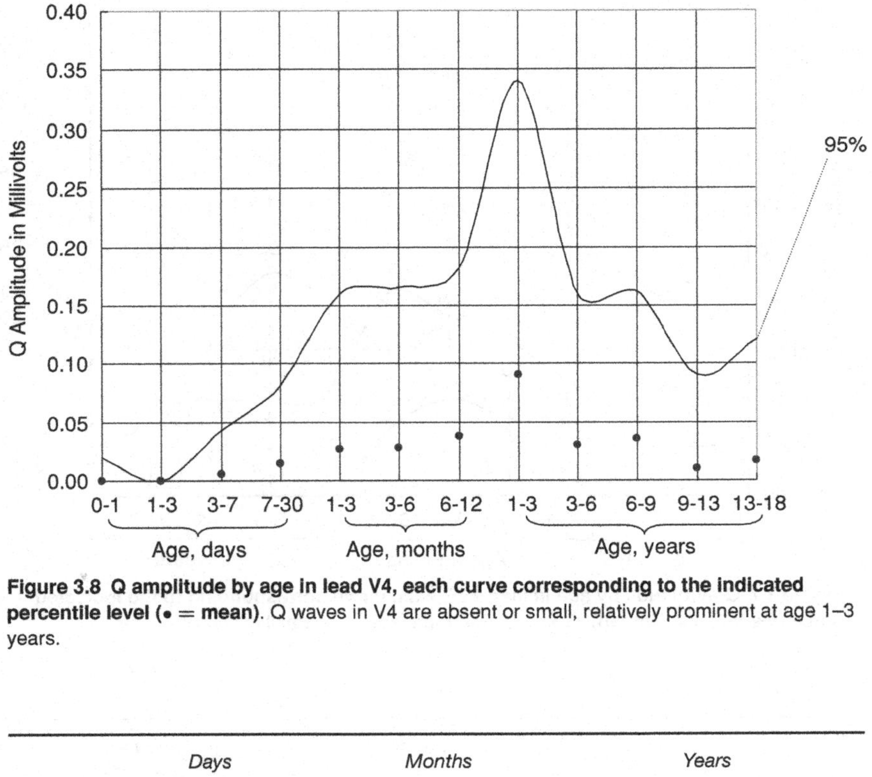

Figure 3.8 Q amplitude by age in lead V4, each curve corresponding to the indicated percentile level (• = mean). Q waves in V4 are absent or small, relatively prominent at age 1–3 years.

	Days				*Months*			*Years*				
Age	*0–1*	*1–3*	*3–7*	*7–30*	*1–3*	*3–6*	*6–12*	*1–3*	*3–6*	*6–9*	*9–13*	*13–18*
95%	0.02	0.00	0.04	0.08	0.16	0.17	0.18	0.34	0.16	0.16	0.09	0.12
Mean	**0**	**0**	**0.01**	**0.01**	**0.03**	**0.03**	**0.04**	**0.09**	**0.03**	**0.03**	**0.01**	**0.02**
(±SD)	**0.00**	**0.00**	**0.02**	**0.04**	**0.06**	**0.06**	**0.08**	**0.11**	**0.05**	**0.08**	**0.00**	**0.05**
5%	0	0	0	0	0	0	0	0	0	0	0	0
(N)	109	128	95	100	113	91	97	113	107	99	289	510

Q amplitude by age in lead V5

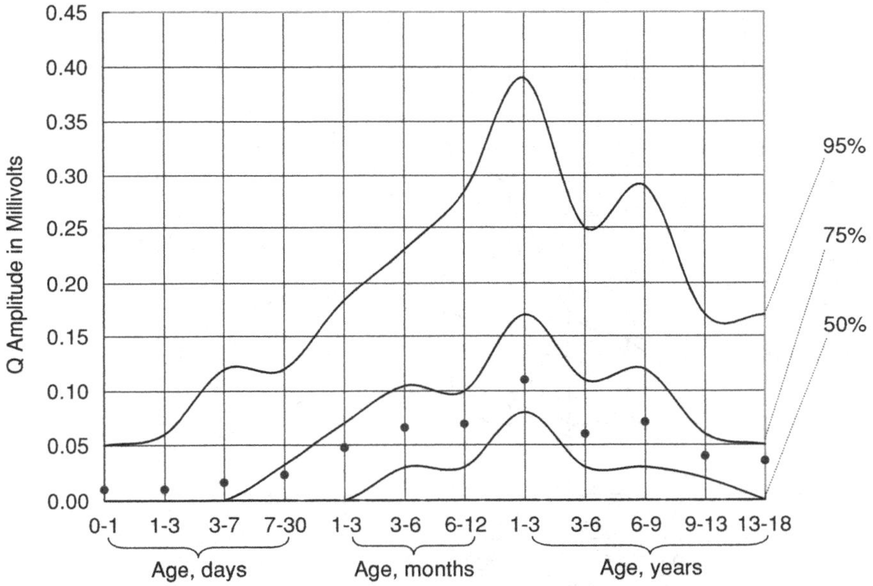

Figure 3.9 Q amplitude by age in lead V5, each curve corresponding to the indicated percentile level (• = mean). Q waves in V5 are generally absent or small during infancy. The Q amplitudes can be large, up to 3.9 mm, at age 1–3 years.

	Days				*Months*			*Years*				
Age	*0–1*	*1–3*	*3–7*	*7–30*	*1–3*	*3–6*	*6–12*	*1–3*	*3–6*	*6–9*	*9–13*	*13–18*
95%	0.05	0.06	0.12	0.12	0.18	0.23	0.28	0.39	0.25	0.29	0.17	0.17
Mean	**0.01**	**0.01**	**0.02**	**0.02**	**0.05**	**0.07**	**0.07**	**0.11**	**0.06**	**0.07**	**0.04**	**0.04**
(±SD)	**0.00**	**0.00**	**0.04**	**0.05**	**0.07**	**0.08**	**0.10**	**0.11**	**0.11**	**0.10**	**0.09**	**0.06**
5%	0	0	0	0	0	0	0	0	0	0	0	0
(N)	109	128	95	100	113	91	97	113	107	99	289	510

Q amplitude by age in lead V6

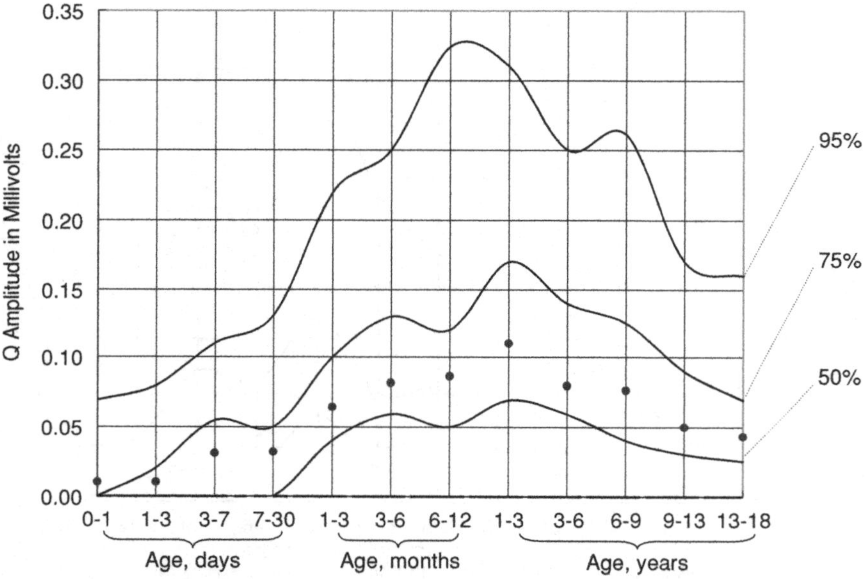

Figure 3.10 Q amplitude by age in lead V6, each curve corresponding to the indicated percentile level (• = mean). Q waves in V6 are absent or small throughout newborn to adolescence. The deflections can be large, up to 3.2 mm, in late infancy and early childhood.

	Days				*Months*			*Years*				
Age	*0–1*	*1–3*	*3–7*	*7–30*	*1–3*	*3–6*	*6–12*	*1–3*	*3–6*	*6–9*	*9–13*	*13–18*
95%	0.07	0.08	0.11	0.13	0.22	0.25	0.32	0.31	0.25	0.26	0.17	0.16
Mean	**0.01**	**0.01**	**0.03**	**0.03**	**0.06**	**0.08**	**0.09**	**0.11**	**0.08**	**0.08**	**0.05**	**0.04**
(±SD)	**0.05**	**0.06**	**0.05**	**0.05**	**0.08**	**0.08**	**0.11**	**0.11**	**0.11**	**0.10**	**0.09**	**0.06**
5%	0	0	0	0	0	0	0	0	0	0	0	0
(N)	109	128	95	100	113	91	97	113	107	99	289	510

R amplitude by age in lead aVR

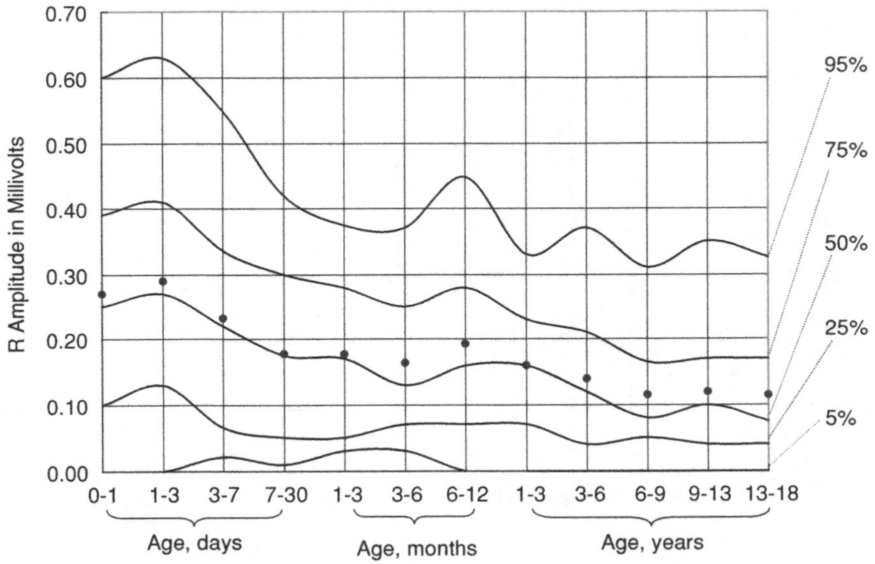

Figure 3.11 R amplitude by age in lead aVR, each curve corresponding to the indicated percentile level (• = mean). R waves in aVR are prominent from birth to late infancy. The R wave amplitude increases in the first 3 days, then decreases strikingly thereafter, reaching a plateau by age 6–9 years.

	Days				*Months*			*Years*				
Age	*0–1*	*1–3*	*3–7*	*7–30*	*1–3*	*3–6*	*6–12*	*1–3*	*3–6*	*6–9*	*9–13*	*13–18*
95%	0.60	0.63	0.55	0.42	0.37	0.37	0.45	0.33	0.37	0.31	0.35	0.33
Mean	**0.27**	**0.29**	**0.23**	**0.18**	**0.18**	**0.16**	**0.19**	**0.16**	**0.14**	**0.12**	**0.12**	**0.11**
(±SD)	**0.21**	**0.17**	**0.17**	**0.14**	**0.12**	**0.13**	**0.15**	**0.11**	**0.11**	**0.10**	**0.09**	**0.11**
5%	0.00	0.00	0.02	0.01	0.03	0.03	0.00	0.00	0.00	0.00	0.00	0.00
(N)	109	128	95	100	113	91	97	113	107	99	289	510

R amplitude by age in lead V1

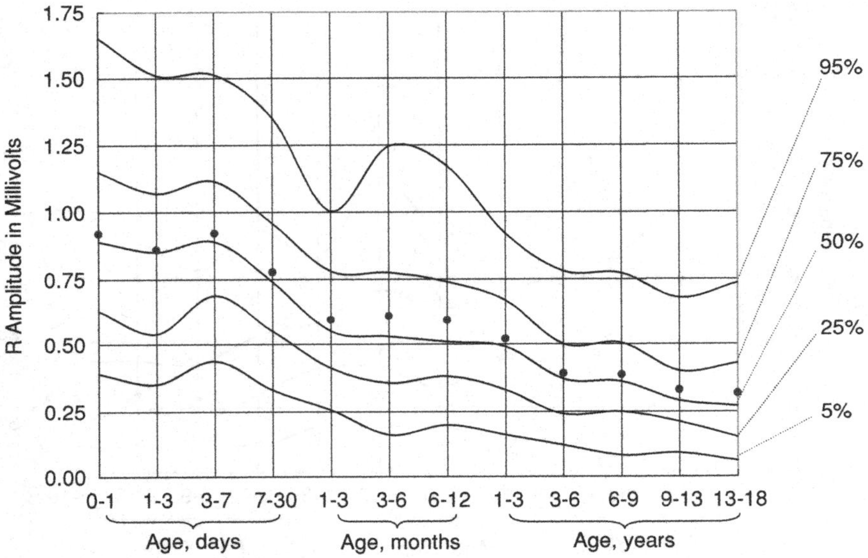

Figure 3.12 R amplitude by age in lead V1, each curve corresponding to the indicated percentile level (• = mean). R waves amplitude in V1 declines strikingly then gradually from birth to adolescence. An R wave in V1 of 16.5 mm can be normal in term newborns.

	Days				*Months*			*Years*				
Age	*0–1*	*1–3*	*3–7*	*7–30*	*1–3*	*3–6*	*6–12*	*1–3*	*3–6*	*6–9*	*9–13*	*13–18*
95%	1.65	1.51	1.51	1.35	1.00	1.25	1.17	0.92	0.78	0.77	0.68	0.74
Mean	**0.92**	**0.86**	**0.92**	**0.78**	**0.60**	**0.61**	**0.59**	**0.52**	**0.39**	**0.38**	**0.33**	**0.32**
(±SD)	**0.37**	**0.35**	**0.32**	**0.32**	**0.24**	**0.33**	**0.32**	**0.27**	**0.21**	**0.20**	**0.17**	**0.22**
5%	0.39	0.35	0.44	0.33	0.26	0.16	0.20	0.16	0.12	0.08	0.09	0.06
(N)	109	128	95	100	113	91	97	113	107	99	289	510

R amplitude by age in lead V2

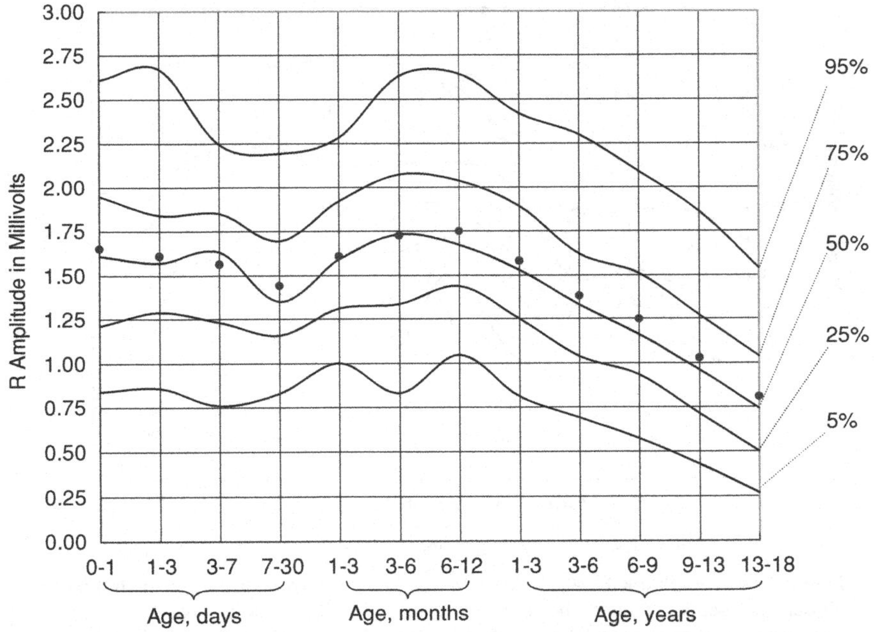

Figure 3.13 R amplitude by age in lead V2, each curve corresponding to the indicated percentile level (• = mean). R waves in V2 are most prominent. The amplitude can be high, up to 26.7 mm, after birth. It decreases strikingly with increasing age throughout early childhood to adolescence.

	Days				*Months*			*Years*				
Age	*0–1*	*1–3*	*3–7*	*7–30*	*1–3*	*3–6*	*6–12*	*1–3*	*3–6*	*6–9*	*9–13*	*13–18*
95%	2.61	2.67	2.25	2.19	2.28	2.63	2.64	2.42	2.30	2.09	1.86	1.54
Mean	**1.65**	**1.61**	**1.56**	**1.44**	**1.61**	**1.72**	**1.75**	**1.58**	**1.38**	**1.25**	**1.03**	**0.81**
(±SD)	**0.53**	**0.52**	**0.45**	**0.43**	**0.42**	**0.55**	**0.50**	**0.49**	**0.47**	**0.50**	**0.43**	**0.40**
5%	0.84	0.86	0.76	0.83	1.00	0.83	1.05	0.81	0.69	0.57	0.43	0.27
(N)	109	128	95	100	113	91	97	113	107	99	289	510

R amplitude by age in lead V4

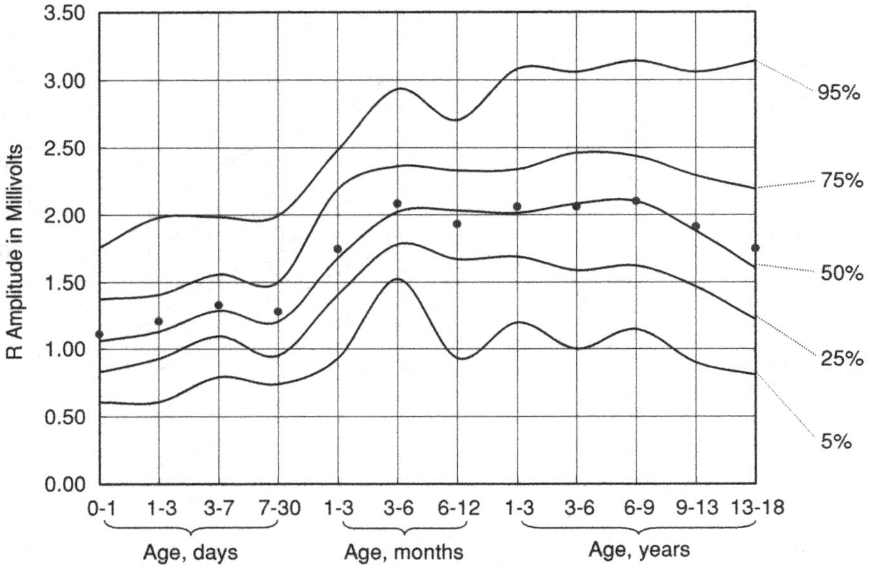

Figure 3.14 R amplitude by age in lead V4, each curve corresponding to the indicated percentile level (• = mean). The R wave amplitude in V4 increases strikingly after age 1–3 months, reaching a plateau by age 6–12 months, and starts to decline by age 9–13 years and thereafter.

	Days				*Months*			*Years*				
Age	*0–1*	*1–3*	*3–7*	*7–30*	*1–3*	*3–6*	*6–12*	*1–3*	*3–6*	*6–9*	*9–13*	*13–18*
95%	1.76	1.98	1.98	1.99	2.48	2.94	2.70	3.08	3.06	3.14	3.06	3.14
Mean	**1.11**	**1.21**	**1.33**	**1.28**	**1.75**	**2.08**	**1.93**	**2.06**	**2.06**	**2.10**	**1.91**	**1.75**
(±SD)	**0.37**	**0.40**	**0.39**	**0.44**	**0.51**	**0.50**	**0.60**	**0.54**	**0.63**	**0.63**	**0.69**	**0.73**
5%	0.61	0.61	0.79	0.74	0.93	1.53	0.93	1.20	1.00	1.15	0.90	0.81
(N)	109	128	95	100	113	91	97	113	107	99	289	510

R amplitude by age in lead V5

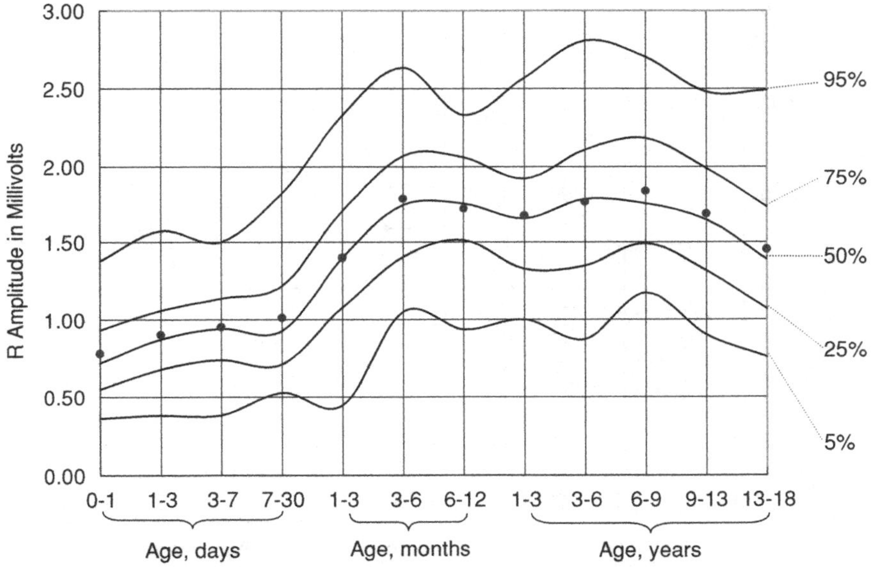

Figure 3.15 R amplitude by age in lead V5, each curve corresponding to the indicated percentile level (• = mean). The amplitude of R wave in V5 strikingly increases at age 1–3 months, reaching a plateau by age 3–6 months, and starts declining by age 9–13 years and thereafter. The normal highest amplitude can be up to 28.1 mm at age 3–6 years.

	Days				*Months*			*Years*				
Age	*0–1*	*1–3*	*3–7*	*7–30*	*1–3*	*3–6*	*6–12*	*1–3*	*3–6*	*6–9*	*9–13*	*13–18*
95%	1.38	1.57	1.50	1.82	2.33	2.64	2.33	2.57	2.81	2.70	2.48	2.49
Mean	**0.78**	**0.9**	**0.95**	**1.01**	**1.40**	**1.78**	**1.72**	**1.67**	**1.76**	**1.84**	**1.68**	**1.45**
(±SD)	**0.32**	**0.35**	**0.33**	**0.42**	**0.54**	**0.49**	**0.44**	**0.49**	**0.58**	**0.51**	**0.52**	**0.53**
5%	0.36	0.38	0.38	0.53	0.44	1.05	0.93	1.00	0.87	1.18	0.90	0.76
(N)	109	128	95	100	113	91	97	113	107	99	289	510

R amplitude by age in lead V6

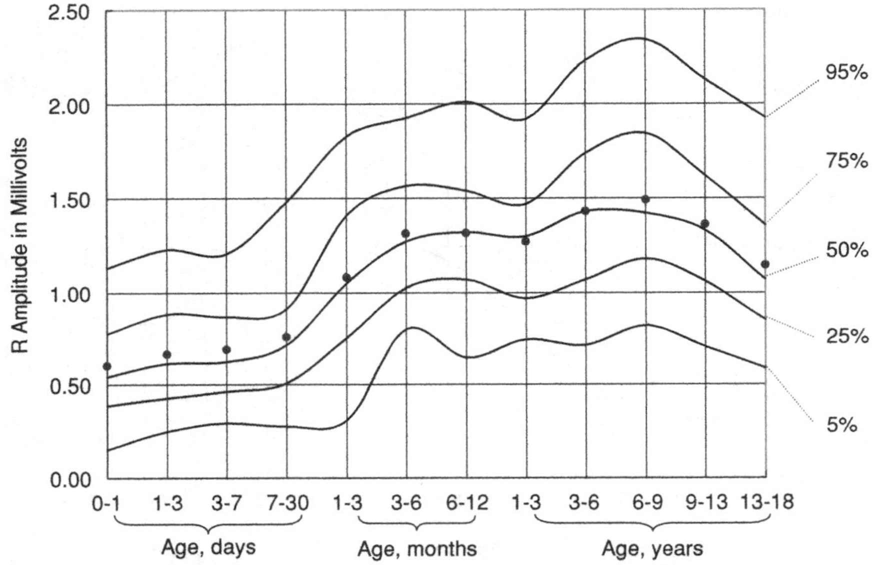

Figure 3.16 R amplitude by age in lead V6, each curve corresponding to the indicated percentile level (• = mean). A typical progression of R amplitude changes from birth to adolescence is seen here. The R amplitude in V6 increases gradually after birth, rapidly from age 1–3 months, reaching a plateau by age 3–6 months, increases again from 3–6 years up to 6–9 years of age, followed by a decrease at 9–13 years until 13–18 years of age.

	Days				*Months*			*Years*				
Age	*0–1*	*1–3*	*3–7*	*7–30*	*1–3*	*3–6*	*6–12*	*1–3*	*3–6*	*6–9*	*9–13*	*13–18*
95%	1.13	1.23	1.21	1.48	1.83	1.93	2.01	1.92	2.23	2.34	2.13	1.93
Mean	**0.6**	**0.66**	**0.69**	**0.75**	**1.08**	**1.31**	**1.32**	**1.27**	**1.43**	**1.49**	**1.36**	**1.15**
(±SD)	**0.32**	**0.29**	**0.30**	**0.35**	**0.46**	**0.38**	**0.41**	**0.38**	**0.47**	**0.49**	**0.43**	**0.41**
5%	0.15	0.25	0.30	0.28	0.31	0.80	0.64	0.74	0.71	0.82	0.70	0.58
(N)	109	128	95	100	113	91	97	113	107	99	289	510

S amplitude by age in lead I

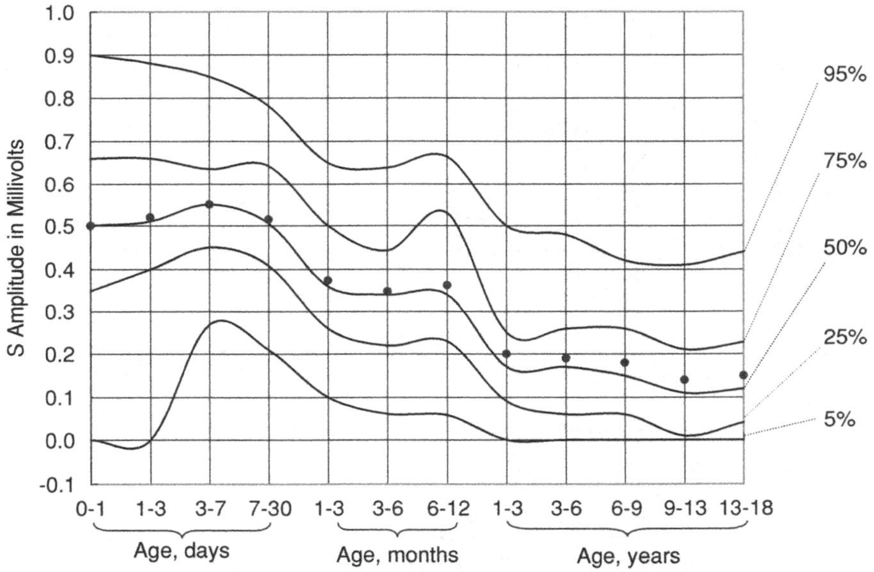

Figure 3.17 S amplitude by age in lead I, each curve corresponding to the indicated percentile level (• = mean). S waves in lead I are prominent after birth. The S wave deflection becomes shallow after age 7–30 days, becoming smaller or absent after age 1–3 years.

	Days				*Months*			*Years*				
Age	*0–1*	*1–3*	*3–7*	*7–30*	*1–3*	*3–6*	*6–12*	*1–3*	*3–6*	*6–9*	*9–13*	*13–18*
95%	0.9	0.9	0.8	0.8	0.7	0.6	0.7	0.5	0.5	0.4	0.4	0.4
Mean	**0.5**	**0.52**	**0.55**	**0.51**	**0.37**	**0.35**	**0.36**	**0.2**	**0.19**	**0.18**	**0.14**	**0.15**
(±SD)	**0.27**	**0.23**	**0.17**	**0.19**	**0.17**	**0.20**	**0.20**	**0.16**	**0.16**	**0.15**	**0.17**	**0.14**
5%	0.0	0.0	0.3	0.2	0.1	0.1	0.1	0.0	0.0	0.0	0.0	0.0
(N)	109	128	95	100	120	92	97	113	107	100	289	510

S amplitude by age in lead II

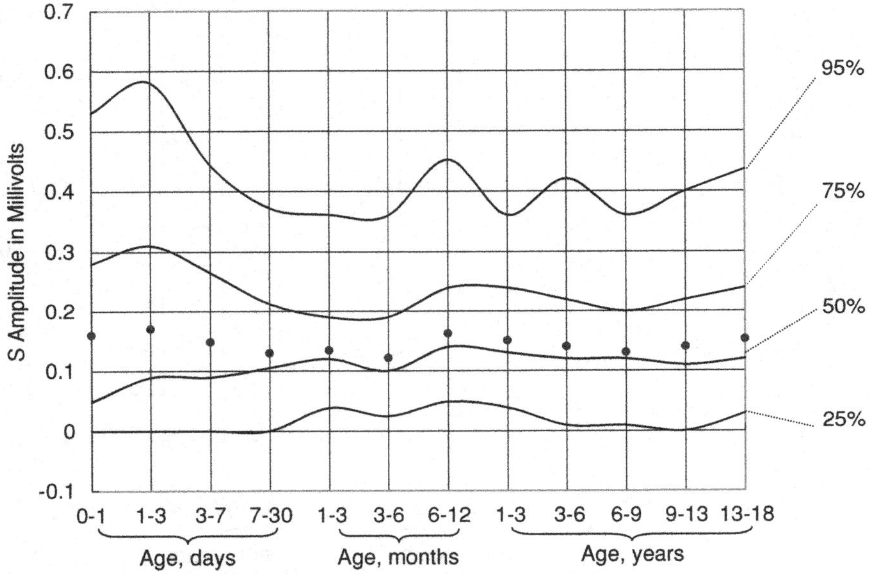

Figure 3.18 S amplitude by age in lead II, each curve corresponding to the indicated percentile level (• = mean). S waves in II are relatively shallow or absent, and change little during the entire pediatric ages.

	Days				*Months*			*Years*				
Age	*0–1*	*1–3*	*3–7*	*7–30*	*1–3*	*3–6*	*6–12*	*1–3*	*3–6*	*6–9*	*9–13*	*13–18*
95%	0.53	0.58	0.44	0.37	0.36	0.36	0.45	0.36	0.42	0.36	0.40	0.44
Mean	**0.16**	**0.17**	**0.15**	**0.13**	**0.13**	**0.12**	**0.16**	**0.15**	**0.14**	**0.13**	**0.14**	**0.15**
(±SD)	**0.21**	**0.17**	**0.17**	**0.14**	**0.12**	**0.12**	**0.14**	**0.11**	**0.16**	**0.10**	**0.17**	**0.15**
5%	0	0	0	0	0	0	0	0	0	0	0	0
(N)	109	128	95	100	120	92	97	113	107	100	289	510

S amplitude by age in lead III

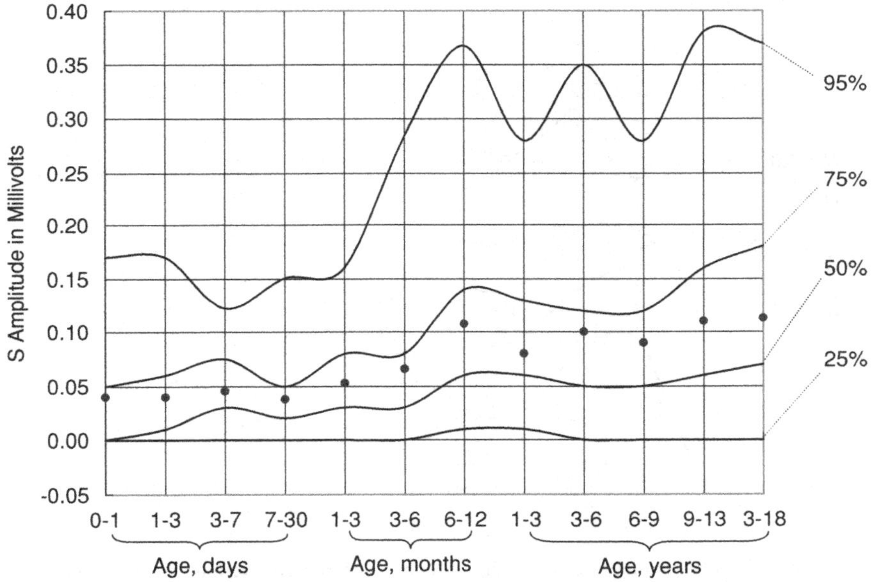

Figure 3.19 S amplitude by age in lead III, each curve corresponding to the indicated percentile level (• = mean). S waves in lead III are shallow or absent after birth, becoming more prominent after age 3–6 months, reaching the adult pattern by age 9–13 years.

	Days				*Months*			*Years*				
Age	*0–1*	*1–3*	*3–7*	*7–30*	*1–3*	*3–6*	*6–12*	*1–3*	*3–6*	*6–9*	*9–13*	*13–18*
95%	0.17	0.17	0.12	0.15	0.16	0.28	0.37	0.28	0.35	0.28	0.38	0.37
Mean	**0.04**	**0.04**	**0.05**	**0.04**	**0.05**	**0.07**	**0.11**	**0.08**	**0.1**	**0.09**	**0.11**	**0.11**
(±SD)	**0.05**	**0.06**	**0.05**	**0.06**	**0.06**	**0.11**	**0.14**	**0.11**	**0.16**	**0.10**	**0.09**	**0.13**
5%	0	0	0	0	0	0	0	0	0	0	0	0
(N)	109	128	95	100	120	92	97	113	107	100	289	510

S amplitude by age in lead aVL

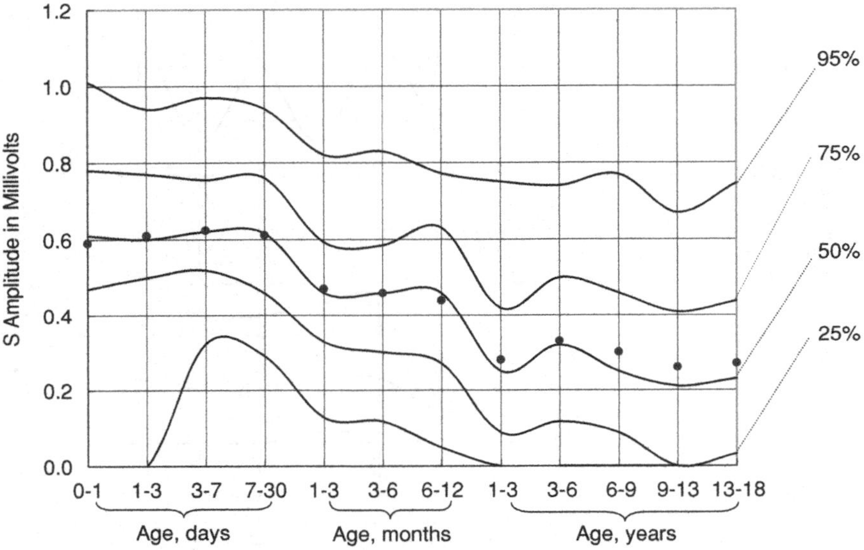

Figure 3.20 S amplitude by age in lead aVL, each curve corresponding to the indicated percentile level (• = mean). S waves in aVL can be deep or absent during the neonatal period. The S deflection decreases gradually and steadily after age 7–3 days, becoming adult pattern by 9–13 years.

	Days				*Months*			*Years*				
Age	*0–1*	*1–3*	*3–7*	*7–30*	*1–3*	*3–6*	*6–12*	*1–3*	*3–6*	*6–9*	*9–13*	*13–18*
95%	1.0	0.9	1.0	0.9	0.8	0.8	0.8	0.8	0.7	0.8	0.7	0.7
Mean	**0.59**	**0.61**	**0.62**	**0.61**	**0.47**	**0.46**	**0.44**	**0.28**	**0.33**	**0.3**	**0.26**	**0.27**
(±SD)	**0.27**	**0.23**	**0.21**	**0.21**	**0.21**	**0.23**	**0.24**	**0.22**	**0.26**	**0.26**	**0.26**	**0.25**
5%	0.0	0.0	0.3	0.3	0.1	0.1	0.1	0.0	0.0	0.0	0.0	0.0
(N)	109	128	95	100	120	92	97	113	107	100	289	510

S amplitude by age in lead aVF

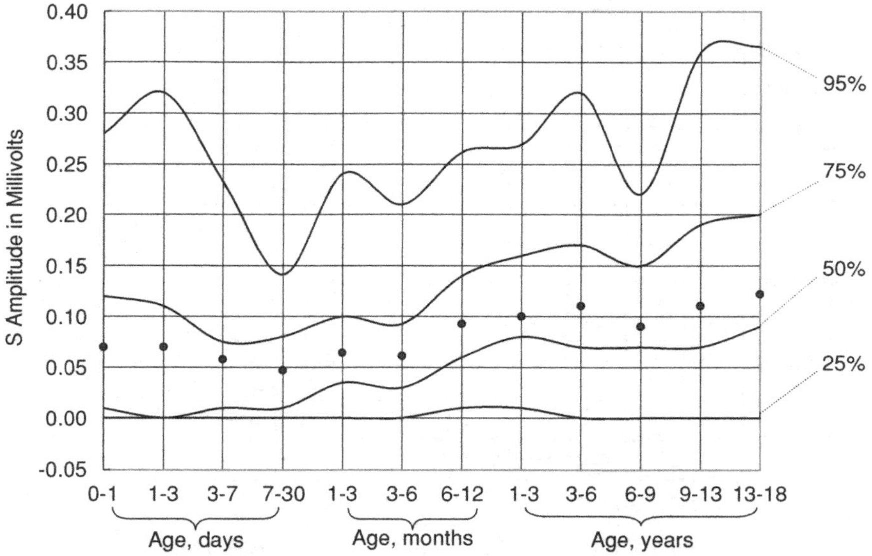

Figure 3.21 S amplitude by age in lead aVF, each curve corresponding to the indicated percentile level (• = mean). S waves in aVF are small or absent. The S amplitude increases little, however, after age 1–3 months until adolescence.

	Days				*Months*			*Years*				
Age	*0–1*	*1–3*	*3–7*	*7–30*	*1–3*	*3–6*	*6–12*	*1–3*	*3–6*	*6–9*	*9–13*	*13–18*
95%	0.28	0.32	0.23	0.14	0.24	0.21	0.26	0.27	0.32	0.22	0.36	0.37
Mean	**0.07**	**0.07**	**0.06**	**0.05**	**0.06**	**0.06**	**0.09**	**0.1**	**0.11**	**0.09**	**0.11**	**0.12**
(±SD)	**0.11**	**0.12**	**0.09**	**0.07**	**0.08**	**0.08**	**0.10**	**0.11**	**0.11**	**0.10**	**0.09**	**0.13**
5%	0	0	0	0	0	0	0	0	0	0	0	0
(N)	109	128	95	100	120	92	97	113	107	100	289	510

S amplitude by age in lead V1

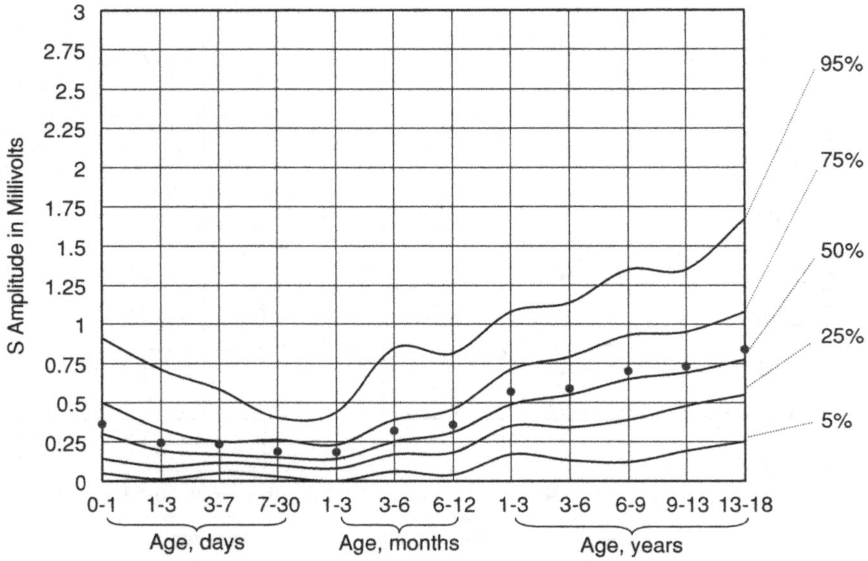

Figure 3.22 S amplitude by age in lead V1, each curve corresponding to the indicated percentile level (• = mean). S waves in lead V1 are small or absent after birth, increasing their depth little during infancy, then are more prominent thereafter until age 13–18 years.

	Days				*Months*			*Years*				
Age	*0–1*	*1–3*	*3–7*	*7–30*	*1–3*	*3–6*	*6–12*	*1–3*	*3–6*	*6–9*	*9–13*	*13–18*
95%	0.91	0.71	0.59	0.40	0.44	0.85	0.81	1.08	1.14	1.35	1.35	1.67
Mean	**0.36**	**0.24**	**0.23**	**0.19**	**0.18**	**0.32**	**0.36**	**0.57**	**0.59**	**0.7**	**0.73**	**0.84**
(±SD)	**0.32**	**0.17**	**0.21**	**0.14**	**0.16**	**0.23**	**0.28**	**0.33**	**0.32**	**0.41**	**0.35**	**0.44**
5%	0.1	0.0	0.1	0.0	0.0	0.1	0.0	0.2	0.1	0.1	0.2	0.2
(N)	109	128	95	100	120	92	97	113	107	100	289	510

S amplitude by age in lead V2

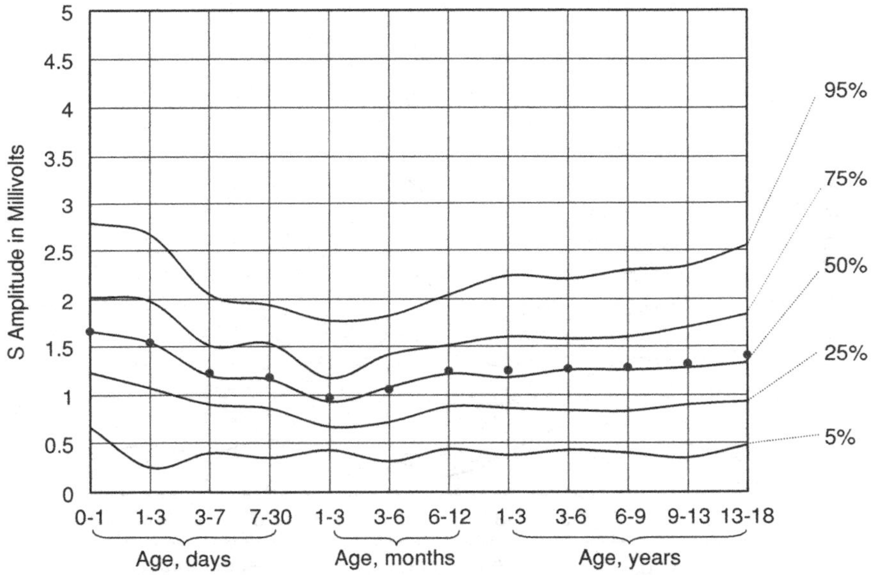

Figure 3.23 S amplitude by age in lead V2, each curve corresponding to the indicated percentile level (• = mean). S waves deflection in V2 decreases slightly after birth until age 1–3 months. From this age on, the deflection increases, but very little, until adolescence.

	Days				*Months*			*Years*				
Age	*0–1*	*1–3*	*3–7*	*7–30*	*1–3*	*3–6*	*6–12*	*1–3*	*3–6*	*6–9*	*9–13*	*13–18*
95%	2.79	2.67	2.05	1.94	1.77	1.83	2.04	2.24	2.21	2.30	2.34	2.56
Mean	**1.66**	**1.54**	**1.22**	**1.18**	**0.97**	**1.06**	**1.25**	**1.25**	**1.27**	**1.28**	**1.32**	**1.41**
(±SD)	**0.59**	**0.69**	**0.47**	**0.49**	**0.41**	**0.48**	**0.57**	**0.60**	**0.63**	**0.56**	**0.61**	**0.64**
5%	0.66	0.25	0.40	0.35	0.43	0.32	0.44	0.38	0.43	0.40	0.35	0.48
(N)	109	128	95	100	120	92	97	113	107	100	289	510

S amplitude by age in lead V4

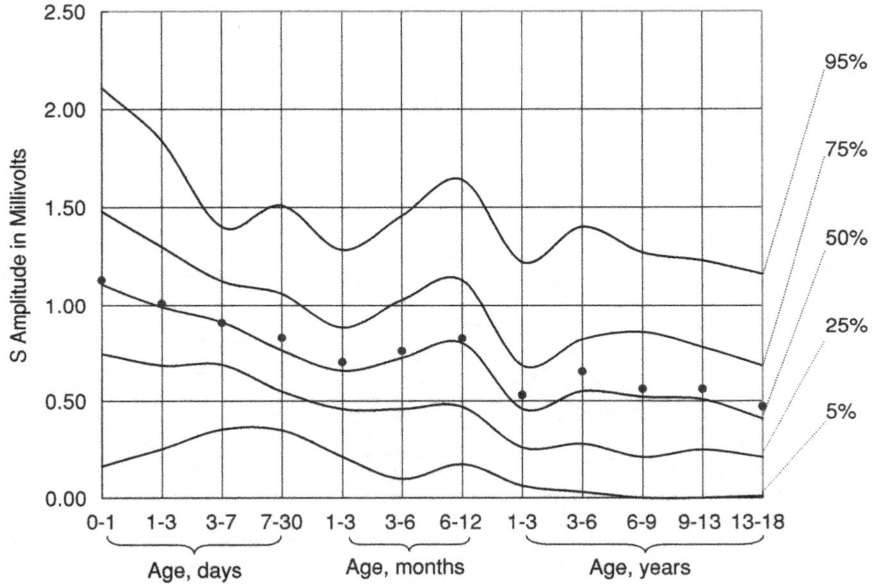

Figure 3.24 S amplitude by age in lead V4, each curve corresponding to the indicated percentile level (• = mean). S waves in V4 are prominent after birth, and become shallower and less prominent thereafter until age 13–18 years.

	Days				*Months*			*Years*				
Age	*0–1*	*1–3*	*3–7*	*7–30*	*1–3*	*3–6*	*6–12*	*1–3*	*3–6*	*6–9*	*9–13*	*13–18*
95%	2.11	1.84	1.40	1.51	1.28	1.46	1.64	1.22	1.40	1.27	1.23	1.16
Mean	**1.13**	**1.01**	**0.91**	**0.83**	**0.70**	**0.76**	**0.82**	**0.53**	**0.65**	**0.56**	**0.56**	**0.47**
(±SD)	**0.59**	**0.46**	**0.37**	**0.36**	**0.34**	**0.47**	**0.49**	**0.38**	**0.58**	**0.41**	**0.43**	**0.35**
5%	0.16	0.25	0.35	0.35	0.21	0.10	0.17	0.06	0.03	0.00	0.00	0.01
(N)	109	128	95	100	120	92	97	113	107	100	289	510

CHAPTER 3.25

S amplitude by age in lead V5

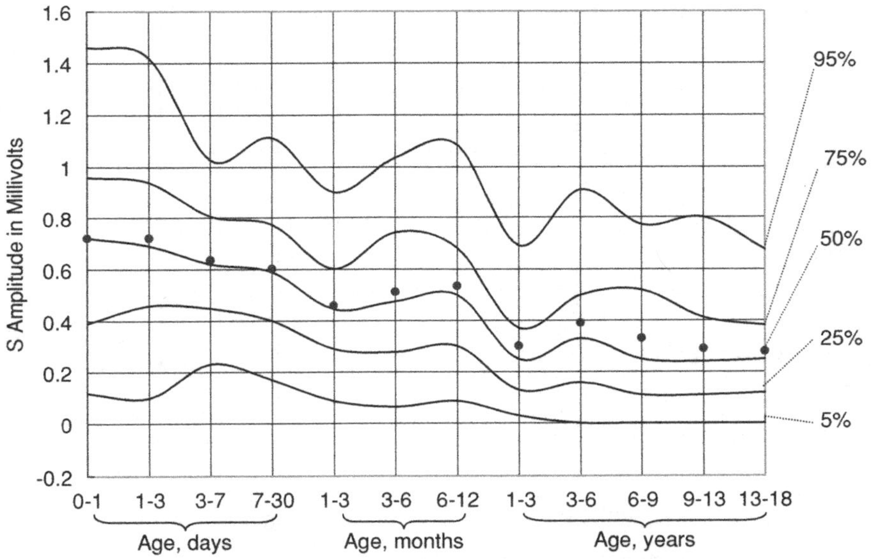

Figure 3.25 S amplitude by age in lead V5, each curve corresponding to the indicated percentile level (• = mean). S waves are present after birth, becoming shallower gradually thereafter until adolescence. The changing patterns are quite comparable to those of lead V4.

	Days				*Months*			*Years*				
Age	*0–1*	*1–3*	*3–7*	*7–30*	*1–3*	*3–6*	*6–12*	*1–3*	*3–6*	*6–9*	*9–13*	*13–18*
95%	1.46	1.42	1.03	1.11	0.90	1.03	1.08	0.69	0.91	0.77	0.80	0.68
Mean	**0.72**	**0.72**	**0.63**	**0.60**	**0.46**	**0.51**	**0.53**	**0.3**	**0.39**	**0.33**	**0.29**	**0.28**
(±SD)	**0.43**	**0.40**	**0.28**	**0.28**	**0.25**	**0.35**	**0.33**	**0.22**	**0.37**	**0.26**	**0.26**	**0.22**
5%	0.12	0.10	0.23	0.17	0.09	0.07	0.09	0.03	0.00	0.00	0.00	0.00
(N)	109	128	95	100	120	92	97	113	107	100	289	510

S amplitude by age in lead V6

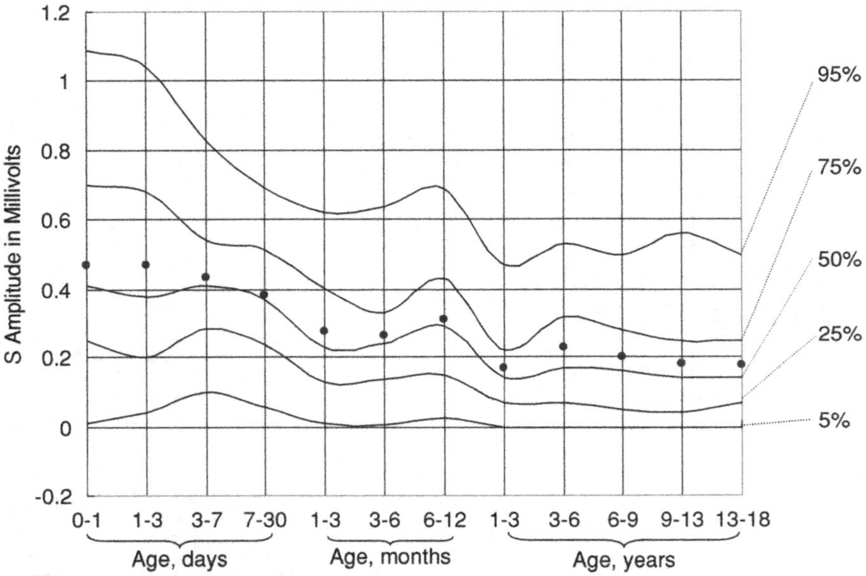

Figure 3.26 S amplitude by age in lead V6, each curve corresponding to the indicated percentile level (• = mean). S waves in V6 are prominent after birth, and their amplitude decreases gradually along with increasing age until adolescence.

	Days				*Months*			*Years*				
Age	*0–1*	*1–3*	*3–7*	*7–30*	*1–3*	*3–6*	*6–12*	*1–3*	*3–6*	*6–9*	*9–13*	*13–18*
95%	1.09	1.04	0.83	0.69	0.62	0.64	0.69	0.47	0.53	0.50	0.56	0.50
Mean	**0.47**	**0.47**	**0.43**	**0.38**	**0.27**	**0.26**	**0.31**	**0.17**	**0.23**	**0.2**	**0.18**	**0.18**
(±SD)	**0.32**	**0.35**	**0.23**	**0.21**	**0.20**	**0.21**	**0.23**	**0.16**	**0.26**	**0.15**	**0.17**	**0.16**
5%	0.01	0.04	0.10	0.06	0.01	0.01	0.03	0.00	0.00	0.00	0.00	0.00
(N)	109	128	95	100	120	92	97	113	107	100	289	510

CHAPTER 3.27

T amplitude by age in lead I

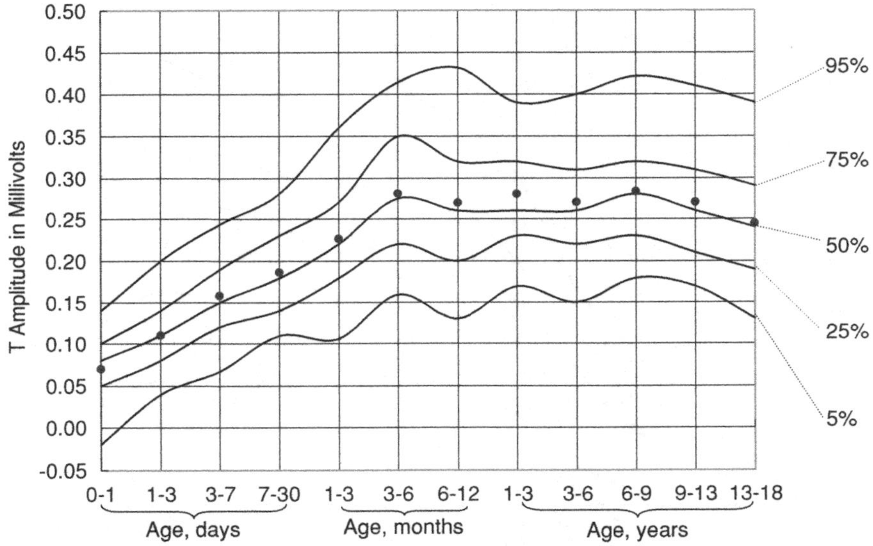

Figure 3.27 T amplitude by age in lead I, each curve corresponding to the indicated percentile level (• = mean). T waves in lead I are small, absent, or even negative, shortly after birth and their amplitude increases gradually, reaching a plateau by age 3–6 months, and stays little changed until adolescence.

	Days				*Months*			*Years*				
Age	*0–1*	*1–3*	*3–7*	*7–30*	*1–3*	*3–6*	*6–12*	*1–3*	*3–6*	*6–9*	*9–13*	*13–18*
95%	0.14	0.20	0.24	0.28	0.36	0.41	0.43	0.39	0.40	0.42	0.41	0.39
Mean	**0.07**	**0.11**	**0.16**	**0.19**	**0.23**	**0.28**	**0.27**	**0.28**	**0.27**	**0.28**	**0.27**	**0.24**
(±SD)	**0.05**	**0.06**	**0.07**	**0.06**	**0.07**	**0.08**	**0.10**	**0.05**	**0.05**	**0.08**	**0.09**	**0.08**
5%	−0.02	0.04	0.07	0.11	0.11	0.16	0.13	0.17	0.15	0.18	0.17	0.13
(N)	109	128	95	100	113	91	97	113	107	99	289	510

T amplitude by age in lead II

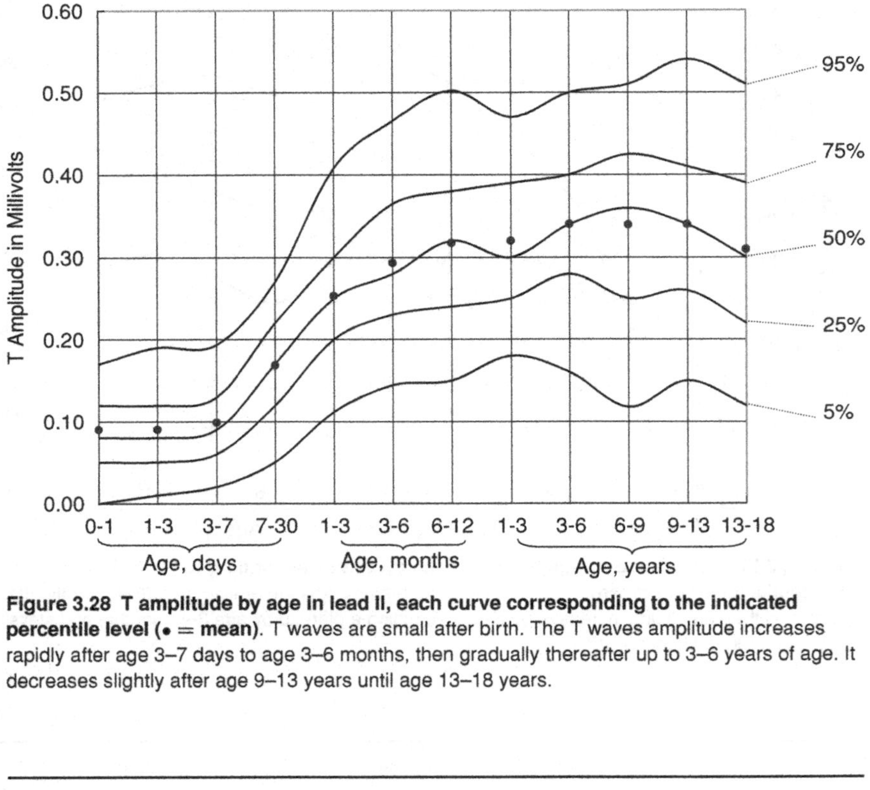

Figure 3.28 T amplitude by age in lead II, each curve corresponding to the indicated percentile level (• = mean). T waves are small after birth. The T waves amplitude increases rapidly after age 3–7 days to age 3–6 months, then gradually thereafter up to 3–6 years of age. It decreases slightly after age 9–13 years until age 13–18 years.

	Days				*Months*			*Years*				
Age	*0–1*	*1–3*	*3–7*	*7–30*	*1–3*	*3–6*	*6–12*	*1–3*	*3–6*	*6–9*	*9–13*	*13–18*
95%	0.17	0.19	0.19	0.27	0.41	0.47	0.50	0.47	0.50	0.51	0.54	0.51
Mean	**0.09**	**0.09**	**0.10**	**0.17**	**0.25**	**0.29**	**0.32**	**0.32**	**0.34**	**0.34**	**0.34**	**0.31**
(±SD)	**0.05**	**0.06**	**0.06**	**0.07**	**0.09**	**0.11**	**0.12**	**0.11**	**0.11**	**0.12**	**0.09**	**0.12**
5%	0.00	0.01	0.02	0.05	0.11	0.15	0.15	0.18	0.16	0.12	0.15	0.12
(N)	109	128	95	100	113	91	97	113	107	99	289	510

T amplitude by age in lead III

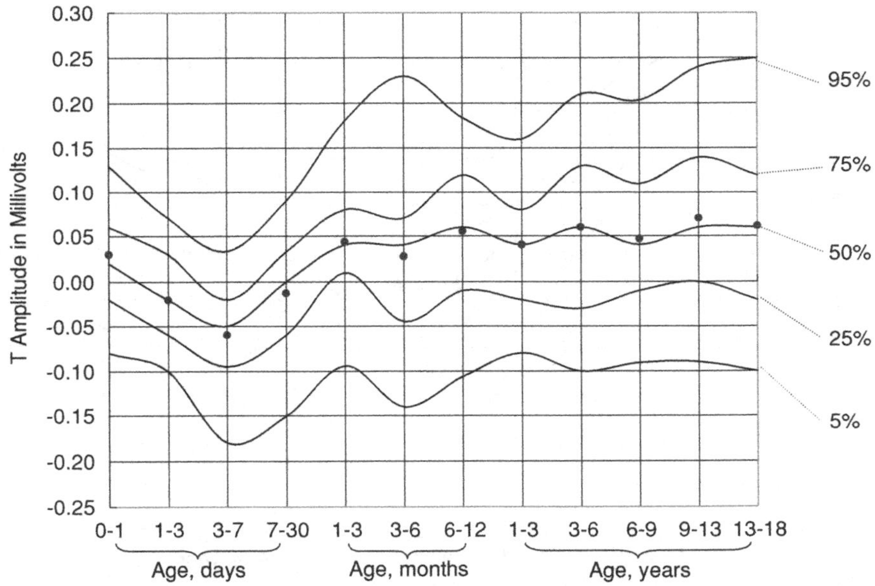

Figure 3.29 T amplitude by age in lead III, each curve corresponding to the indicated percentile level (• = mean). T waves changes in lead III during the newborn period are very characteristic. The T amplitude decreases even becomes negative, reaching a nadir at age 3–7 days. It increases thereafter, up to a plateau by age 6–12 months until adolescence.

	Days				*Months*			*Years*				
Age	*0–1*	*1–3*	*3–7*	*7–30*	*1–3*	*3–6*	*6–12*	*1–3*	*3–6*	*6–9*	*9–13*	*13–18*
95%	0.13	0.07	0.03	0.09	0.18	0.23	0.18	0.16	0.21	0.20	0.24	0.25
Mean	**0.03**	**−0.02**	**−0.06**	**−0.01**	**0.04**	**0.03**	**0.06**	**0.04**	**0.06**	**0.05**	**0.07**	**0.06**
(±SD)	**0.05**	**0.06**	**0.07**	**0.07**	**0.07**	**0.11**	**0.09**	**0.05**	**0.11**	**0.10**	**0.09**	**0.11**
5%	−0.08	−0.10	−0.18	−0.15	−0.09	−0.14	−0.11	−0.08	−0.10	−0.09	−0.09	−0.10
(N)	109	128	95	100	113	91	97	113	107	99	289	510

T amplitude by age in lead aVR

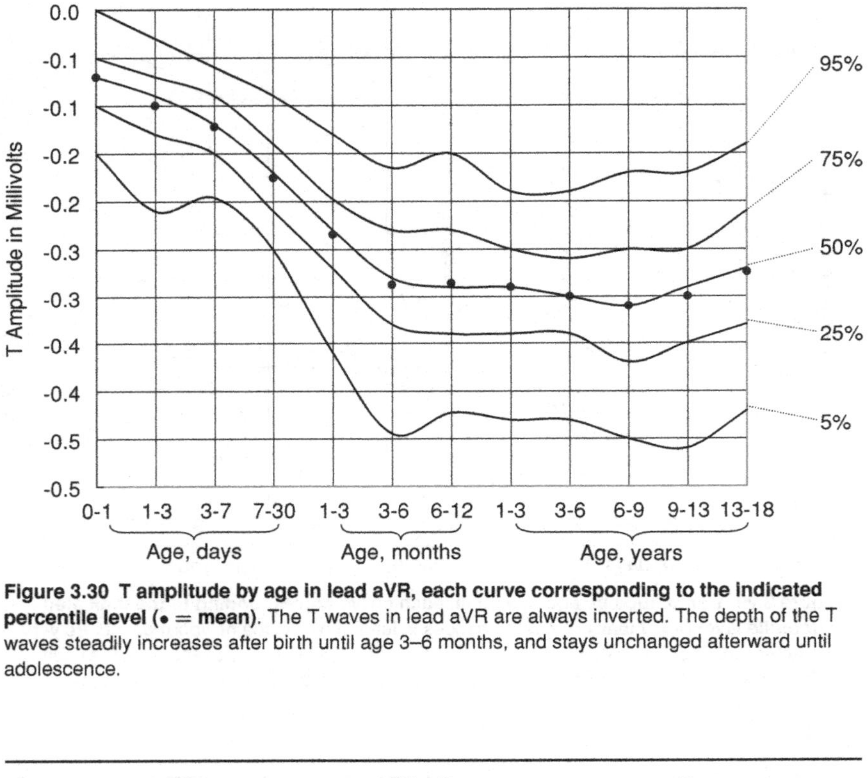

Figure 3.30 T amplitude by age in lead aVR, each curve corresponding to the indicated percentile level (• = mean). The T waves in lead aVR are always inverted. The depth of the T waves steadily increases after birth until age 3–6 months, and stays unchanged afterward until adolescence.

	Days				*Months*			*Years*				
Age	*0–1*	*1–3*	*3–7*	*7–30*	*1–3*	*3–6*	*6–12*	*1–3*	*3–6*	*6–9*	*9–13*	*13–18*
95%	0.0	0.0	−0.1	−0.1	−0.1	−0.2	−0.2	−0.2	−0.2	−0.2	−0.2	−0.1
Mean	**−0.07**	**−0.1**	**−0.12**	**−0.18**	**−0.23**	**−0.29**	**−0.29**	**−0.29**	**−0.3**	**−0.31**	**−0.3**	**−0.27**
(±SD)	**0.05**	**0.06**	**0.05**	**0.05**	**0.07**	**0.08**	**0.09**	**0.05**	**0.05**	**0.10**	**0.09**	**0.09**
5%	−0.2	−0.2	−0.2	−0.3	−0.4	−0.4	−0.4	−0.4	−0.4	−0.5	−0.5	−0.4
(N)	109	128	95	100	120	92	97	113	107	100	289	510

T amplitude by age in lead aVL

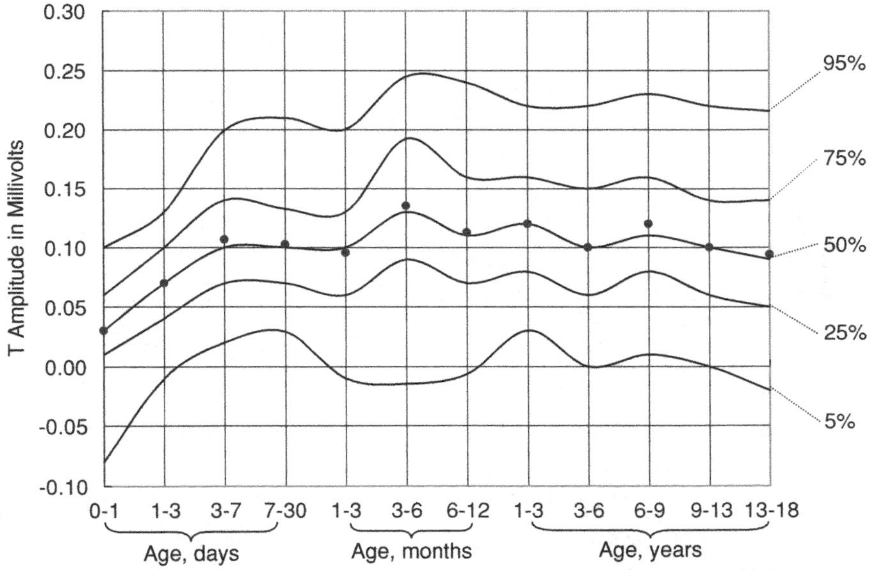

Figure 3.31 T amplitude by age in lead aVL, each curve corresponding to the indicated percentile level (• = mean). The T waves amplitude in aVL increases after birth reaching a plateau at age 3–7 days, then increases slightly with a wider range, at age 3–6 months and thereafter.

	Days				*Months*			*Years*				
Age	*0–1*	*1–3*	*3–7*	*7–30*	*1–3*	*3–6*	*6–12*	*1–3*	*3–6*	*6–9*	*9–13*	*13–18*
95%	0.10	0.13	0.20	0.21	0.20	0.24	0.24	0.22	0.22	0.23	0.22	0.22
Mean	**0.03**	**0.07**	**0.11**	**0.10**	**0.10**	**0.14**	**0.11**	**0.12**	**0.1**	**0.12**	**0.1**	**0.09**
(±SD)	**0.05**	**0.06**	**0.06**	**0.05**	**0.07**	**0.08**	**0.08**	**0.05**	**0.05**	**0.05**	**0.09**	**0.07**
5%	−0.08	−0.01	0.02	0.03	−0.01	−0.01	−0.01	0.03	0.00	0.01	0.00	−0.02
(N)	109	128	95	100	120	92	97	113	107	100	289	510

T amplitude by age in lead aVF

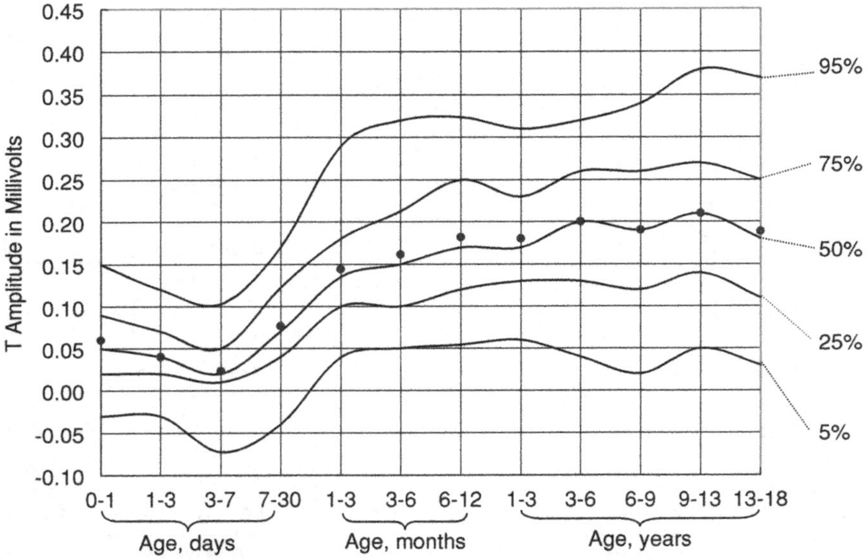

Figure 3.32 T amplitude by age in lead aVF, each curve corresponding to the indicated percentile level (• = mean). The T waves in aVF are low, flat or inverted at birth. The T waves amplitude decreases during the first days of life, followed by a rapid increase until age 1–3 months, then steady and gradual increase until adolescence.

	Days				*Months*			*Years*				
Age	*0–1*	*1–3*	*3–7*	*7–30*	*1–3*	*3–6*	*6–12*	*1–3*	*3–6*	*6–9*	*9–13*	*13–18*
95%	0.15	0.12	0.10	0.17	0.29	0.32	0.32	0.31	0.32	0.34	0.38	0.37
Mean	**0.06**	**0.04**	**0.02**	**0.08**	**0.14**	**0.16**	**0.18**	**0.18**	**0.2**	**0.19**	**0.21**	**0.19**
(±SD)	**0.05**	**0.06**	**0.06**	**0.06**	**0.07**	**0.10**	**0.09**	**0.05**	**0.11**	**0.10**	**0.09**	**0.11**
5%	−0.03	−0.03	−0.07	−0.04	0.04	0.05	0.05	0.06	0.04	0.02	0.05	0.03
(N)	109	128	95	100	120	92	97	113	107	100	289	510

T amplitude by age in lead V1

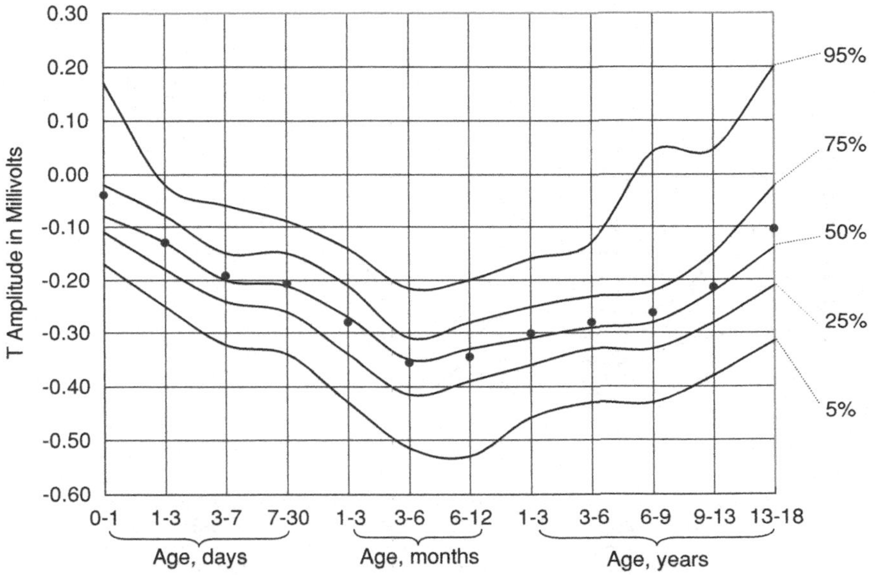

Figure 3.33 T amplitude by age in lead V1, each curve corresponding to the indicated percentile level (• = mean). T waves in V1 are characteristically upright, low or only slightly inverted during the first day of life. They all become inverted with increased depth until age 3–6 months, then turning to be less inverted or even upright thereafter along with increasing age.

	Days				*Months*			*Years*				
Age	*0–1*	*1–3*	*3–7*	*7–30*	*1–3*	*3–6*	*6–12*	*1–3*	*3–6*	*6–9*	*9–13*	*13–18*
95%	0.17	−0.02	−0.06	−0.09	−0.14	−0.22	−0.20	−0.16	−0.13	0.04	0.05	0.20
Mean	**−0.04**	**−0.13**	**−0.19**	**−0.21**	**−0.28**	**−0.36**	**−0.35**	**−0.30**	**−0.28**	**−0.26**	**−0.21**	**−0.11**
(±SD)	**0.11**	**0.06**	**0.08**	**0.08**	**0.09**	**0.11**	**0.12**	**0.10**	**0.11**	**0.12**	**0.12**	**0.16**
5%	−0.17	−0.25	−0.32	−0.34	−0.43	−0.52	−0.53	−0.46	−0.43	−0.43	−0.38	−0.32
(N)	109	128	95	100	113	91	97	113	107	99	289	510

T amplitude by age in lead V2

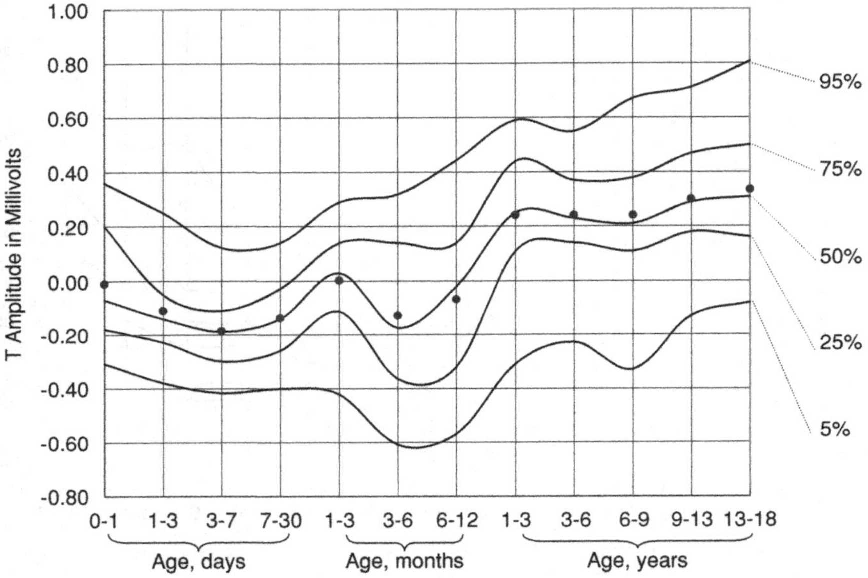

Figure 3.34 T amplitude by age in lead V2, each curve corresponding to the indicated percentile level (• = mean). T wave changes by age in lead V2 are not as spectacular and characteristic as those registered in lead V1.

	Days				*Months*			*Years*				
Age	*0–1*	*1–3*	*3–7*	*7–30*	*1–3*	*3–6*	*6–12*	*1–3*	*3–6*	*6–9*	*9–13*	*13–18*
95%	0.36	0.25	0.12	0.14	0.29	0.32	0.44	0.59	0.55	0.67	0.71	0.81
Mean	**−0.01**	**−0.11**	**−0.19**	**−0.14**	**0.00**	**−0.13**	**−0.07**	**0.24**	**0.24**	**0.24**	**0.3**	**0.34**
(±SD)	**0.21**	**0.17**	**0.18**	**0.17**	**0.21**	**0.32**	**0.35**	**0.27**	**0.21**	**0.26**	**0.26**	**0.26**
5%	−0.31	−0.38	−0.42	−0.40	−0.42	−0.61	−0.57	−0.31	−0.23	−0.33	−0.13	−0.08
(N)	109	128	95	100	120	92	97	113	107	100	289	510

CHAPTER 3.35

T amplitude by age in lead V4

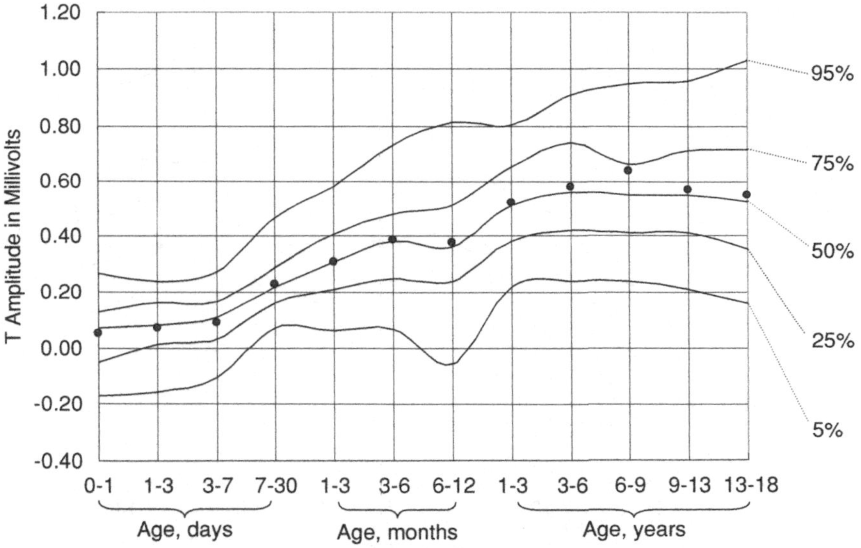

Figure 3.35 T amplitude by age in lead V4, each curve corresponding to the indicated percentile level (• = mean). T waves registered in V4 during the first week of life are low, flat or slightly inverted. They turn upright and taller from age 7–30 days and thereafter with a wider range along with increasing age.

	Days				*Months*			*Years*				
Age	*0–1*	*1–3*	*3–7*	*7–30*	*1–3*	*3–6*	*6–12*	*1–3*	*3–6*	*6–9*	*9–13*	*13–18*
95%	0.27	0.24	0.28	0.46	0.58	0.73	0.81	0.80	0.91	0.95	0.96	1.03
Mean	**0.05**	**0.07**	**0.09**	**0.23**	**0.31**	**0.39**	**0.37**	**0.52**	**0.58**	**0.64**	**0.57**	**0.55**
(±SD)	**0.11**	**0.12**	**0.14**	**0.12**	**0.16**	**0.22**	**0.26**	**0.16**	**0.21**	**0.87**	**0.26**	**0.28**
5%	−0.17	−0.16	−0.10	0.07	0.06	0.07	−0.06	0.22	0.24	0.24	0.21	0.16
(N)	109	128	95	100	120	92	97	113	107	100	289	510

T amplitude by age in lead V5

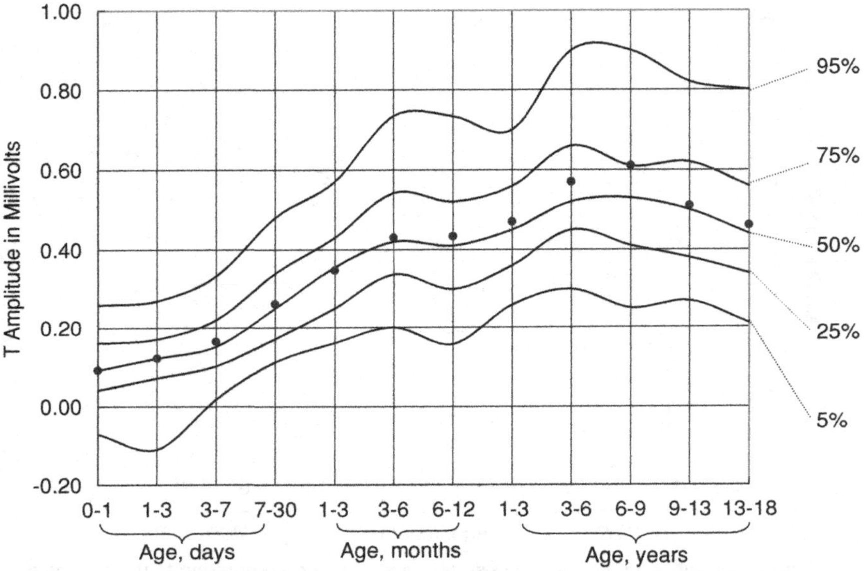

Figure 3.36 T amplitude by age in lead V5, each curve corresponding to the indicated percentile level (• = mean). The T waves changes recorded in V5 from birth to adolescence are similar to those recorded in V4, except that the decrease of the T waves amplitude after age 9–13 years are more prominent.

	Days				*Months*			*Years*				
Age	*0–1*	*1–3*	*3–7*	*7–30*	*1–3*	*3–6*	*6–12*	*1–3*	*3–6*	*6–9*	*9–13*	*13–18*
95%	0.26	0.27	0.33	0.48	0.57	0.73	0.73	0.70	0.90	0.90	0.82	0.80
Mean	**0.09**	**0.12**	**0.16**	**0.26**	**0.35**	**0.43**	**0.43**	**0.47**	**0.57**	**0.61**	**0.51**	**0.46**
(±SD)	**0.11**	**0.12**	**0.11**	**0.11**	**0.14**	**0.19**	**0.18**	**0.11**	**0.16**	**0.82**	**0.17**	**0.18**
5%	−0.07	−0.11	0.02	0.11	0.16	0.20	0.16	0.26	0.30	0.25	0.27	0.21
(N)	109	128	95	100	120	92	97	113	107	100	289	510

T amplitude by age in lead V6

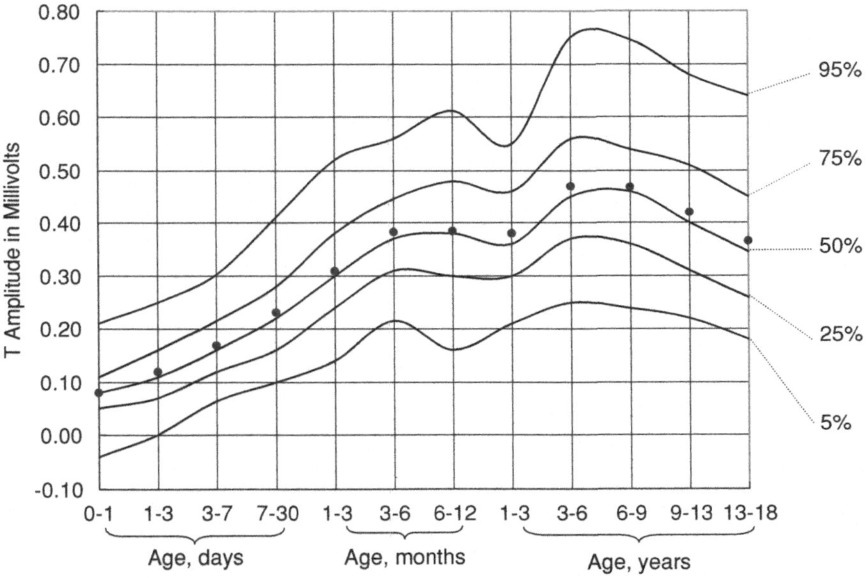

Figure 3.37 T amplitude by age in lead V6, each curve corresponding to the indicated percentile level (• = mean). Normal T wave changes registered in lead V6 are more striking and characteristic than those registered in V5.

	Days				*Months*			*Years*				
Age	*0–1*	*1–3*	*3–7*	*7–30*	*1–3*	*3–6*	*6–12*	*1–3*	*3–6*	*6–9*	*9–13*	*13–18*
95%	0.21	0.25	0.30	0.41	0.52	0.56	0.61	0.55	0.75	0.75	0.68	0.64
Mean	**0.08**	**0.12**	**0.17**	**0.23**	**0.31**	**0.38**	**0.38**	**0.38**	**0.47**	**0.47**	**0.42**	**0.37**
(±SD)	**0.05**	**0.06**	**0.09**	**0.09**	**0.11**	**0.12**	**0.14**	**0.11**	**0.16**	**0.19**	**0.17**	**0.15**
5%	−0.04	0.00	0.06	0.10	0.14	0.22	0.16	0.21	0.25	0.24	0.22	0.18
(N)	109	128	95	100	113	91	97	113	107	99	289	510

PART 4

Calculated values on RS amplitude and ventricular activation time by age

R/S amplitude ratio by age in lead I

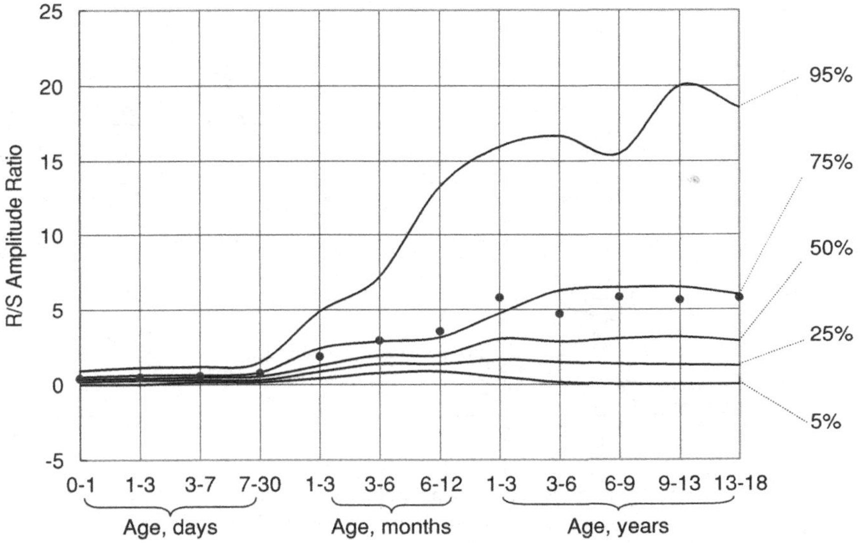

Figure 4.1 R/S amplitude ratio by age in lead I, each curve corresponding to the indicated percentile level (• = mean). R/S amplitude ratio of lead I is small from birth to age 7–30 days. From that age on, the ratio increases steadily and gradually with dominant R waves until adolescence.

	Days				*Months*			*Years*				
Age	*0–1*	*1–3*	*3–7*	*7–30*	*1–3*	*3–6*	*6–12*	*1–3*	*3–6*	*6–9*	*9–13*	*13–18*
95%	0.9	1.1	1.2	1.4	4.9	7.2	13.3	16.0	16.7	15.5	20.0	18.6
Mean	**0.36**	**0.47**	**0.51**	**0.73**	**1.81**	**2.90**	**3.48**	**5.81**	**4.68**	**5.84**	**5.63**	**5.78**
(±SD)	**0.34**	**0.41**	**0.34**	**1.00**	**1.62**	**3.81**	**5.04**	**12.51**	**5.29**	**10.45**	**8.43**	**10.50**
5%	0.00	0.00	0.15	0.15	0.40	0.74	0.85	0.50	0.16	0.00	0.00	0.00
(N)	109	128	95	100	113	91	97	113	107	99	289	510

R/S amplitude ratio by age in lead II

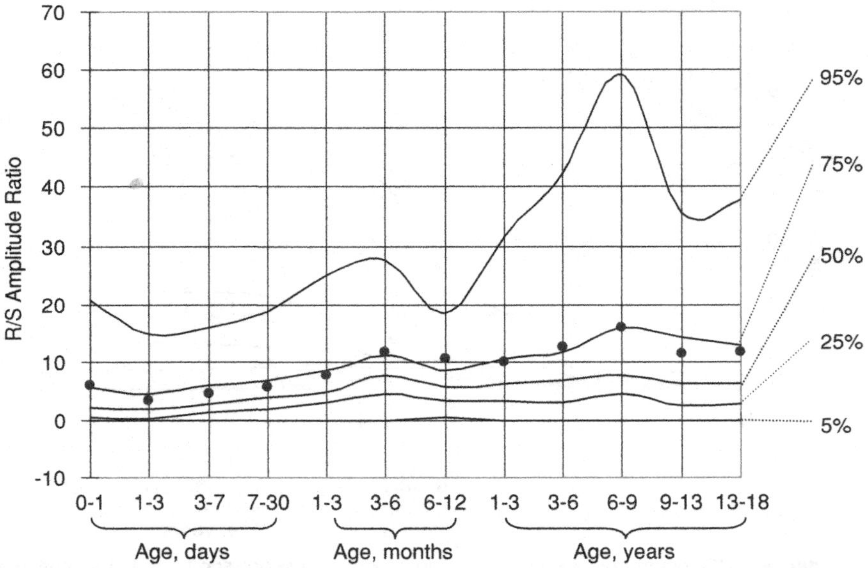

Figure 4.2 R/S amplitude ratio by age in lead II, each curve corresponding to the indicated percentile level (• = mean). The R/S ratio in II decreases slightly after birth, followed by gradual and steady increase from age 1–3 days and thereafter until adolescence.

	Days				*Months*			*Years*				
Age	*0–1*	*1–3*	*3–7*	*7–30*	*1–3*	*3–6*	*6–12*	*1–3*	*3–6*	*6–9*	*9–13*	*13–18*
95%	20.67	14.67	15.82	18.68	25.02	27.46	18.50	31.66	42.33	59.10	35.50	37.89
Mean	**5.82**	**3.45**	**4.39**	**5.76**	**7.61**	**11.67**	**10.49**	**9.92**	**12.36**	**15.94**	**11.45**	**11.50**
(±SD)	**12.37**	**5.32**	**5.09**	**6.17**	**9.22**	**21.21**	**22.85**	**14.67**	**21.35**	**24.90**	**16.48**	**19.71**
5%	0.00	0.00	0.00	0.00	0.00	0.00	0.63	0.00	0.00	0.00	0.00	0.00
(N)	109	128	95	100	113	91	97	113	107	99	289	510

R/S amplitude ratio by age in lead III

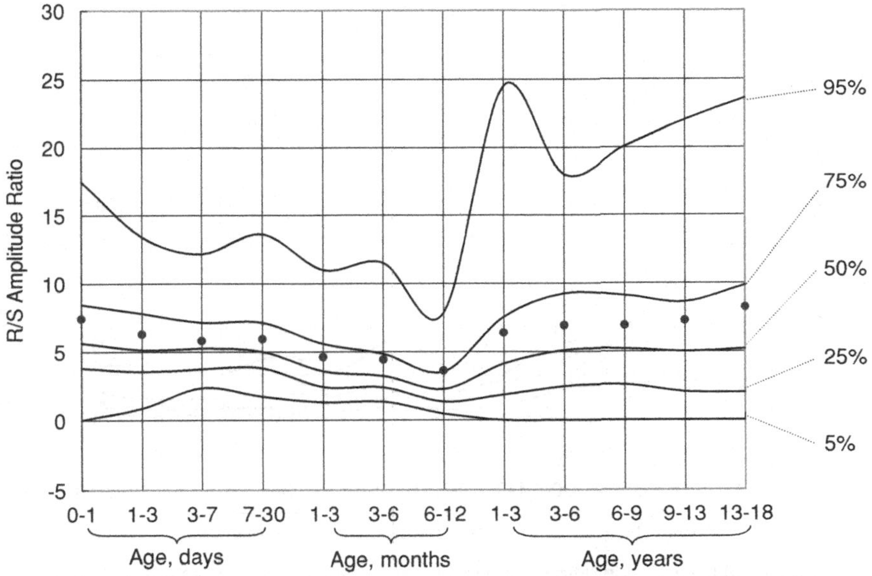

Figure 4.3 R/S amplitude ratio by age in lead III, each curve corresponding to the indicated percentile level (• = mean). Dominant R waves are registered in lead III throughout the pediatric ages.

	Days				*Months*			*Years*				
Age	*0–1*	*1–3*	*3–7*	*7–30*	*1–3*	*3–6*	*6–12*	*1–3*	*3–6*	*6–9*	*9–13*	*13–18*
95%	17.50	13.40	12.15	13.61	11.00	11.50	7.80	24.50	18.00	20.07	22.00	23.59
Mean	**7.41**	**6.30**	**5.80**	**5.94**	**4.62**	**4.45**	**3.63**	**6.39**	**6.90**	**6.89**	**7.25**	**8.19**
(±SD)	**9.17**	**4.72**	**3.08**	**3.68**	**3.28**	**4.38**	**7.88**	**7.65**	**7.12**	**6.63**	**9.76**	**12.52**
5%	0.00	0.91	2.41	1.76	1.34	1.39	0.50	0.00	0.00	0.00	0.00	0.00
(N)	109	128	95	100	113	91	97	113	107	99	289	510

R/S amplitude ratio by age in lead aVR

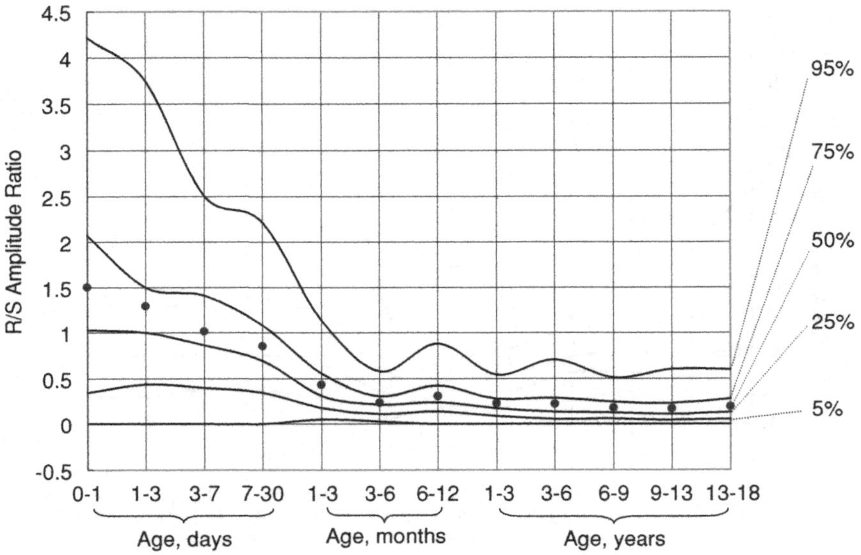

Figure 4.4 R/S amplitude ratio by age in lead aVR, each curve corresponding to the indicated percentile level (• = mean). Dominant R waves are registered in aVR from birth until age 3–6 months. The R/S ratio stays little changed thereafter until adolescence.

	Days				*Months*			*Years*				
Age	*0–1*	*1–3*	*3–7*	*7–30*	*1–3*	*3–6*	*6–12*	*1–3*	*3–6*	*6–9*	*9–13*	*13–18*
95%	4.21	3.75	2.51	2.22	1.14	0.58	0.88	0.54	0.71	0.51	0.60	0.60
Mean	**1.50**	**1.30**	**1.01**	**0.85**	**0.43**	**0.24**	**0.31**	**0.23**	**0.22**	**0.18**	**0.17**	**0.20**
(±SD)	**1.67**	**1.34**	**0.83**	**0.86**	**0.48**	**0.18**	**0.24**	**0.20**	**0.27**	**0.17**	**0.18**	**0.19**
5%	0.00	0.00	0.00	0.00	0.05	0.03	0.00	0.00	0.00	0.00	0.00	0.00
(N)	109	128	95	100	113	91	97	113	107	99	289	510

R/S amplitude ratio by age in lead aVL

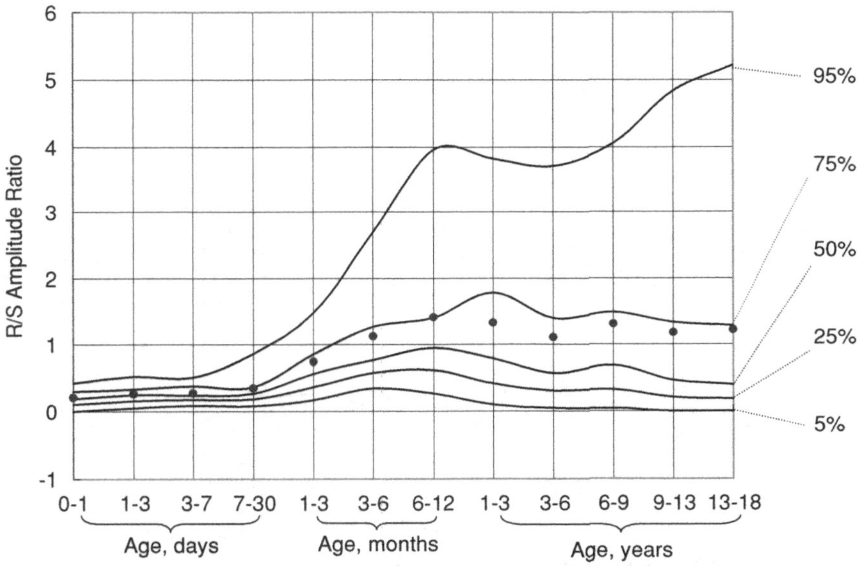

Figure 4.5 R/S amplitude ratio by age in lead aVL, each curve corresponding to the indicated percentile level (• = mean). The R/S ratio of aVL is small after birth until age 7–30 days, then increases typically with increasing age.

	Days				*Months*			*Years*				
Age	*0–1*	*1–3*	*3–7*	*7–30*	*1–3*	*3–6*	*6–12*	*1–3*	*3–6*	*6–9*	*9–13*	*13–18*
95%	0.43	0.53	0.52	0.86	1.49	2.69	3.96	3.83	3.71	4.06	4.83	5.21
Mean	**0.22**	**0.27**	**0.28**	**0.35**	**0.75**	**1.13**	**1.41**	**1.33**	**1.11**	**1.31**	**1.18**	**1.22**
(±SD)	**0.13**	**0.16**	**0.14**	**0.39**	**0.71**	**1.07**	**1.85**	**1.71**	**1.39**	**2.01**	**2.01**	**2.13**
5%	0.00	0.05	0.09	0.09	0.18	0.36	0.28	0.11	0.05	0.05	0.00	0.00
(N)	109	128	95	100	113	91	97	113	107	99	289	510

R/S amplitude ratio by age in lead aVF

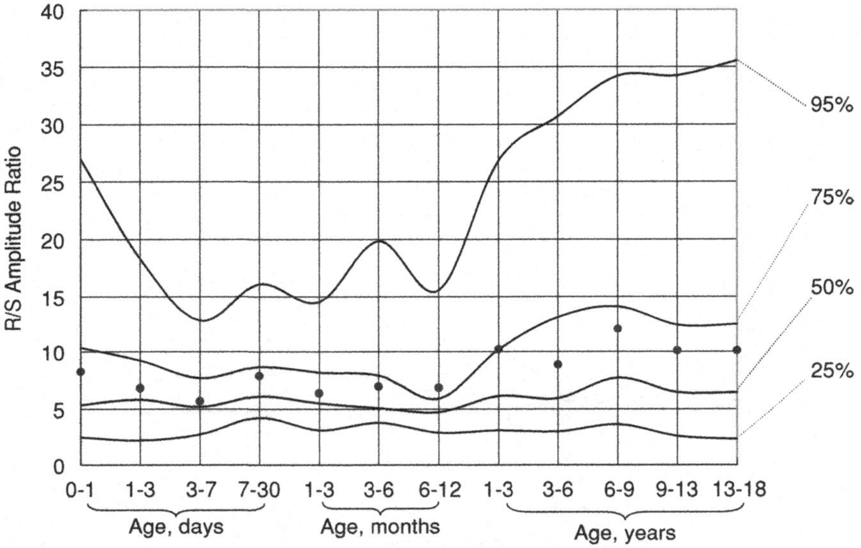

Figure 4.6 R/S amplitude ratio by age in lead aVF, each curve corresponding to the indicated percentile level (• = mean). The R waves in aVF stay dominant through birth to adolescence. The R/S ratio increases substantially after age 6–12 months until adolescence.

	Days				*Months*			*Years*				
Age	*0–1*	*1–3*	*3–7*	*7–30*	*1–3*	*3–6*	*6–12*	*1–3*	*3–6*	*6–9*	*9–13*	*13–18*
95%	27.00	18.29	12.83	16.08	14.52	19.85	15.56	26.85	30.67	34.20	34.25	35.53
Mean	**8.20**	**6.77**	**5.66**	**7.84**	**6.36**	**6.91**	**6.79**	**10.17**	**8.80**	**12.03**	**10.07**	**10.07**
(±SD)	**10.81**	**6.73**	**5.98**	**10.38**	**6.14**	**8.08**	**12.44**	**17.53**	**8.82**	**16.35**	**14.70**	**14.30**
5%	0.00	0.00	0.00	0.09	0.00	0.00	0.00	0.00	0.00	0.00	0.00	0.00
(N)	109	128	95	100	113	91	97	113	107	99	289	510

R/S amplitude ratio by age in lead V1

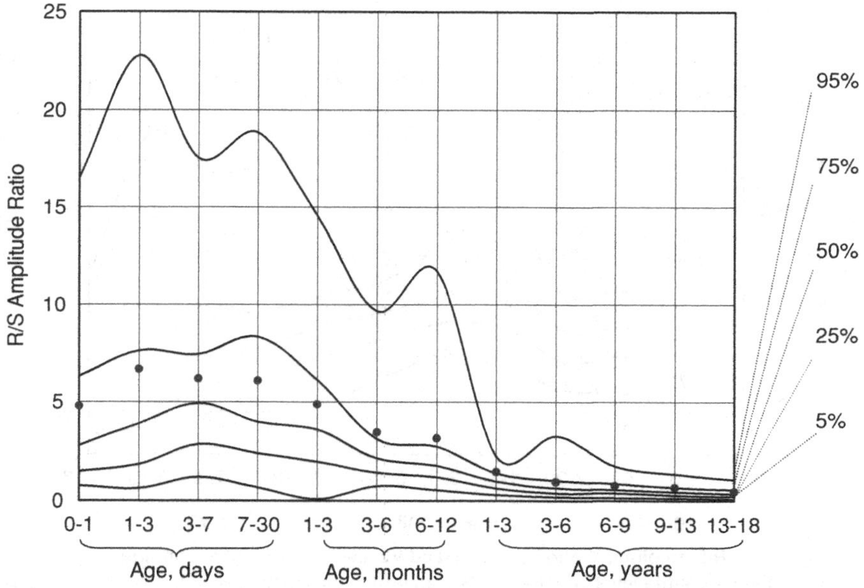

Figure 4.7 R/S amplitude ratio by age in lead V1, each curve corresponding to the indicated percentile level (• = mean). R/S amplitude ratio in V1 reflects the structural changes of the heart occurring from birth to adolescence. The ratio increases slightly after birth, then decreases strikingly throughout infancy, childhood and adolescence.

	Days				*Months*			*Years*				
Age	*0–1*	*1–3*	*3–7*	*7–30*	*1–3*	*3–6*	*6–12*	*1–3*	*3–6*	*6–9*	*9–13*	*13–18*
95%	16.55	22.75	17.53	18.83	14.51	9.67	11.72	2.23	3.25	1.74	1.34	1.06
Mean	**4.79**	**6.69**	**6.20**	**6.10**	**4.88**	**3.44**	**3.14**	**1.45**	**0.95**	**0.77**	**0.67**	**0.47**
(±SD)	**5.11**	**9.09**	**5.30**	**5.82**	**4.91**	**6.06**	**4.82**	**4.10**	**1.05**	**0.96**	**1.56**	**0.48**
5%	0.75	0.64	1.20	0.68	0.09	0.75	0.55	0.31	0.20	0.15	0.12	0.09
(N)	109	128	95	100	113	91	97	113	107	99	289	510

R/S amplitude ratio by age in lead V2

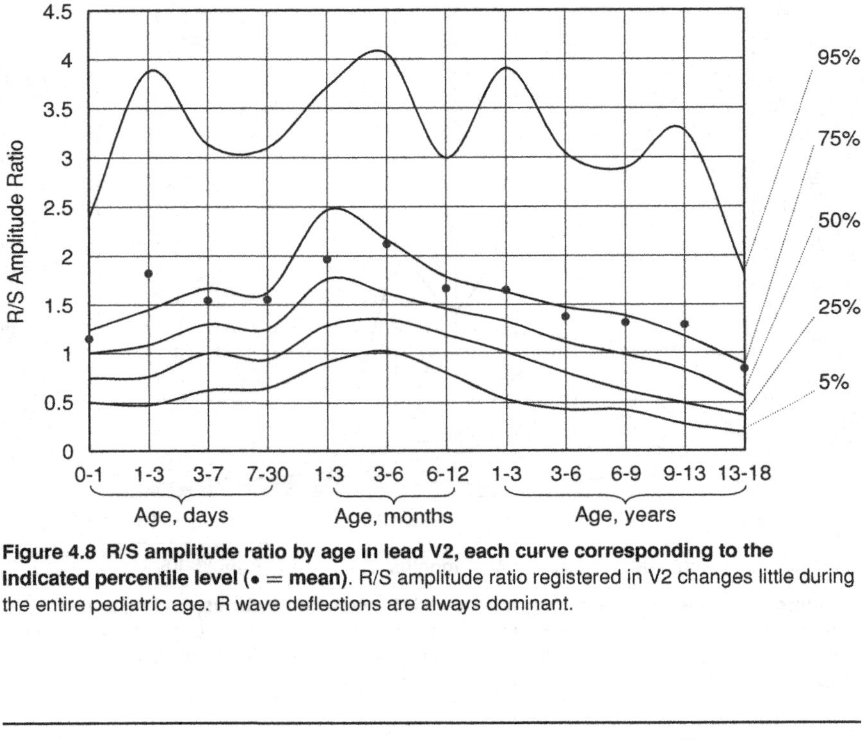

Figure 4.8 R/S amplitude ratio by age in lead V2, each curve corresponding to the indicated percentile level (• = mean). R/S amplitude ratio registered in V2 changes little during the entire pediatric age. R wave deflections are always dominant.

	Days				*Months*			*Years*				
Age	*0–1*	*1–3*	*3–7*	*7–30*	*1–3*	*3–6*	*6–12*	*1–3*	*3–6*	*6–9*	*9–13*	*13–18*
95%	2.39	3.88	3.14	3.10	3.71	4.06	3.00	3.91	3.04	2.89	3.28	1.82
Mean	**1.14**	**1.82**	**1.55**	**1.56**	**1.96**	**2.12**	**1.67**	**1.65**	**1.37**	**1.31**	**1.29**	**0.84**
(±SD)	**0.67**	**4.01**	**1.05**	**1.57**	**0.93**	**2.32**	**1.03**	**1.51**	**1.14**	**1.39**	**3.19**	**1.79**
5%	0.51	0.48	0.63	0.65	0.90	1.02	0.80	0.54	0.43	0.43	0.28	0.19
(N)	109	128	95	100	113	91	97	113	107	99	289	510

R/S amplitude ratio by age in lead V3

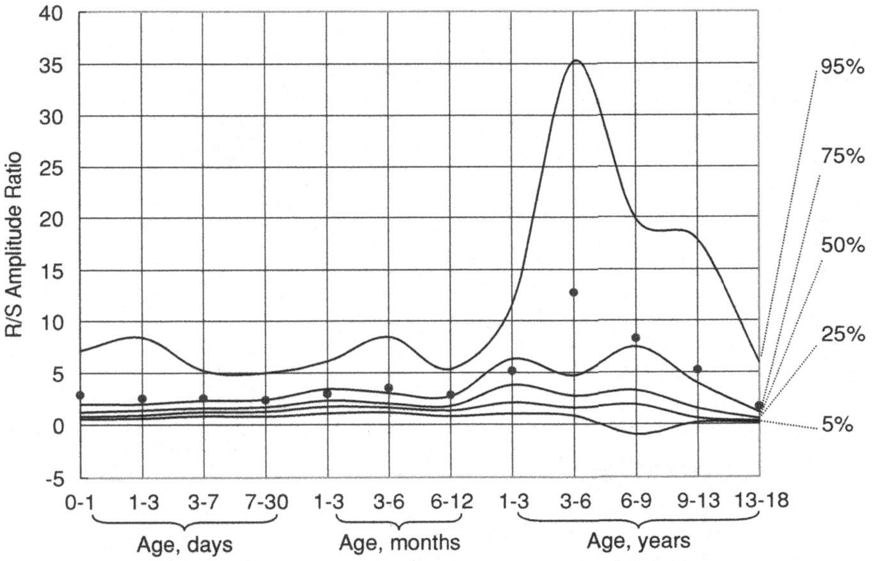

Figure 4.9 R/S amplitude ratio by age in lead V3, each curve corresponding to the indicated percentile level (• = mean). R/S amplitude ratio remains unchanged during infancy. It starts to increase by age 1 year and forward, followed by a decrease after age 6–9 years.

	Days				*Months*			*Years*				
Age	*0–1*	*1–3*	*3–7*	*7–30*	*1–3*	*3–6*	*6–12*	*1–3*	*3–6*	*6–9*	*9–13*	*13–18*
95%	7.20	8.43	5.23	5.04	6.12	8.47	5.37	11.54	35.19	19.84	17.86	5.96
Mean	**2.90**	**2.55**	**2.54**	**2.39**	**2.98**	**3.53**	**2.84**	**5.18**	**12.73**	**8.24**	**5.22**	**1.70**
(±SD)	**7.16**	**4.73**	**5.15**	**2.81**	**2.26**	**5.41**	**6.73**	**5.68**	**51.57**	**25.30**	**14.97**	**4.65**
5%	0.58	0.62	0.82	0.80	1.10	1.19	0.80	1.06	0.85	−1.00	0.17	0.14
(N)	109	128	95	100	113	91	97	113	107	99	289	510

R/S amplitude ratio by age in lead V4

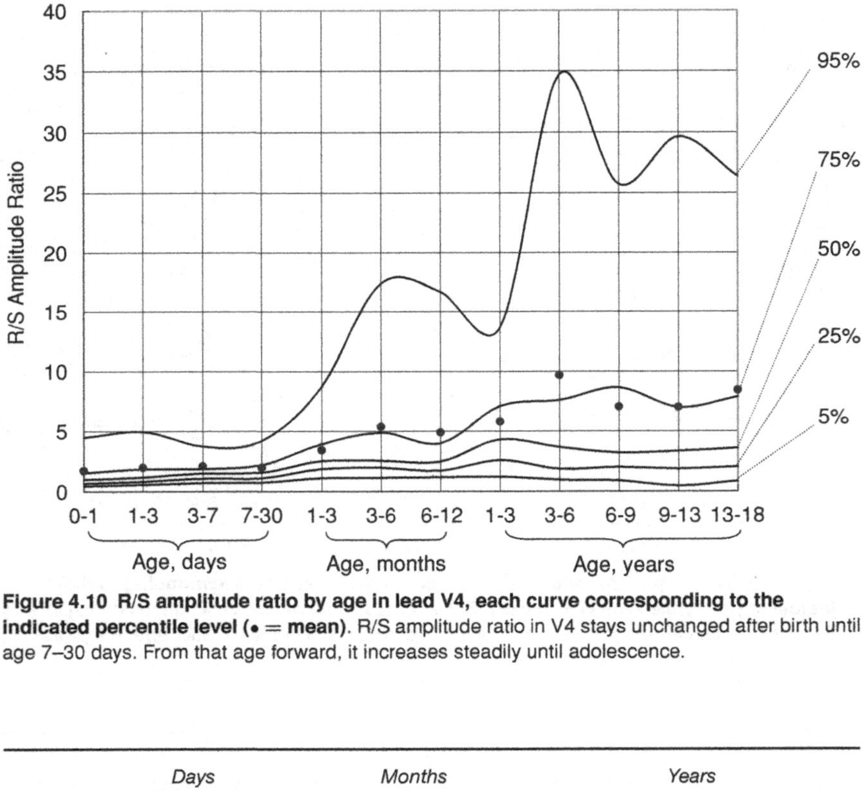

Figure 4.10 R/S amplitude ratio by age in lead V4, each curve corresponding to the indicated percentile level (• = mean). R/S amplitude ratio in V4 stays unchanged after birth until age 7–30 days. From that age forward, it increases steadily until adolescence.

	Days				*Months*			*Years*				
Age	*0–1*	*1–3*	*3–7*	*7–30*	*1–3*	*3–6*	*6–12*	*1–3*	*3–6*	*6–9*	*9–13*	*13–18*
95%	4.47	4.95	3.73	4.20	8.77	17.40	16.69	13.67	34.67	25.70	29.64	26.34
Mean	**1.72**	**1.95**	**2.06**	**1.98**	**3.40**	**5.38**	**4.90**	**5.84**	**9.70**	**7.09**	**7.05**	**8.46**
(±SD)	**2.88**	**3.76**	**3.70**	**2.06**	**2.79**	**7.97**	**8.92**	**5.44**	**21.99**	**11.43**	**13.00**	**19.77**
5%	0.48	0.57	0.73	0.75	1.11	1.15	1.18	1.20	0.98	0.91	0.46	0.86
(N)	109	128	95	100	113	91	97	113	107	99	289	510

R/S amplitude ratio by age in lead V5

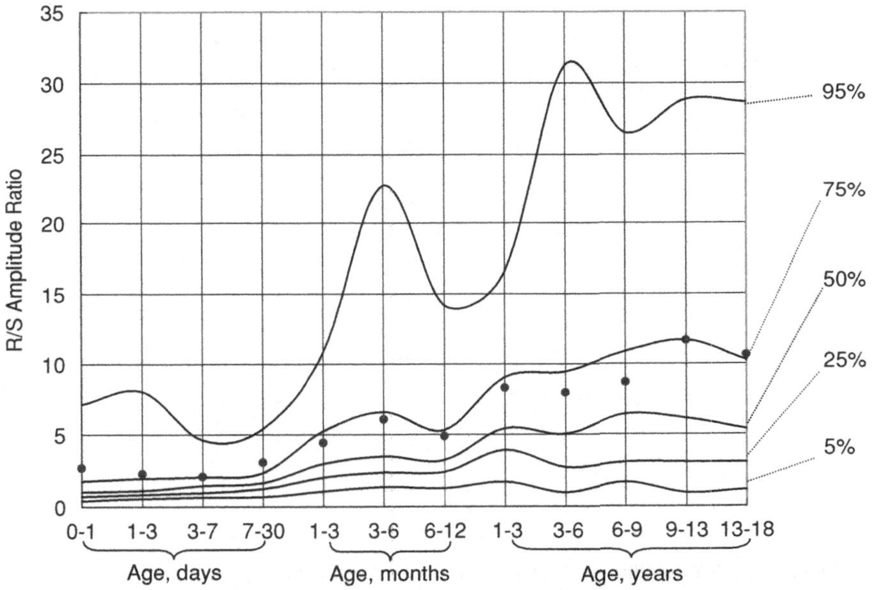

Figure 4.11 R/S amplitude ratio by age in lead V5, each curve corresponding to the indicated percentile level (• = mean). R/S amplitude ratio in V5 stays little changed after birth. It starts to increase from 7–30 days of age until age 13–18 years.

	Days				*Months*			*Years*				
Age	*0–1*	*1–3*	*3–7*	*7–30*	*1–3*	*3–6*	*6–12*	*1–3*	*3–6*	*6–9*	*9–13*	*13–18*
95%	7.14	8.09	4.62	5.42	10.83	22.79	14.19	16.56	31.22	26.52	28.88	28.66
Mean	**2.72**	**2.28**	**2.09**	**3.07**	**4.44**	**6.07**	**4.89**	**8.35**	**8.01**	**8.72**	**11.66**	**10.63**
(±SD)	**8.24**	**3.54**	**2.63**	**10.39**	**4.26**	**6.36**	**4.76**	**15.03**	**8.35**	**9.13**	**22.88**	**22.24**
5%	0.41	0.56	0.67	0.70	1.08	1.38	1.29	1.73	0.99	1.70	0.94	1.16
(N)	109	128	95	100	113	91	97	113	107	99	289	510

R/S amplitude ratio by age in lead V6

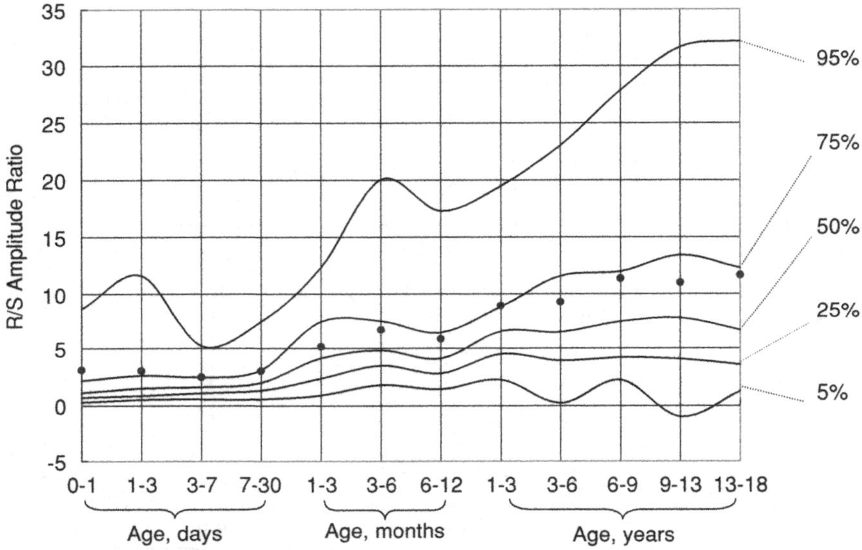

Figure 4.12 R/S amplitude ratio by age in lead V6, each curve corresponding to the indicated percentile level (• = mean). The progress of R/S amplitude ratio in lead V6 is striking. The ratio stays little changed after birth, then increases from age 1 month, then continues to increase forward until age 13–18 years.

	Days				*Months*			*Years*				
Age	*0–1*	*1–3*	*3–7*	*7–30*	*1–3*	*3–6*	*6–12*	*1–3*	*3–6*	*6–9*	*9–13*	*13–18*
95%	8.69	11.60	5.21	7.48	12.35	20.03	17.29	19.50	23.00	27.86	31.67	32.17
Mean	**3.06**	**2.97**	**2.42**	**2.98**	**5.16**	**6.69**	**5.85**	**8.93**	**9.27**	**11.35**	**11.00**	**11.66**
(±SD)	**8.34**	**4.21**	**3.77**	**4.25**	**4.19**	**6.43**	**5.59**	**11.62**	**11.92**	**16.37**	**13.29**	**19.18**
5%	0.29	0.52	0.57	0.56	0.90	1.75	1.39	2.21	0.21	2.20	−1.00	1.27
(N)	109	128	95	100	113	91	97	113	107	99	289	510

R amplitude in lead V3 + S amplitude in lead V3 by age

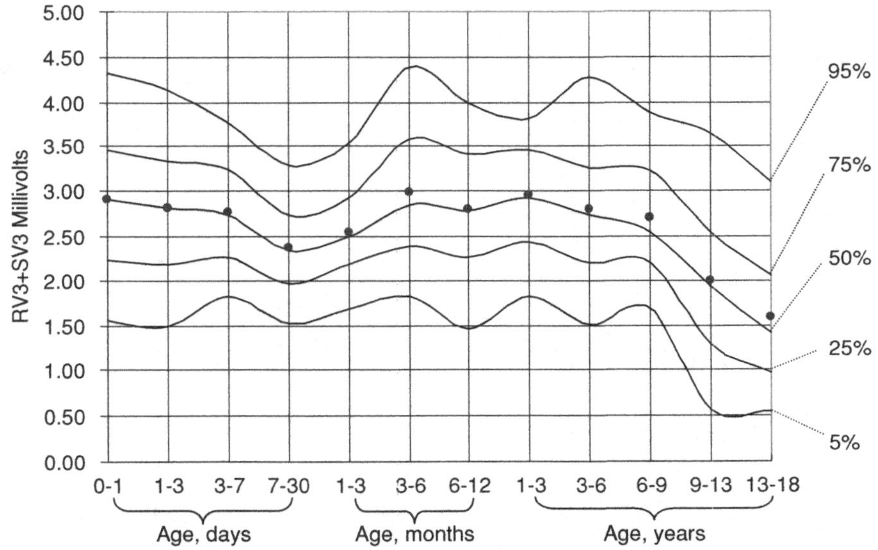

Figure 4.13 R amplitude in lead V3+ S amplitude in lead V3 by age, each curve corresponding to the indicated percentile level (• = mean). The sum of R wave amplitude in lead V3 and S wave amplitude in V3 decreases slightly after birth. It increases after age 7–30 days, reaching the highest value at ages 3–6 months and 1–3 years, then decreases thereafter up to age 13–18 years.

	Days				*Months*			*Years*				
Age	*0–1*	*1–3*	*3–7*	*7–30*	*1–3*	*3–6*	*6–12*	*1–3*	*3–6*	*6–9*	*9–13*	*13–18*
95%	4.32	4.13	3.77	3.28	3.54	4.38	4.00	3.82	4.28	3.88	3.65	3.10
Mean	**2.91**	**2.81**	**2.77**	**2.38**	**2.55**	**2.99**	**2.80**	**2.95**	**2.8**	**2.7**	**1.99**	**1.59**
(±SD)	**0.91**	**0.81**	**0.67**	**0.62**	**0.60**	**0.79**	**0.85**	**0.65**	**0.90**	**0.71**	**0.95**	**0.81**
5%	1.55	1.50	1.83	1.53	1.69	1.83	1.47	1.83	1.51	1.69	0.56	0.55
(N)	109	128	95	100	120	92	97	113	107	100	289	510

R amplitude in lead V6 + S amplitude in lead V1 by age

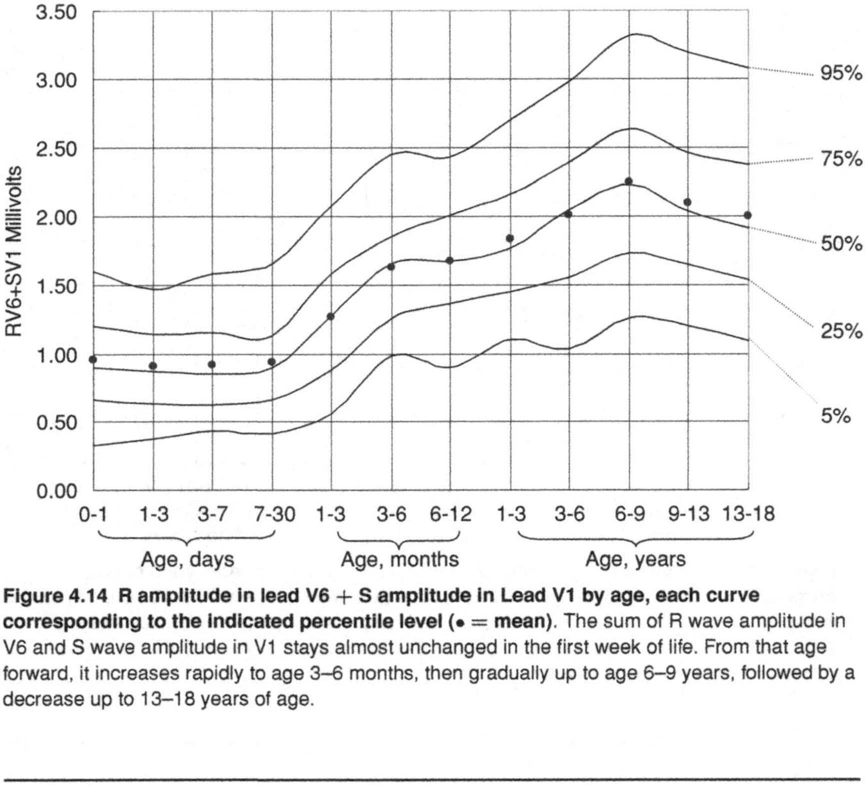

Figure 4.14 R amplitude in lead V6 + S amplitude in Lead V1 by age, each curve corresponding to the indicated percentile level (• = mean). The sum of R wave amplitude in V6 and S wave amplitude in V1 stays almost unchanged in the first week of life. From that age forward, it increases rapidly to age 3–6 months, then gradually up to age 6–9 years, followed by a decrease up to 13–18 years of age.

	Days				*Months*			*Years*					
Age	*0–1*	*1–3*	*3–7*	*7–30*	*1–3*	*3–6*	*6–12*	*1–3*	*3–6*	*6–9*	*9–13*	*13–18*
95%	1.60	1.47	1.58	1.66	2.08	2.45	2.43	2.70	2.98	3.32	3.19	3.08
Mean	**0.96**	**0.91**	**0.92**	**0.94**	**1.27**	**1.63**	**1.68**	**1.84**	**2.01**	**2.25**	**2.1**	**2.00**
(±SD)	**0.43**	**0.35**	**0.39**	**0.37**	**0.49**	**0.47**	**0.50**	**0.49**	**0.58**	**0.71**	**0.61**	**0.63**
5%	0.33	0.37	0.43	0.41	0.56	0.99	0.90	1.10	1.04	1.26	1.20	1.09
(N)	109	128	95	100	120	92	97	113	107	100	289	510

R amplitude in lead V6 + S amplitude in lead V2 by age

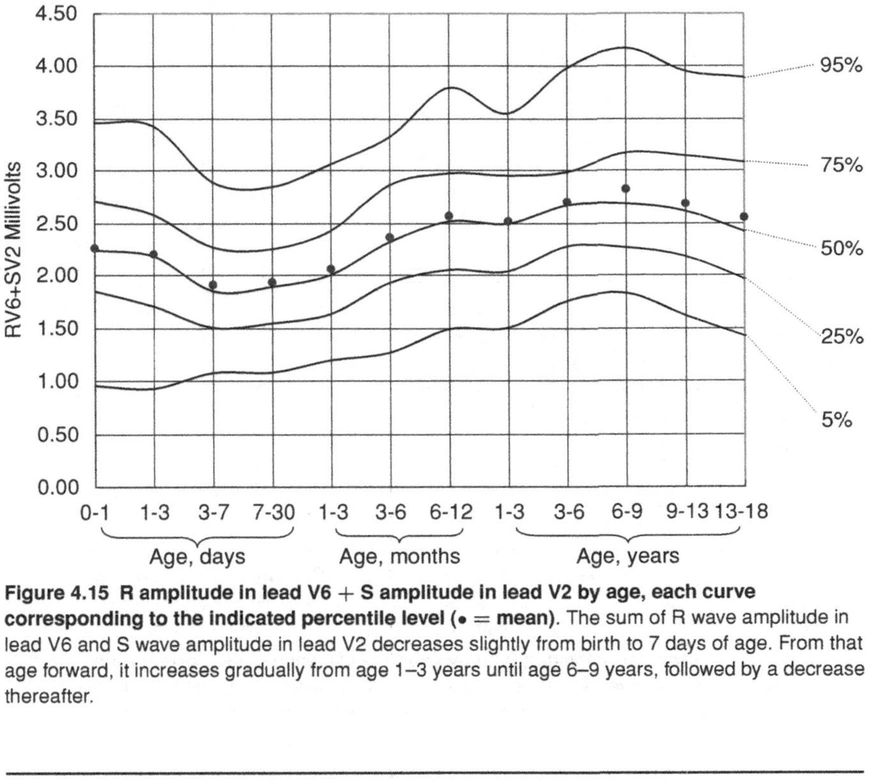

Figure 4.15 R amplitude in lead V6 + S amplitude in lead V2 by age, each curve corresponding to the indicated percentile level (• = mean). The sum of R wave amplitude in lead V6 and S wave amplitude in lead V2 decreases slightly from birth to 7 days of age. From that age forward, it increases gradually from age 1–3 years until age 6–9 years, followed by a decrease thereafter.

	Days				*Months*			*Years*				
Age	*0–1*	*1–3*	*3–7*	*7–30*	*1–3*	*3–6*	*6–12*	*1–3*	*3–6*	*6–9*	*9–13*	*13–18*
95%	3.46	3.43	2.89	2.85	3.06	3.32	3.79	3.55	3.98	4.17	3.95	3.89
Mean	**2.26**	**2.2**	**1.91**	**1.94**	**2.06**	**2.37**	**2.57**	**2.52**	**2.7**	**2.82**	**2.68**	**2.55**
(±SD)	**0.75**	**0.75**	**0.55**	**0.55**	**0.59**	**0.62**	**0.73**	**0.65**	**0.63**	**0.77**	**0.69**	**0.79**
5%	0.96	0.93	1.08	1.08	1.20	1.27	1.50	1.51	1.76	1.83	1.62	1.43
(N)	109	128	95	100	120	92	97	113	107	100	289	510

Ventricular activation time by age in lead I

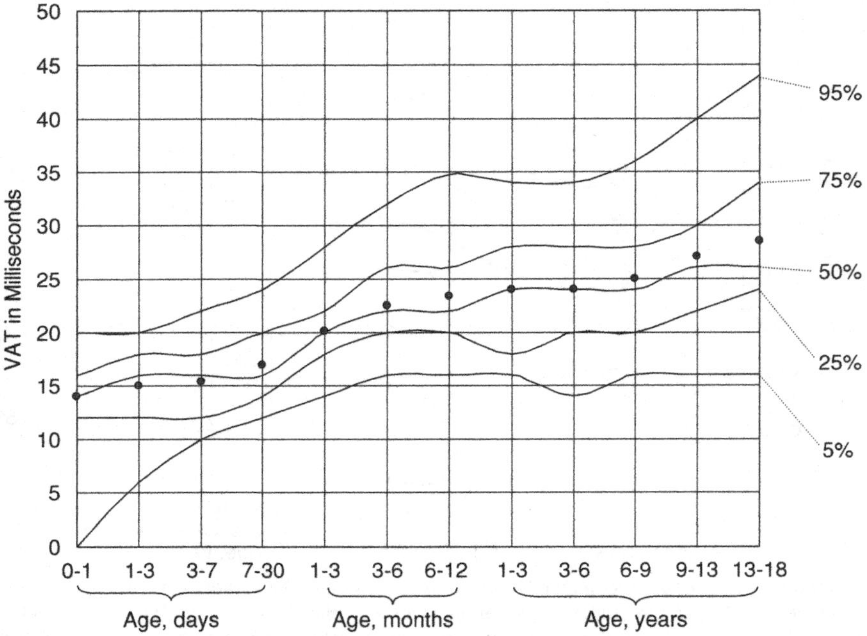

Figure 4.16 Ventricular activation time by age in lead I, each curve corresponding to the indicated percentile level (• = mean). The ventricular activation time recorded in lead I becomes longer with increasing age, more strikingly during infancy and adolescence.

	Days				*Months*			*Years*				
Age	*0–1*	*1–3*	*3–7*	*7–30*	*1–3*	*3–6*	*6–12*	*1–3*	*3–6*	*6–9*	*9–13*	*13–18*
95%	20	20	22	24	28	32	35	34	34	36	40	44
Mean	**14**	**15**	**15**	**17**	**20**	**22**	**23**	**24**	**24**	**25**	**27**	**29**
(±SD)	**5.33**	**5.77**	**3.87**	**4.86**	**4.72**	**5.45**	**6.00**	**5.42**	**5.28**	**10.20**	**8.67**	**8.26**
5%	0	6	10	12	14	16	16	16	14	16	16	16
(N)	109	128	95	100	120	92	97	113	107	100	289	510

Ventricular activation time by age in lead II

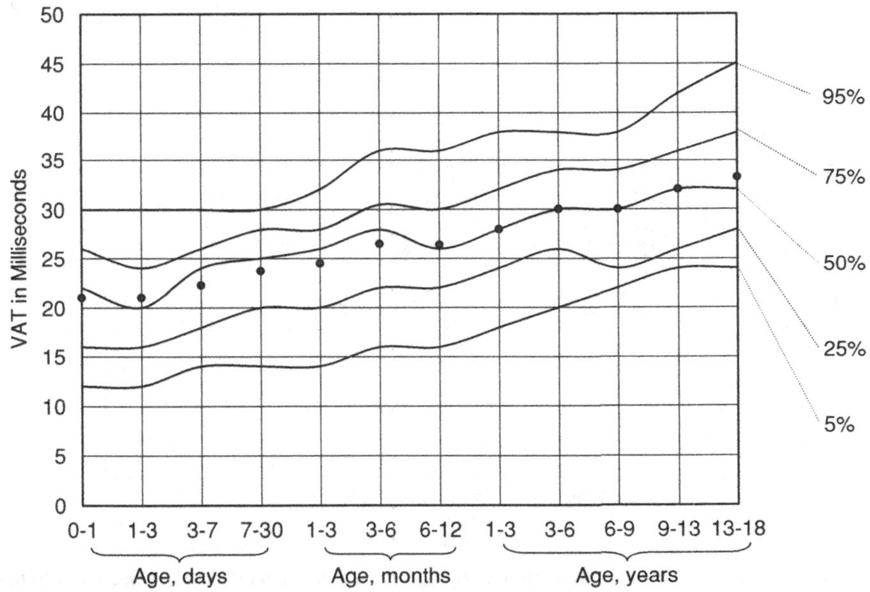

Figure 4.17 Ventricular activation time by age in lead II, each curve corresponding to the indicated percentile level (• = mean). The ventricular activation time registered in lead II becomes longer gradually and steadily with increasing age from birth to adolescence.

	Days				*Months*			*Years*				
Age	*0–1*	*1–3*	*3–7*	*7–30*	*1–3*	*3–6*	*6–12*	*1–3*	*3–6*	*6–9*	*9–13*	*13–18*
95%	30	30	30	30	32	36	36	38	38	38	42	45
Mean	**21**	**21**	**22**	**24**	**24**	**27**	**26**	**28**	**30**	**30**	**32**	**33**
(±SD)	**5.33**	**5.77**	**5.44**	**5.00**	**5.59**	**6.94**	**7.05**	**5.42**	**5.28**	**5.10**	**8.67**	**7.11**
5%	12	12	14	14	14	16	16	18	20	22	24	24
(N)	109	128	95	100	120	92	97	113	107	100	289	510

Ventricular activation time by age in lead III

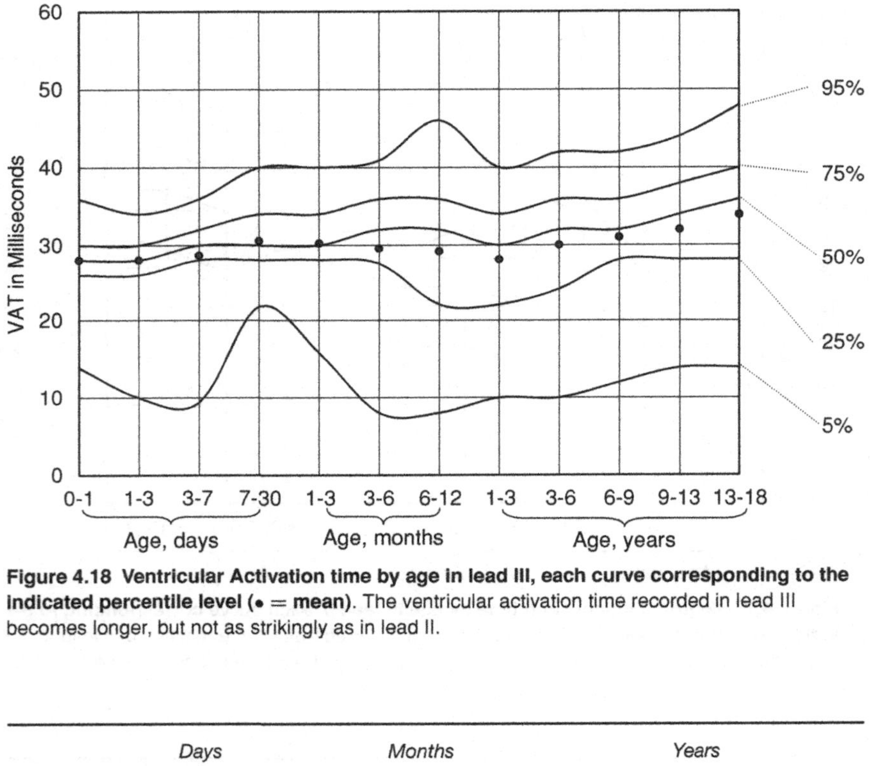

Figure 4.18 Ventricular Activation time by age in lead III, each curve corresponding to the indicated percentile level (• = mean). The ventricular activation time recorded in lead III becomes longer, but not as strikingly as in lead II.

	Days				*Months*			*Years*				
Age	*0–1*	*1–3*	*3–7*	*7–30*	*1–3*	*3–6*	*6–12*	*1–3*	*3–6*	*6–9*	*9–13*	*13–18*
95%	36	34	36	40	40	41	46	40	42	42	44	48
Mean	**28**	**28**	**29**	**31**	**30**	**30**	**29**	**28**	**30**	**31**	**32**	**34**
(±SD)	**5.33**	**5.77**	**6.95**	**6.38**	**7.23**	**9.83**	**11.76**	**10.85**	**10.56**	**10.20**	**8.67**	**10.26**
5%	14	10	9	22	16	8	8	10	10	12	14	14
(N)	109	128	95	100	120	92	97	113	107	100	289	510

Ventricular activation time by age in lead aVR

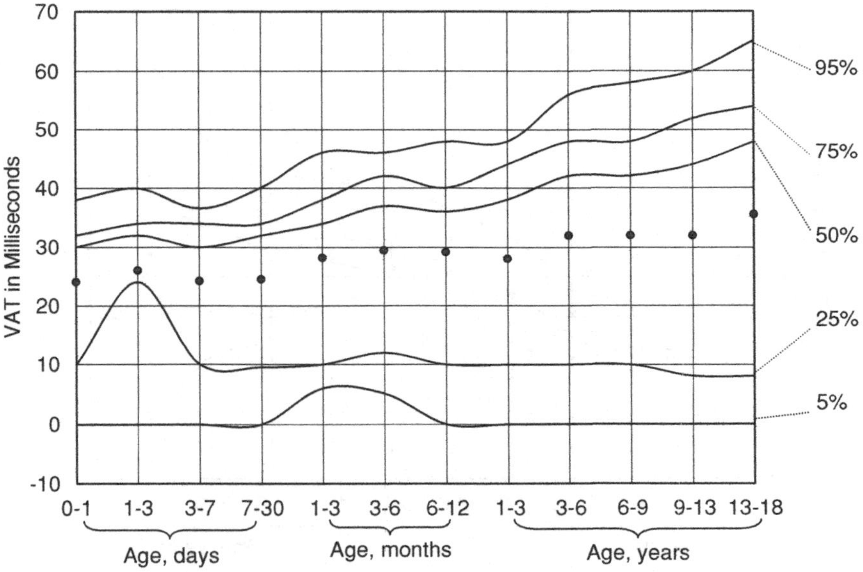

Figure 4.19 Ventricular activation time by age in lead aVR, each curve corresponding to the indicated percentile level (• = mean). Ventricular activation time recorded in lead aVR becomes longer with a wider range along with increasing age.

	Days				*Months*			*Years*				
Age	*0–1*	*1–3*	*3–7*	*7–30*	*1–3*	*3–6*	*6–12*	*1–3*	*3–6*	*6–9*	*9–13*	*13–18*
95%	38	40	37	40	46	46	48	48	56	58	60	65
Mean	**24**	**26**	**24**	**24**	**28**	**29**	**29**	**28**	**32**	**32**	**32**	**35**
(±SD)	**10.65**	**11.54**	**12.15**	**13.82**	**14.46**	**15.47**	**16.31**	**16.27**	**21.11**	**20.41**	**26.02**	**24.61**
5%	0	0	0	0	6	5	0	0	0	0	0	0
(N)	109	128	95	100	120	92	97	113	107	100	289	510

Ventricular activation time by age in lead aVL

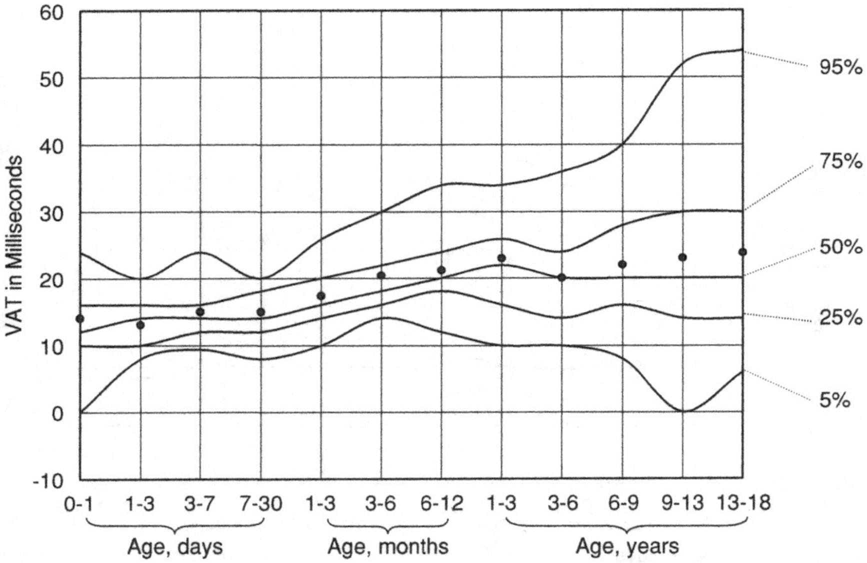

Figure 4.20 Ventricular activation time by age in lead aVL, each curve corresponding to the indicated percentile level (• = mean). The ventricular activation time interval increases with a wider range from birth to adolescence, particularly during late adolescence.

	Days				*Months*			*Years*					
Age	*0–1*	*1–3*	*3–7*	*7–30*	*1–3*	*3–6*	*6–12*	*1–3*	*3–6*	*6–9*	*9–13*	*13–18*
95%	24	20	24	20	26	30	34	34	36	40	52	54
Mean	**14**	**13**	**15**	**15**	**17**	**20**	**21**	**23**	**20**	**22**	**23**	**24**
(±SD)	**10.65**	**5.77**	**6.68**	**4.96**	**6.35**	**7.54**	**6.73**	**10.85**	**10.56**	**10.20**	**17.35**	**15.37**
5%	0	8	9	8	10	14	12	10	10	8	0	6
(N)	109	128	95	100	120	92	97	113	107	100	289	510

Ventricular activation time by age in lead aVF

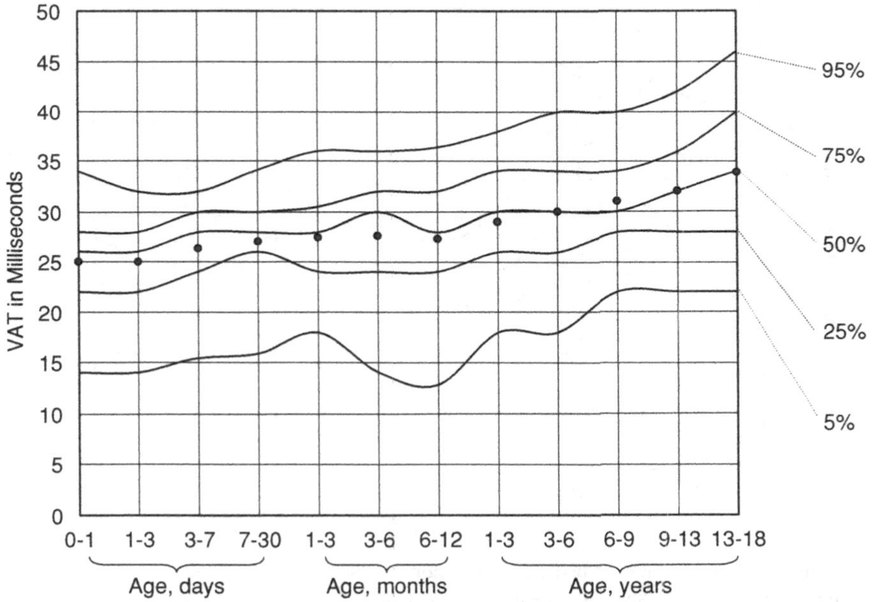

Figure 4.21 Ventricular activation time by age in lead aVF, each curve corresponding to the indicated percentile level (• = mean). The lengthening of ventricular activation time recorded in aVF is gradual and steady during aging from birth to adolescence.

	Days				*Months*			*Years*				
Age	*0–1*	*1–3*	*3–7*	*7–30*	*1–3*	*3–6*	*6–12*	*1–3*	*3–6*	*6–9*	*9–13*	*13–18*
95%	34	32	32	34	36	36	36	38	40	40	42	46
Mean	**25**	**25**	**26**	**27**	**27**	**28**	**27**	**29**	**30**	**31**	**32**	**34**
(±SD)	**5.33**	**5.77**	**5.77**	**5.79**	**5.37**	**7.17**	**7.96**	**5.42**	**5.28**	**5.10**	**8.67**	**7.30**
5%	14	14	15	16	18	14	13	18	18	22	22	22
(N)	109	128	95	100	120	92	97	113	107	100	289	510

CHAPTER 4.22

Ventricular activation time by age in lead V1

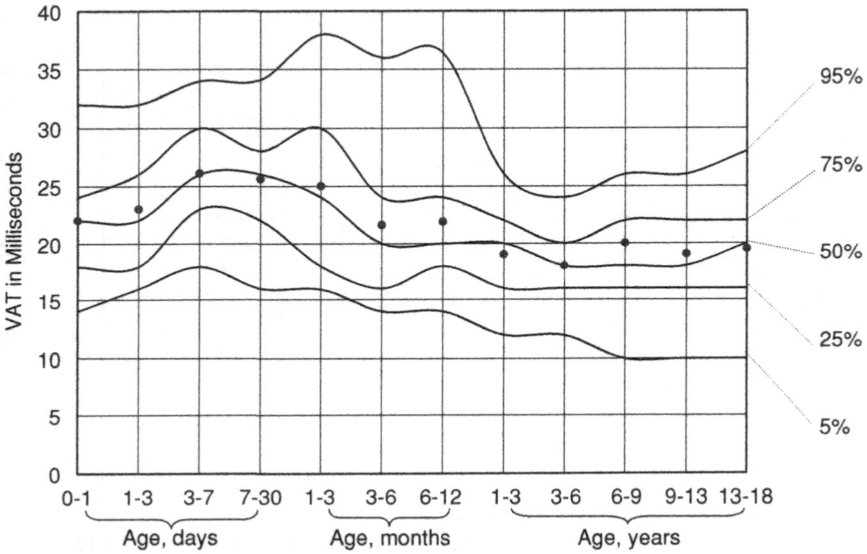

Figure 4.22 Ventricular activation time by age in lead V1, each curve corresponding to the indicated percentile level (• = mean). The ventricular activation time interval recorded in lead V1 increases after birth up to age 3–7 days, then decreases during infancy, reaching a plateau level by age 1–3 years, until adolescence.

	Days				*Months*			*Years*					
Age	*0–1*	*1–3*	*3–7*	*7–30*	*1–3*	*3–6*	*6–12*	*1–3*	*3–6*	*6–9*	*9–13*	*13–18*
95%	32	32	34	34	38	36	36	26	24	26	26	28
Mean	**22**	**23**	**26**	**26**	**25**	**22**	**22**	**19**	**18**	**20**	**19**	**19**
(±SD)	**5.33**	**5.77**	**4.90**	**5.67**	**8.52**	**6.56**	**6.99**	**5.42**	**5.28**	**5.10**	**8.67**	**6.87**
5%	14	16	18	16	16	14	14	12	12	10	10	10
(N)	109	128	95	100	120	92	97	113	107	100	289	510

Ventricular activation time by age in lead V2

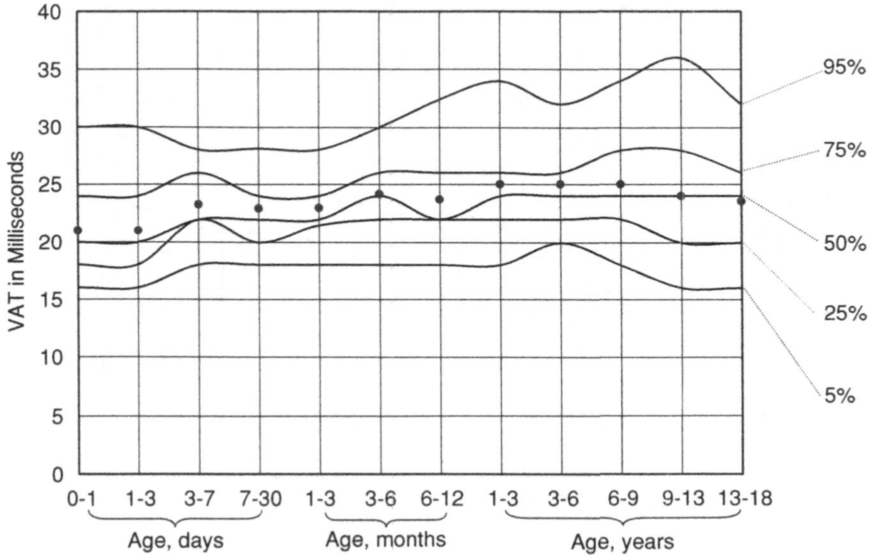

Figure 4.23 Ventricular activation time by age in lead V2, each curve corresponding to the indicated percentile level (• = mean). The average ventricular activation time registered in lead V2 varies little throughout the pediatric age from birth to adolescence.

	Days				*Months*			*Years*				
Age	*0–1*	*1–3*	*3–7*	*7–30*	*1–3*	*3–6*	*6–12*	*1–3*	*3–6*	*6–9*	*9–13*	*13–18*
95%	30	30	28	28	28	30	32	34	32	34	36	32
Mean	**21**	**21**	**23**	**23**	**23**	**24**	**24**	**25**	**25**	**25**	**24**	**24**
(±SD)	**5.33**	**5.77**	**4.54**	**3.15**	**2.97**	**4.16**	**4.26**	**5.42**	**5.28**	**5.10**	**8.67**	**5.15**
5%	16	16	18	18	18	18	18	18	20	18	16	16
(N)	109	128	95	100	120	92	97	113	107	100	289	510

Ventricular activation time by age in lead V4

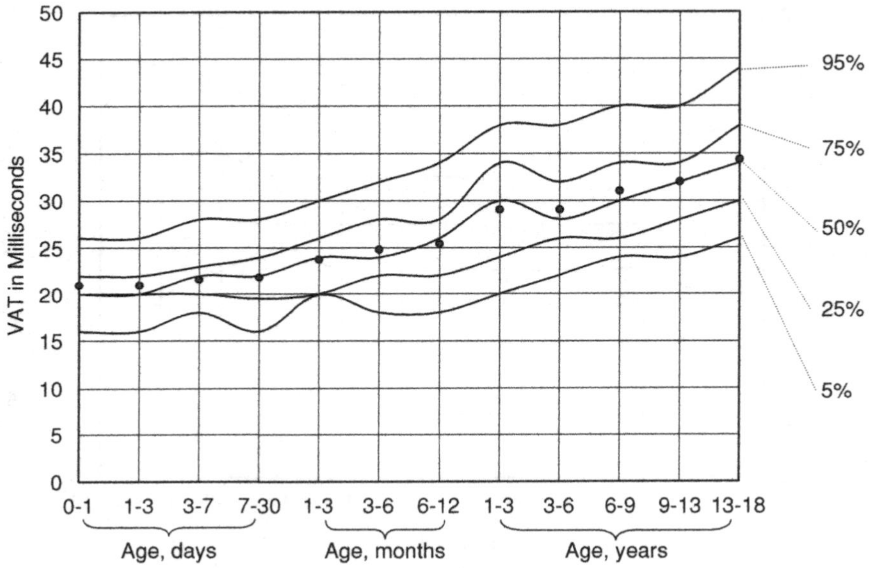

Figure 4.24 Ventricular activation time by age in lead V4, each curve corresponding to the indicated percentile level (• = mean). Lengthening of the ventricular activation time recorded in lead V4 is gradual and strikingly steady from birth to adolescence.

	Days				*Months*			*Years*					
Age	*0–1*	*1–3*	*3–7*	*7–30*	*1–3*	*3–6*	*6–12*	*1–3*	*3–6*	*6–9*	*9–13*	*13–18*
95%	26	26	28	28	30	32	34	38	38	40	40	44
Mean	**21**	**21**	**21.56**	**21.8**	**23.73**	**24.83**	**25.4**	**29**	**29**	**31**	**32**	**34.34**
(±SD)	**5.33**	**5.77**	**3.06**	**4.29**	**3.63**	**5.41**	**6.02**	**5.42**	**5.28**	**5.10**	**8.67**	**6.00**
5%	16	16	18	16	20	18	18	20	22	24	24	26
(N)	109	128	95	100	120	92	97	113	107	100	289	510

Ventricular activation time by age in lead V5

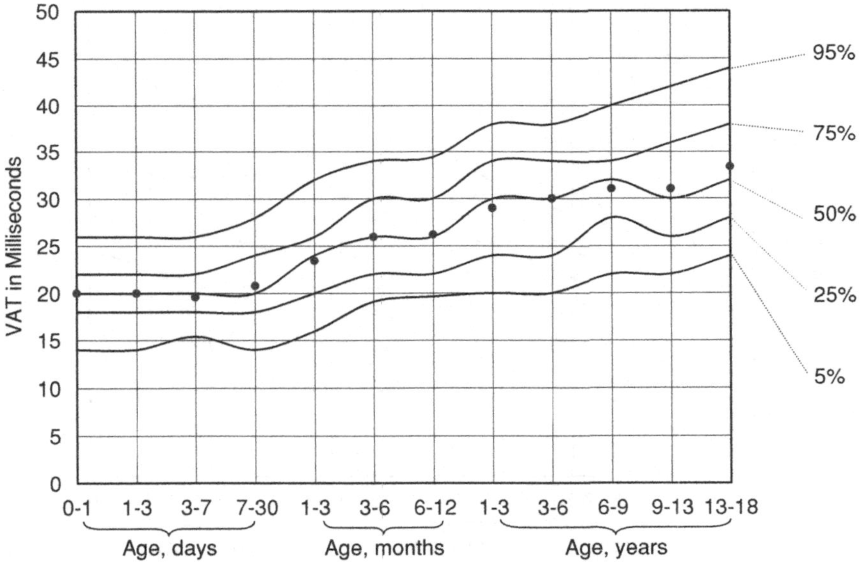

Figure 4.25 Ventricular activation time by age in lead V5, each curve corresponding to the indicated percentile level (• = mean). The ventricular activation time registered in V5 stays unchanged during the first 7 days after birth. From that age forward, the ventricular activation time becomes longer along with increasing age.

	Days				*Months*			*Years*				
Age	*0–1*	*1–3*	*3–7*	*7–30*	*1–3*	*3–6*	*6–12*	*1–3*	*3–6*	*6–9*	*9–13*	*13–18*
95%	26	26	26	28	32	34	34	38	38	40	42	44
Mean	**20**	**20**	**19.56**	**20.74**	**23.4**	**26**	**26.23**	**29**	**30**	**31**	**31**	**33.34**
(±SD)	**5.33**	**5.77**	**3.70**	**4.08**	**5.16**	**5.11**	**5.36**	**5.42**	**5.28**	**5.10**	**8.67**	**6.26**
5%	14	14	15	14	16	19	20	20	20	22	22	24
(N)	109	128	95	100	120	92	97	113	107	100	289	510

Ventricular activation time by age in lead V6

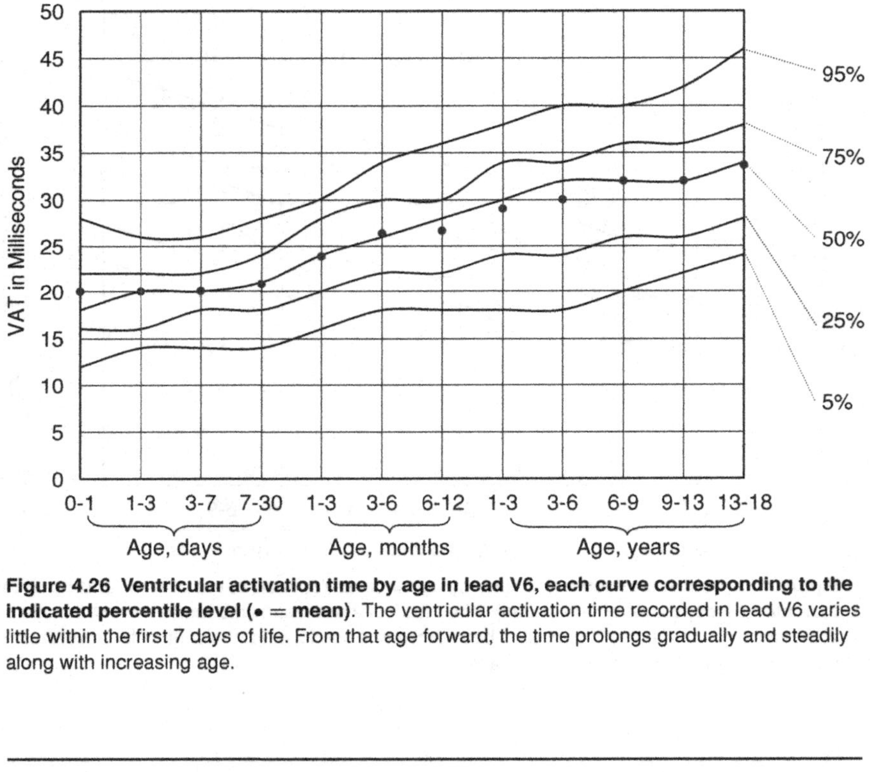

Figure 4.26 Ventricular activation time by age in lead V6, each curve corresponding to the indicated percentile level (• = mean). The ventricular activation time recorded in lead V6 varies little within the first 7 days of life. From that age forward, the time prolongs gradually and steadily along with increasing age.

	Days				*Months*			*Years*				
Age	*0–1*	*1–3*	*3–7*	*7–30*	*1–3*	*3–6*	*6–12*	*1–3*	*3–6*	*6–9*	*9–13*	*13–18*
95%	28	26	26	28	30	34	36	38	40	40	42	46
Mean	**20**	**20**	**20**	**21**	**24**	**26**	**27**	**29**	**30**	**32**	**32**	**34**
(±SD)	**5.33**	**5.77**	**4.25**	**4.62**	**4.80**	**4.75**	**6.17**	**5.42**	**5.28**	**10.20**	**8.67**	**6.99**
5%	12	14	14	14	16	18	18	18	18	20	22	24
(N)	109	128	95	100	120	92	97	113	107	100	289	510

VLSI DESIGN OF WAVELET TRANSFORM

Analysis, Architecture, and Design Examples

VLSI DESIGN OF WAVELET TRANSFORM

Analysis, Architecture, and Design Examples

Liang-Gee Chen

Chao-Tsung Huang

Ching-Yeh Chen

Chih-Chi Cheng

National Taiwan University, Taiwan

ICP

Imperial College Press

Published by

Imperial College Press
57 Shelton Street
Covent Garden
London WC2H 9HE

Distributed by

World Scientific Publishing Co. Pte. Ltd.
5 Toh Tuck Link, Singapore 596224
USA office: 27 Warren Street, Suite 401-402, Hackensack, NJ 07601
UK office: 57 Shelton Street, Covent Garden, London WC2H 9HE

British Library Cataloguing-in-Publication Data
A catalogue record for this book is available from the British Library.

VLSI DESIGN OF WAVELET TRANSFORM
Analysis, Architecture, and Design Examples

ISBN-13 978-1-86094-673-8
ISBN-10 1-86094-673-9

Printed in Singapore

To my family

Preface

Aims

The rapid and successful evolution of digital multimedia systems is indispensable in today's digital world. Ubiquitous multimedia access is no longer a dream and has become a future goal of current technology development. Now, many electronic products and multimedia applications are developed to reach this goal, such as mobile broadcast TV, mobile multimedia services, video phones, digital cameras and camcorders.

In this book, we introduce an important technique of multimedia applications, Discrete Wavelet Transform (DWT), which not only is the key algorithm of signal processing but has also led to revolutions in image and video coding algorithms. This book provides a comprehensive analysis and discussion of DWT and its applications, including the important material and the newest development of wavelet processing. We discuss DWT from its theories, algorithms, to related architectures. The architecture designs of DWT in JPEG 2000 are given as a practical example, and the latest development of DWT, Motion-Compensated Temporal Filtering (MCTF), is also explored in this book. We believe it is an important reference book for related research or courses on DWT.

Organization

This book is organized as follows. Chapters 1, 2, and 6 are introductions. Chapter 1 describes the roles of DWT in image and video coding systems. Chapters 2 and 6 give the basic introductions of DWT and MCTF. Chapters 3, 4, and 8 are the related analyses and architectures of 1-D DWT, 2-D DWT, and MCTF. Chapter 5 is a practical design of DWT, which is an image encoding system. Chapter 7 is the introduction of motion estimation

(ME), which is the background knowledge of MCTF. Except Chapters 1, 2, and 6, all other chapters focus on specific topics related to DWT or MCTF, so that readers can understand specific topics in one chapter without the knowledge of other chapters.

In Chapter 2, the fundamental theories of DWT are presented and its characteristics are also interpreted from various theorems. In Chapter 3, various VLSI architectures of 1-D DWT are introduced and compared; we focus on area and speed efficiency. VLSI architecture designs for 2-D DWT are presented in Chapter 4. The trade-off between off-chip memory bandwidth and on-chip memory area is the critical issue. After introducing the architectures of 1-D and 2-D DWT, Chapter 5 contains a real design of DWT in the JPEG 2000 encoding system. The design issues of 2-D DWT under the constraints of system scheduling are discussed.

Chapter 6 introduces the algorithms of MCTF and related scalable video coding. Similar to most video coding algorithms, ME is the most critical part of MCTF, and various algorithms, VLSI architectures, and memory management schemes of ME are reviewed in Chapter 7. Finally, some important hardware design issues of MCTF, like memory bandwidth, computation complexity, and so on, are discussed and formulated in Chapter 8.

Use of the Book

This book is suitable for readers with various knowledge and interests. If the readers are not familiar with the basic theorems of DWT, we suggest the readers can study from Chapters 1 to Chapter 8. If the readers only want to study the image applications of DWT, only Chapters 1–5 need to be studied. If the readers are interested in the temporal filtering of DWT, only Chapters 6–8 are required to be read.

For those readers who have understood the basic theorems of DWT, Chapter 2 can be skipped before reading Chapter 3–5. If the reader wants to study the architecture of 1-D DWT, all related materials are shown in Chapter 3. All materials about 2-D DWT are discussed in Chapter 4. Chapter 5 presents design examples of 2-D DWT in JPEG 2000 coding system, so Chapter 5 is recommended to be read after Chapter 4 or for those readers who are familiar with 2-D DWT.

For researchers in video processing, Chapter 6 is a good introduction and survey of temporal filtering and scalable video coding. Chapter 7 is a basic introduction to Motion-Estimation (ME) from algorithms to architectures, which is a background knowledge of Motion-Compensated Temporal Filtering (MCTF). If the readers are familiar with ME, they can skip this chapter. Chapter 8 discusses the hardware design issues of MCTF, which is recommended to be read after the readers understand the material in Chapters 6 and 7.

Acknowledgement

Finally, many people have contributed to the creation of this book. The author is grateful for the help of his current students and many former students, especially for Yu-Wen Huang, Hung-Chi Fang, and Yu-Wei Chang. They have provided many important materials and suggestions in this book. The author also appreciates the support of National Science Council in Taiwan. Most of the author's research programs included in this book have been funded by it. I also want to thank my family. I thank my wife for her encouragement. I thank my two sons for their support. This is your book, too. Last, but definitely not least, I would like to thank Laurent Chaminade for inviting me to write this book and thank the editors, Lenore Betts and Kaite Lydon, at Imperial College Press for their help in publication of this book.

L.-G. Chen

Contents

Chapter 1

Introduction

Digital multimedia systems play a more and more important role in today's digital world. Ubiquitous multimedia has become one of the major goals of current technology development. In this chapter, we will first introduce the trends in image and video coding algorithms, which presents how image coding is evolved from discrete cosine transform (DCT)-based block coding to discrete wavelet transform (DWT)-based bit-plane coding, and how video coding is evolved from close-loop motion compensated prediction (MCP) to open-loop motion-compensated temporal filtering (MCTF). Then general design considerations and methodologies of VLSI implementation for multimedia systems are discussed. Lastly, the operation hierarchy of DWT and MCTF is identified, which is a guideline of the VLSI architecture and memory analysis for DWT and MCTF.

1.1 Trends in Image Coding Algorithm

1.1.1 *DCT-based block coding*

Before this century, image coding algorithms were mainly based on DCT block coding as shown in Fig. 1.1(a), such as the popular JPEG standard [1]. Usually, the image is separated into 8×8 blocks, and DCT is performed on them. The two-dimensional (2-D) DCT can analyze 2-D image signals into nearly uncorrelated 2-D frequencies to reduce source redundancy. The performance of DCT is very close to the optimum Karhunen-Loeve Transform (KLT) but requires less computational complexity [2]. For a higher compression ratio, a lossy image coding is usually applied by quantizing DCT coefficients. The quantization is the only component that results in image quality distortion. However, the distortion can be made visually unnoticed by considering human visual perceptibility. For example, people are more sensitive to low frequency distortion than high frequency distortion, such that the quantization steps for higher frequencies can be enlarged more for a better compression capability. After quantization, the redundancy among frequency coefficients is further reduced by entropy coding. The coding symbols are usually established by zig-zag scanning the quantized frequency coefficients. Then they are encoded by variable length coding (VLC), such as Huffman coding or arithmetic coding.

For increasing the coding performance, the DC frequency coefficients are usually through differential pulse code modulation (DPCM) first before quantization and entropy coding. The DCT-based block coding highly utilizes the correlation and data dependency among DCT coefficients to achieve acceptable coding gain for popular manipulation. However, it is hard to provide many other functionalities, such as spatial or quality scalable coding and error-immune transmission. If some part of bitstream is missed, the image is very likely to be crashed because of DPCM and zig-zag scanned VLC.

1.1.2 *DWT-based bit-plane coding*

In the last decade, the DWT-based image coding matured to provide excellent coding gain and many other functionalities. The DWT transform is basically a frame-based computation. The image can be separated into many tiles, on which DWT are performed independently. The tile size is an encoding issue and could be large than 256×256 for avoiding blocking artifacts [3]. As shown in Fig. 1.1(b), the tile (or image) is transformed into hierarchically structured DWT subbands. The subband coefficients are encoded in a bitplane-by-bitplane way, instead of the word-by-word way in JPEG. There are two kinds of subband coding schemes that exploit inter- and intra-subband redundancy, respectively. The inter-subband coding is to explore the redundancy among subbands. They usually use a tree structure to utilize the similarity for high coding performance, such as EZW [4] and SPIHT [5]. On the other hand, the intra-subband scheme only utilizes the local redundancy inside each subband by context-adaptive coding, like EBCOT [6]. The EBCOT algorithm is also adopted in the JPEG 2000 standard [7], which can achieve about 2dB peak-signal-to-noise-ratio (PSNR) gain than JPEG [3]. Moreover, one DWT-based coding algorithm that combines both intra- and inter-subband schemes, called EZBC, can achieve about 0.5dB coding gain more than EBCOT [8].

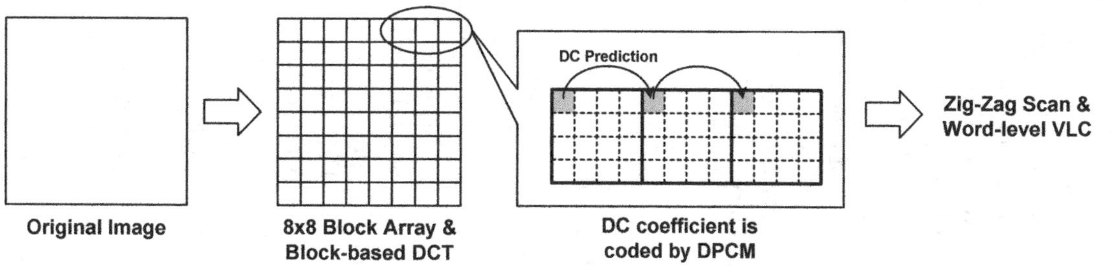

(a)

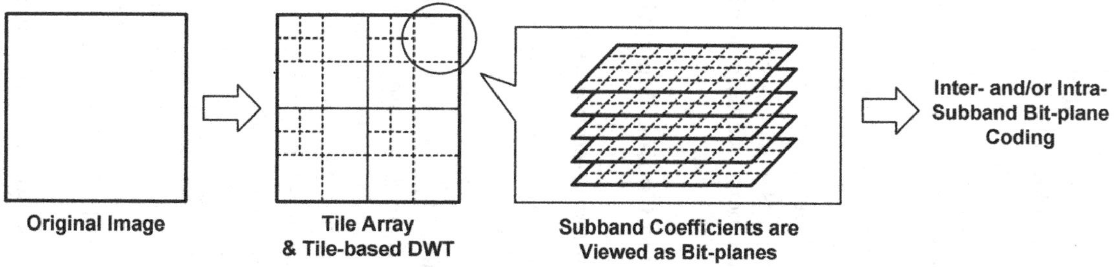

(b)

Fig. 1.1 Transform-based image coding flows. (a) DCT-based block coding. An image is separated into small blocks, and DCT is performed on them. For higher coding performance, the DC coefficients cross blocks are usually through DPCM before quantization and word-level entropy coding. (b) DWT-based bit-plane coding. An image is separated into large tiles. After performing DWT on them, the DWT coefficients are encoded by bit-plane-based entropy coding algorithms.

All above-mentioned DWT-based bit-plane coding algorithms can produce embedded bitstreams for quality scalability. The bit-planes can be refined from the most significant bit (MSB) to the least significant bit (LSB) sequentially. They can produce single bitstream when encoding, and the decoder derives more visual quality when receiving more bitstream for more bit-planes. Besides, the intra-subband coding can also provide spatially scalable bitstreams that utilize the time-frequency decomposition property of DWT. For example, the decoder can derive the one-fourth size image by only receiving the bitstream of the low-pass-low-pass (LL) subband. Furthermore, the independent coding unit of EBCOT, a code-block, can be smaller than a subband, which is usually of size 32×32 or 64×64. Thus, one missed code-block will not hurt the decoding of other independent code-blocks, which makes a robust error-immune transmission. The high quality embedded bitstream of great error immunity is the reason why JPEG 2000 can provide better communication capability than JPEG.

1.2 Trends in Video Coding Algorithm

1.2.1 *Close-loop motion-compensated prediction*

Existing hybrid video standards, such as MPEG-1/2/4 [9, 10, 11] and the emerging H.264/AVC [12], mainly consist of a close-loop motion-compensated prediction (MCP) scheme and a transform-based texture coder. The MCP is used to reduce temporal redundancy of video frames, and the texture transform is adopted to reduce spatial redundancy. The "close-loop" means it uses the reconstructed frames to predict the current frame, which forms a feedback loop as shown in Fig. 1.2(a). The "MCP" means image signals of the current frame are compensated by those in the previously reconstructed frames with proper motion models. The block-based motion model is usually used because of the rigid object motion assumption. The close-loop MCP scheme has been highly optimized for the compression efficiency in the last decade, and the H.264/AVC is a landmark of this development. However, for many video applications in the present and the future, the spatial, temporal, and quality scalabilities are more in demand.

The scalability means we can have multiple adaptations for one video bitstream, such as different frame sizes, frame rates, and visual qualities. The close-loop MCP scheme is hard to provide scalabilities while maintaining a high compression efficiency because of the drift problem, like

MPEG-4 FGS. The drift occurs when the encoder and decoder have different reconstructed frames, which can create serious error propagation in the close-loop MCP scheme. But the encoder and decoder inevitably have different video sequences, when the scalability is provided. For overcoming the drift problem, the compression efficiency will be greatly degraded and become unacceptable when there are many scalability layers. This is due to using the base layer that has worse visual quality as reference frames and adopting DCT coefficients for scalable quality coding.

1.2.2 *Open-loop motion-compensated temporal filtering*

The open-loop interframe wavelet coding scheme becomes a good alternative for scalable video coding. The concept is to perform wavelet transform in the temporal direction. But the coding performance is unacceptable without motion compensation (MC). In 1993, Ohm introduced a block-based displacement interframe scheme using the Haar filter [13]. However, the compression efficiency is still not comparable to existing MCP video standards until the lifting-based motion-compensated temporal filtering (MCTF) is proposed and the longer tap wavelet filters, like 5/3 filter, are used [14, 15]. The details of the development of MCTF can be found in [16]. The MCTF is a breakthrough of video coding algorithms, which breaks the close loop for efficient scalable coding as shown in Fig. 1.2(b). It uses original frames or filtered frames, instead of reconstructed or coded frames, as reference frames for MC. Any drifted mismatch will only propagate locally.

MPEG has identified a set of applications that require scalable and reliable video coding technologies. After evaluating the response to call for proposals on Scalable Video Coding (SVC) [17], it has been shown that there is a new and innovative video technology that MPEG can bring to industry in a future video standard [18]. The scalable extension of H.264/AVC with MCTF has been adopted in the Working Draft (WD) 1.0 of SVC [19]. It is a hybrid open-loop and close-loop video coding scheme. The lifting-based MCTF is the core technology to provide scalable video coding. The MCTF can provide a variety of efficient scalabilities because the drift problem of traditional close-loop prediction scheme is prevented by the open-loop structure. It also can further increase the compression efficiency of H.264/AVC [20, 21].

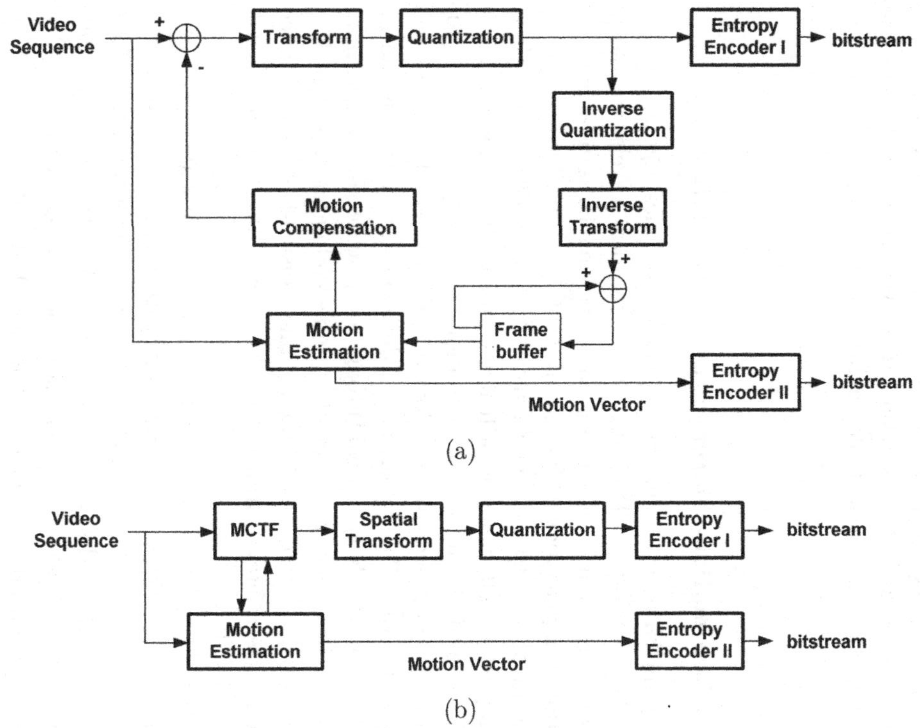

Fig. 1.2 Hybrid video coding flows. (a) Close-loop MCP scheme. The MCP forms a close-loop that also includes forward/inverse texture transform and forward/inverse quantization. (b) Open-loop MCTF scheme. The temporal redundancy is reduced by temporal filtering with motion compensation. No feedback loop is required.

1.3 VLSI Design Consideration of Multimedia Systems

Low cost and low power hardware with sufficiently high performance is extremely essential for image and video coding applications to be popular. Thus, efficient hardware implementations in VLSI are of vital importance. However, image and video coding algorithms usually require very high computational complexity and data access. In the following, the design methodologies for hardware architectures of image and video coding are introduced.

The optimization of hardware design for image and video coding systems can be achieved by considering two different levels of architecture design: system design and module design. The former decides the whole system architecture and the relationship between modules. The latter is to optimize each module according to the allocated resource and constraints.

1.3.1 *System design consideration*

The system architecture is usually designed by use of computation analysis and data access analysis that consider computing and data issues, respectively.

1.3.1.1 *Computation analysis*

The computation analysis is to classify the coding tools of the adopted coding algorithm into different level computational characteristics and choose the suitable implementation types. It further includes computational characteristic and complexity analysis.

Figure 1.3 shows the computational characteristic analysis, which categorizes computation into three different levels of operations. On the other hand, the computational complexity analysis is to evaluate the complexity of each coding tool by task profiling. The general result is that low-level operations require more complexity. The low-level operation represents highly regular computation and predictable computational flow. It is suitable to be implemented by a dedicated hardware, because its complexity is usually very high and the regular computation can be easily accelerated via parallel processing. The high-level operation represents highly irregular computation and unpredictable computational flow. However, its complexity is usually much lower than the low-level operation. Thus, it is suitable to be implemented using programmable design. Between these two extremes, the medium-level operation is preferred to be implemented by use of configurable architecture that can be on-the-fly adapted according to data-dependent decisions.

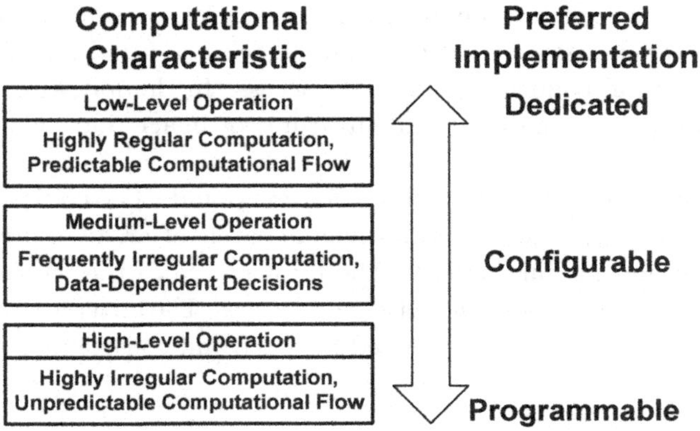

Fig. 1.3 Computational characteristic analysis and the corresponding preferred implementation.

1.3.1.2 *Data access analysis*

The data access analysis is used to decide how data are transferred in the system. It analyzes how data should be stored for access (memory management) and how data are transferred between modules (bus interconnect). The storage and access issue is to provide a good memory management. As described in [22], memory bandwidth and on-chip memory capacity are limited factors for many multimedia applications, and today on-chip memory already occupies more than 50% of total chip area in many applications. Good memory management becomes necessary for successful system-on-a-chip solutions.

The memory management is to provide an efficient and balanced memory hierarchy that consists of off-chip memory, on-chip memory, and registers [23], as shown in Fig. 1.4. Different memory types have different features. Off-chip memory, usually DRAM, offers a large amount of storage size but consumes the most power. The off-chip memory and I/O access may dominate the power budget. To solve this problem, many techniques have been developed. For example, embedded DRAM [22] is developed to reduce the I/O access by integrating large on-chip DRAM. However, the embedded DRAM technology is not very mature because the yield issue and many physical design challenges are still needed to be solved. Even integrating large embedded DRAM, the access power is still larger than smaller on-chip SRAM. Besides, embedded compression (EC) is usually adopted to reduce the off-chip memory bandwidth and size for video decoders [24, 25, 26], and few EC algorithms are designed for video encoders [27]. EC is to compress the transmitted data on-the-fly to reduce the data amount, but video quality could be degraded if lossy EC is applied.

The on-chip memory, usually implemented by SRAM, can provide faster access and less power-consumption than off-chip memory, but the memory cell size is larger. It also occupies much on-chip die area for implementing multimedia coding systems. Registers can be faster than on-chip memory and provide the most flexible data storage.

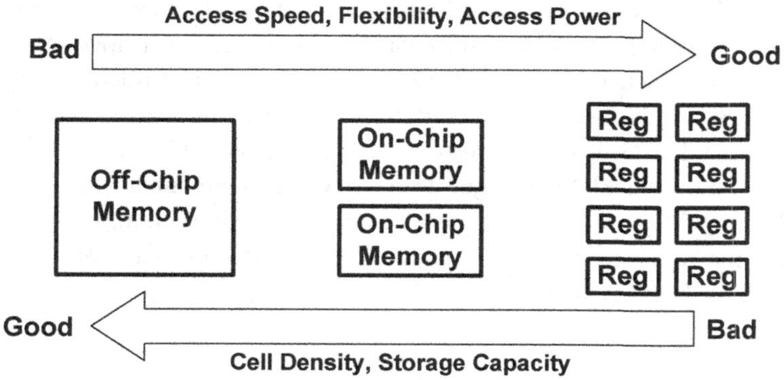

Fig. 1.4 Memory hierarchy consists of off-chip memory, on-chip memory, and registers.

Memory management can be organized from two different levels: algorithm-level and architecture-level. The algorithm-level memory hierarchy optimization is to modify the coding system algorithm to improve some system parameters, like power or area, but some other parameters, like coding performance, become the trade-off. For example, EC belongs to one algorithm-level memory improvement, in which degraded visual quality could be traded by reducing off-chip memory bandwidth. On the other hand, the architecture-level memory organization is to optimize the memory hierarchy from modifying hardware architecture. For example, on-chip memory is usually used as a cache to replace regular off-chip memory access for reducing off-chip memory bandwidth.

The interconnect issue is to decide how to allocate global bus and dedicated connection between modules. The global bus provides flexible configuration and saves the interconnect area. The dedicated interconnect is to provide high throughput and efficient communication between highly related modules.

1.3.2 *Module design consideration*

After the system architecture is defined, every module can be designed by use of algorithm-level and architecture-level optimization. The algorithm-level optimization is mainly to optimize the rate-distortion quality under given complexity constraints, or vice versa. For some coding tools, such as motion estimation (ME) and rate control, more computation power usually results in the better visual quality. How to provide a acceptable quality and minimize the required computational complexity is the design challenge.

The architecture-level optimization is to perform data flow smoothing and to balance scheduling and timing control for determined algorithms. Many VLSI implementation techniques [28], such as pipelining, folding, unfolding, and systolic array mapping, can be used for this purpose. Besides computational consideration, good memory management for some critical module, like ME, is also very important. There have many data re-use schemes for different memory management strategies been proposed for ME, such as Level A to D re-use schemes [29, 30].

1.4 Book Outline

The chapters in this book present VLSI implementation issues for DWT and MCTF that have led revolutions for image and video coding algorithms, in which architecture design and memory analysis will be discussed. Figure 1.5 shows the operation hierarchy and corresponding design challenge for 1-D DWT, 2-D DWT, and MCTF, which is an outline of this book. Chapters 2 and 6 will give detailed introductions to DWT and MCTF.

The 1-D DWT belongs to pixel-level operation, and it is the basic processing element for 2-D DWT. In Chapter 3, various VLSI architectures of 1-D DWT are introduced and compared. The design effort is focused on area and speed efficiency. The different 1-D DWT design categories will be discussed from different mathematical formulations.

The 2-D DWT becomes frame-level operations. VLSI architecture de-

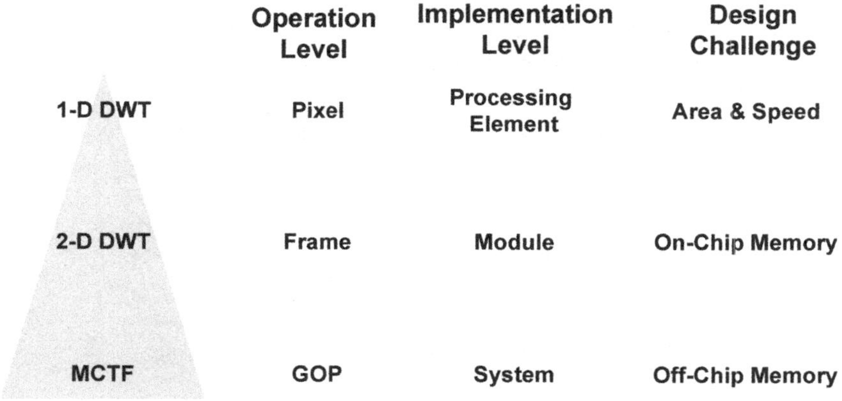

Fig. 1.5 Operation hierarchy and design challenges of 1-D DWT, 2-D DWT, and MCTF.

signs for 2-D DWT are presented in Chapter 4. The trade-off between off-chip memory bandwidth and on-chip memory area is the critical point. When the memory management strategy for 2-D DWT module is decided after considering system requirement, how to optimize the implementation of on-chip memory is the design challenge. We will introduce many memory management schemes for 2-D DWT and discuss on-chip memory implementation issues in detail.

Chapter 5 contains the design examples of 2-D DWT in JPEG 2000 encoding systems. The design issues of 2-D DWT under the constraints of system scheduling will be discussed. Two types of JPEG 2000 encoding scheduling will be shown and the corresponding DWT architecture will be introduced.

Furthermore, the MCTF operates in the group-of-picture (GOP) level, which performs DWT through temporal direction with MC. The ME is the most important computation for finding the best MC blocks in the commonly used block-based motion model of existing video coding standards. In Chapter 7, algorithms, VLSI architectures, and memory management schemes for ME will be reviewed. Chapter 8 considers the design issues for MCTF. Due to the huge amount of data access and computation, the design challenge of MCTF becomes a system-level consideration. The system issues, especially off-chip memory requirement, will be discussed and explored.

Chapter 2

Algorithm Views of Discrete Wavelet Transform

With the great effort of mathematicians, the discrete wavelet transform (DWT) was formulated from continuous wavelet transform (CWT) [31, 32]. In the last decade, researches on wavelet-based signal analysis, image compression [33, 4, 5, 6, 8], and video compression [13, 16], have derived fruitful results because of the good time-frequency decomposition feature. The DWT has been adopted as the transform coder in emerging image coding standards, including JPEG 2000 still image coding [7] and MPEG-4 visual texture coding (VTC) [11], as well as the motion picture compression standard, Motion JPEG 2000 [34]. In this chapter, the algorithms of 1-D DWT and 2-D DWT will be introduced.

2.1 Basic Theoretical View of Discrete Wavelet Transform

In this section, the basic theory of continuous and discrete wavelet transform is presented. More details can be found in [32, 35].

2.1.1 *Properties of a multi-resolution transform*

Wavelet transform is a form of multi-resolution transform since multi-resolution approximations of the input signal are provided. In this section, the properties of a multi-resolution transform proposed by S. G. Mallat [32] are presented.

(1) Let A_{2^j} be a linear operator and $A_{2^j}(f(x))$ be the approximation of some function $f(x)$ at the resolution 2^j. Then $A_{2^j}(f(x))$ will not be changed if it is approximated again in resolution 2^j, that is,

$$A_{2^j} \circ A_{2^j} = A_{2^j} \,. \tag{2.1}$$

We can therefore define a square-integratable vector space $\mathbf{V}_{2^j}$ which comprises all possible approximations at the resolution 2^j of square-integratable functions. The linear operator A_{2^j} thus project function $f(x)$ onto the vector space $\mathbf{V}_{2^j}$.

(2) $A_{2^j}(f(x))$ is function most similar to $f(x)$ in $\mathbf{V}_{s^j}$. That is,

$$\forall g(x) \in \mathbf{V}_{2^j}, \|g(x) - f(x)\| \geq \|A_{2^j} f(x) - f(x)\|. \tag{2.2}$$

(3) The approximation in resolution 2^j is a subset of approximation in resolution 2^{j+1}. That is,

$$\forall j \in \mathbf{Z}, \mathbf{V}_{2^j} \subset \mathbf{V}_{2^{j+1}} \tag{2.3}$$

where $\mathbf{Z}$ is the set of all integers.

(4) The spaces of approximated functions in one resolution should be able to be derived from that in another resolution by scaling in time domain. That is,

$$\forall j \in \mathbf{Z},\ f(x) \in \mathbf{V}_{2^j} \Leftrightarrow f(2x) \in \mathbf{V}_{2^{j+1}}. \tag{2.4}$$

(5) $A_{2^j}(f(x))$ can be characterized by 2^j samples per length unit. When $f(x)$ is translated by 2^{-j}, $A_{2^j}(f(x))$ is translated by the same amount, and the discretized signal is translated by one sample. That is,

(a) There exists an isomorphism $\mathbf{I}$ from $\mathbf{V}_1$ onto the vector space of square summable sequences.

(b) Let $f_k(x) = f(x-k)$, $A_1 f_k(x) = a_1(x)$, $A_1 f(x) = b_1(x)$

$$\forall j \in \mathbf{Z}, a_1(x) = b_1(x-k). \tag{2.5}$$

(c) Let $f_k(x) = f(x-k)$, $\mathbf{I}$ is the isomorphism from $\mathbf{V}_1$ onto the vector space of square summable sequences, then

$$\mathbf{I}(A_1 f(x)) = (\alpha_i)_{i\in\mathbf{Z}} \Leftrightarrow \mathbf{I}(A_1 f_k(x)) = (\alpha_{i-k})_{i\in\mathbf{Z}}. \tag{2.6}$$

(6) As the resolution approaches $+\infty$, the approximated signal converges to the original signal. On the contrary, as the resolution approaches zero, the approximated signal converges to zero function. Combining with Eq. 2.3,

$$\lim_{j\to+\infty} \mathbf{V}_{2^j} = \cup_{j=-\infty}^{j=+\infty} \mathbf{V}_{2^j} \tag{2.7}$$

which is dense in the set of all square-integratable functions

and

$$\lim_{j\to-\infty} \mathbf{V}_{2^j} = \cap_{j=-\infty}^{j=+\infty} \mathbf{V}_{2^j} = \{0\}. \tag{2.8}$$

According to the definition in [32], a multi-resolution approximation satisfies Eq. 2.3–2.8. The approximation operator A_{2^j} is an orthogonal projection to vector space $\mathbf{V}_{2^j}$. The Theorem 1 in [32] shows that an orthonormal basis of $\mathbf{V}_{2^j}$ can be obtained from translating and dilating a unique scaling function.

Theorem 2.1 *Let $\mathbf{V}_{2^j}$ be the vector space comprising multi-resolution approximations of square-integratable functions. There exists a square-integratable function $\phi(x)$, called scaling function. Define $\phi_{2^j}(x) = 2^j\phi(2^j x)$ for $j \in \mathbf{Z}$, then an orthonormal basis of $\mathbf{V}_{2^j}$ is*

$$(\sqrt{2^{-j}}\phi_{2^j}(x - 2^{-j}n)\ , n \in \mathbf{Z}. \tag{2.9}$$

2.1.2 *The pyramid structure of discrete multi-resolution representation*

From Theorem 2.1, an approximated signal $A_{2^j}(f(x))$ can be expressed:

$$\begin{aligned} &A_{2^j}(f(x)) \\ &= 2^{-j}\sum_{n=-\infty}^{\infty} < f(u), \phi_{2^j}(u - 2^{-j}n) > \phi_{2^j}(x - 2^{-j}n). \end{aligned} \tag{2.10}$$

If the scaling function $\phi(x)$ has approximately a low-pass shape, the terms $< f(u), \phi_{2^j}(u - 2^{-j}n) >$ can be regarded as a discrete approximation of $f(x)$.

The discrete approximation of a square-integratable function $f(x)$ at resolution 2^j, $A^d_{2^j}(f)(n)$, is defined as:

$$\begin{aligned} A^d_{2^j}(f)(n) &=< f(u), \phi_{2^j}(u - 2^{-j}n) >, n \in \mathbf{Z} \\ &= (f(u) * \phi(-u))|_{u=2^{-j}}. \end{aligned} \tag{2.11}$$

Because the scaling function $\phi(x)$ is a low-pass filter, the discrete approximation $A^d_{2^j}(f)(n)$ can be interpreted as low-pass filtering of the continuous function $f(x)$ followed by uniformly sampling with rate 2^j.

Let the $A^d_1(f)(n)$ be the discrete approximated signal in the highest resolution. From Eq. 2.3, all approximation $A^d_{2^j}(f)(n)$ with $j \leq 0$ can be obtained from $A^d_1(f)(n)$. For any $n \in \mathbf{Z}$, $\phi_{2^j}(x - 2^{-j}n)$ is a member of $\mathbf{V}_{2^j}$.

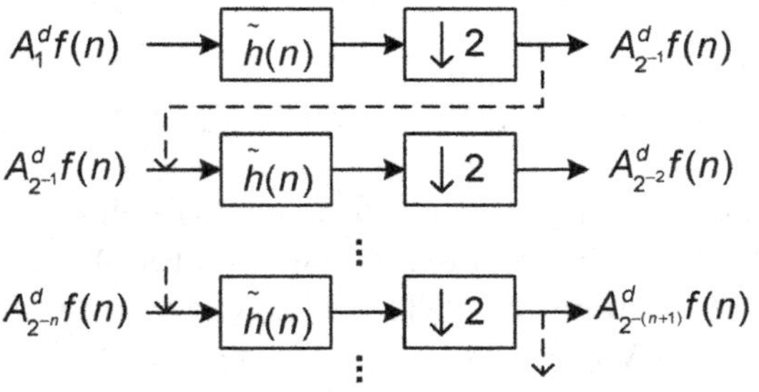

Fig. 2.1 The pyramid structure to derive discrete-time approximated signals in different resolutions.

From Eq. 2.3, $\phi_{2^j}(x - 2^{-j}n)$ is also a member of $\mathbf{V}_{2^{j+1}}$. Therefore,

$$\begin{aligned}
&\phi_{2^j}(x - 2^{-j}n) \\
&= 2^{-(j+1)} \sum_{k=-\infty}^{\infty} (< \phi_{2^j}(u - 2^{-j}n), \phi_{2^{j+1}}(u - 2^{-(j+1)}k) > \\
&\cdot \phi_{2^{j+1}}(u - 2^{-(j+1)}k)) \\
&= \sum_{k=-\infty}^{\infty} < \phi_{2^{-1}}(u), \phi(u - (k - 2n)) > \phi_{2^{j+1}}(u - 2^{-(j+1)}k).
\end{aligned} \tag{2.12}$$

If a discrete-time filter $h(n)$ is defined:

$$< \phi_{2^{-1}}(u), \phi(u - n)) >= h(n) = \widetilde{h}(-n), \forall n \in \mathbf{Z}. \tag{2.13}$$

Therefore, combining Eq. 2.11, Eq. 2.12, and the definition in Eq. 2.13:

$$\begin{aligned}
&A_{2^j}^d(f)(n) \\
&=< f(u), \phi_{2^j}(u - 2^{-j}n > \\
&= \sum_{k=-\infty}^{\infty} < \phi_{2^{-1}}(u), \phi(u - (k - 2n)) >< f(u), \phi_{2^{j+1}}(u - 2^{-(j+1)}k) > \\
&= \sum_{k=-\infty}^{\infty} < \phi_{2^{-1}}(u), \phi(u - (k - 2n)) > A_{2^{j+1}}^d(k) \\
&= \sum_{k=-\infty}^{\infty} \widetilde{h}(2n - k) A_{2^{j+1}}^d(k).
\end{aligned} \tag{2.14}$$

From Eq. 2.14, a pyramid structure to derive discrete-time approximated signals $(A_{2^j}^d(f), j \leq 0)$ from the discrete-time approximated signal in the highest resolution $(A_1^d f)$ is derived. This scheme is illustrated in Fig. 2.1.

In summary, a multi-resolution approximation $\mathbf{V}_{2^j}, \forall j \in \mathbf{Z}$ can be completely characterized by the scaling function $\phi(x)$ which has a low-pass shape. The discrete-time filter $\widetilde{h}(n)$ is defined as Eq. 2.13 and also is a low-pass filter. Any physical device can capture only discrete signals which is defined as discrete-time approximated signals in resolution 2^0, $A_1^d(f)(n)$.

The discrete-time approximated signals in lower resolutions can thus be obtained from the pyramid structure in Eq. 2.14.

2.1.3 *The wavelet decomposition*

In Section 2.1.2, a pyramid structure to approximate a discrete-time signal into multiple resolutions has been derived. However, to transform the signal $A^d_{2^{j+1}}(f)(n)$ to $A^d_{2^j}(f)(n)$ means the degradation of signal resolution. The details beyond the resolution 2^j thus will be discarded. In this section, the methodology to extract those detail signals is presented from continuous case to discrete case. It is also proposed in [32].

The vector space of detail signals between $\mathbf{V}_{2^{j+1}}$ and $\mathbf{V}_{2^j}$ is the orthogonal projection from $\mathbf{V}_{2^{j+1}}$ to $\mathbf{V}_{2^j}$. Any signal in this vector space is in both $\mathbf{V}_{2^{j+1}}$ and the null space of $\mathbf{V}_{2^j}$. Let $\mathbf{O}_{2^j}$ be this orthogonal complement vector space, then

$$\mathbf{O}_{2^j} \bigcup \mathbf{V}_{2^j} = \mathbf{V}_{2^{j+1}} , \tag{2.15}$$

where $\mathbf{O}_{2^j}$ is orthogonal to $\mathbf{V}_{2^j}$.

Therefore, the continuous detail signal in resolution 2^j will be the projection of $f(x)$ into the vector space $\mathbf{O}_{2^j}$. Like Theorem 2.1, a set of orthonormal basis of $\mathbf{O}_{2^j}$ also has to be derived from Theorem 2.2. The proof can be seen in [32].

Theorem 2.2 *Let $\boldsymbol{V}_{2^j}$ be a multi-resolution approximation of square-integratable functions with scaling function $\phi(x)$, and H is the corresponding low-pass discrete-time filter. Define $\psi(x)$ such that its Fourier Transform $\widehat{\Psi}(\omega)$ is:*

$$G(\omega) = e^{-i\omega}\overline{H(\omega + \pi)} \tag{2.16}$$

$$\widehat{\Psi}(\omega) = G(\tfrac{\omega}{2})\widehat{\phi}(\tfrac{\omega}{2}). \tag{2.17}$$

Let $\psi_{2^j}(x) = 2^j\psi(2^j x)$, then an orthonormal basis of $\boldsymbol{O}_{2^j}$ is

$$(\sqrt{2^{-j}}\psi_{2^j}(x - 2^{-j}n) \ , n \in \boldsymbol{Z}. \tag{2.18}$$

Since H is a low-pass filter, from the definition in Eq. 2.16, G is a high-pass filter. The detail signals thus can be derived from this orthonormal basis defined in Eq. 2.18. With the corresponding vectors in $\mathbf{V}_{2^j}$ and $\mathbf{O}_{2^j}$, the higher resolution vector in $\mathbf{V}_{2^{j+1}}$ can be perfect reconstructed.

Let P_{2^j} be the orthogonal projection on the vector space $\mathbf{O}_{2^j}$. From Eq. 2.18, for a square integratable function $f(x)$,

$$P_{2^j}(f)(x) \\ = 2^{-j} \sum_{n=-\infty} +\infty < f(u), \psi_{2^j}(u - 2^{-j}n) > \psi_{2^j}(x - 2^{-j}n). \tag{2.19}$$

As in the process of deriving pyramid structure of multi-resolution approximation in section 2.1.2, the discrete-time detail signal of resolution 2^j can be defined as:

$$D_{2^j}(f)(n) =< f(u), \psi_{2^j}(u - 2^{-j}n) > , n \in \mathbf{Z}. \tag{2.20}$$

$D_{2^j}(f)$ thus comprises the difference of information between $A_{2^{j+1}}(f)$ and $A_{2^j}(f)$. The expression in Eq. 2.20 can be simplified as:

$$< f(u), \psi_{2^j}(u - 2^{-j}n) > = (f(u) * \psi_{2^j}(-u))|_{u=2^{-j}n}. \tag{2.21}$$

Combining Eq. 2.20 and Eq. 2.21,

$$D_{2^j}(f)(n) = (f(u) * \psi_{2^j}(-u))|_{u=2^{-j}n} , n \in \mathbf{Z}. \tag{2.22}$$

As discussed, since H is a low-pass filter, from the definition in Eq. 2.16, G is a high-pass filter. $\psi(x)$ is also a high-pass filter.

Figure 2.2 shows an illustration of frequency response of the defined continuous functions and discrete-time filters. From Eq. 2.13, the scaling function is a low-pass filter, and the approximation filter H will be a discrete-time low-pass filter, as shown in Fig. 2.2(a). From the definition in Eq. 2.16, the frequency response of filter G can be obtained as in Fig. 2.2(b). The frequency of continuous filter $\psi(x)$ can be obtained from Eq. 2.17, and the result is shown in Fig. 2.2(c). Figure 2.2(d) thus can be obtained from the relationship $\psi_{2^j}(x) = 2^j\psi(2^j x)$. The set of orthonormal basis defined in Theorem 2.2 thus can cover the frequency range of absolute value from π to ∞. The frequency from $-\pi$ to π can be covered from the orthonormal basis defined in Theorem 2.1.

The wavelet representation of a continuous signal $f(x)$ thus can be defined as:

$$(A^d_{2^{-J}}(f), D_{2^j} f|_{-J \le j \le -1}). \tag{2.23}$$

From Theorem 2.2, a set of orthonormal basis of $\mathbf{O}_{2^j}$ is:

$$(\sqrt{2^{-j}}\psi_{2^j}(x - 2^{-j}n) = (\sqrt{2^j}\psi(2^j(x - 2^{-j}n)) , n \in \mathbf{Z}. \tag{2.24}$$

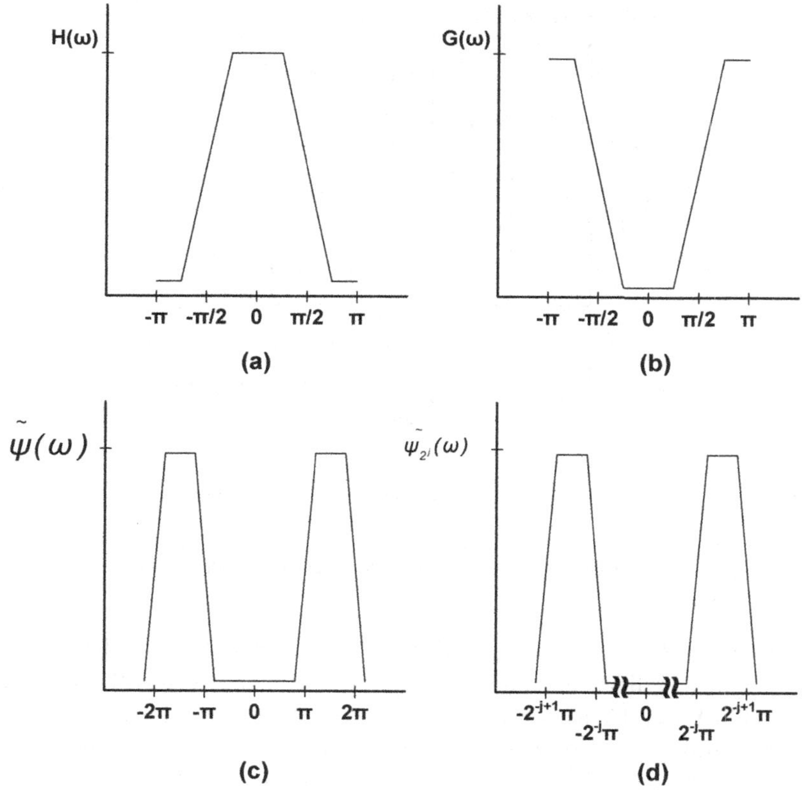

Fig. 2.2 An illustration of frequency response of continuous functions and discrete-time filters.

This basis can develop an interesting time-frequency relationship between frequency resolution j and time resolution n.

The time-frequency decomposition diagram of the basis defined in Theorem 2.2 ($\sqrt{2^j}\psi(2^j(x-2^{-j}n))$) can be shown as Fig. 2.3. As can be seen in Fig. 2.3, for a fixed n, the frequency resolution in low frequency is higher than that in higher frequency. The time resolution is higher in higher frequency. In natural singals, lower frequency components are more steady and can be presented by lower time resolution, and lower frequency is more important to human and has to be presented higher frequency resolution. Therefore, this decomposition characteristic is very suitable for natural signals and human vision.

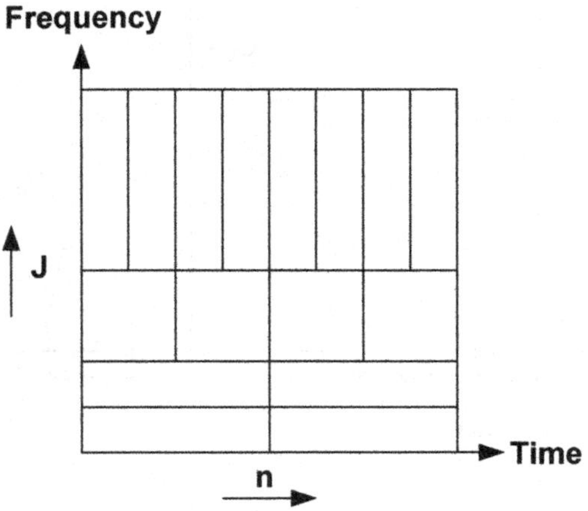

Fig. 2.3 Time-frequency decomposition diagram of CWT coefficients $c_{m,n}$.

2.1.4 *The pyramid structure of computing wavelet transform*

In Section 2.1.2, an approximate filter H is derived, such that the approximated signals in different resolutions can be obtained by use of the structure depicted in Fig. 2.1. In this section, a similar structure is derived to obtain the entire wavelet representation in resolution 2^J.

From Eq. 2.18, $\sqrt{2^{-j}}\psi_{2^j}(x-2^{-j}n)$ is in a set of orthonormal basis of $\mathbf{O}_{2^j}$. Therefore, $\psi_{2^j}(x-2^{-j}n)$ is in vector space $\mathbf{O}_{2^j} \subset \mathbf{V}_{2^{j+1}}$ (Eq. 2.15). Therefore, $\psi_{2^j}(x-2^{-j}n)$ can be expand in $\mathbf{V}_{2^{j+1}}$ by the orthonormal basis in Eq. 2.9. From Eq. 2.10:

$$\begin{aligned}&\psi_{2^j}(x-2^{-j}n)\\&=2^{-(j+1)}\textstyle\sum_{k=-\infty}^{\infty}(<\psi_{2^j}(x-2^{-j}n),\phi_{2^{j+1}}(u-2^{-(j+1)}k)>\\&\cdot\phi_{2^{j+1}}(x-2^{-(j+1)}n)).\end{aligned} \tag{2.25}$$

But it can be shown that:

$$\begin{aligned}&2^{-(j+1)}<\psi_{2^j}(x-2^{-j}n),\phi_{2^{j+1}}(u-2^{-(j+1)}k)>\\&=<\psi_{2^{-1}}(u),\phi(u-(k-2n))>.\end{aligned} \tag{2.26}$$

By defining the filter coefficient of discrete-time filter G:

$$g(n)=\widetilde{g}(-n)=<\psi_{2^{-1}}(u),\phi(u-n)>. \tag{2.27}$$

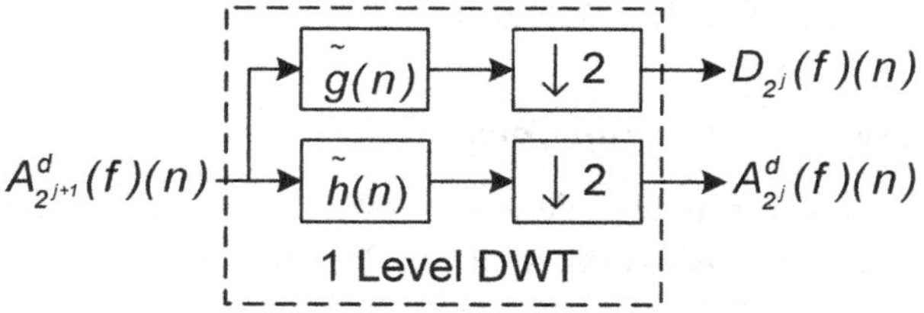

Fig. 2.4 The scheme to decompose signal at resolution 2^{j+1} to approximated signal at resolution 2^j and detail signal at resolution 2^j. This scheme is 1 level DWT.

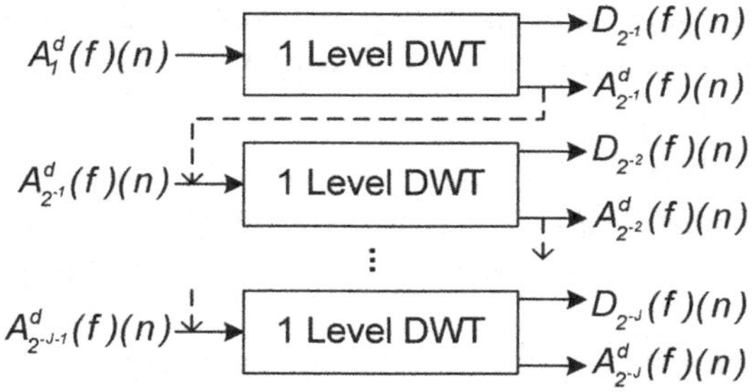

Fig. 2.5 The scheme to of multi-level DWT.

Combining Eq. 2.25, 2.26, and 2.27:

$$
\begin{aligned}
&D_{2^j}(f(x))(n)\\
&=< f(u), \psi_{2^j}(u - 2^{-j}n >\\
&= \sum_{k=-\infty}^{\infty} < \psi_{2^{-1}}(u), \phi(u - (k - 2n)) >< f(u), \phi_{2^{j+1}}(u - 2^{-(j+1)}k) >\\
&= \sum_{k=-\infty}^{\infty} < \psi_{2^{-1}}(u), \phi(u - (k - 2n)) > A^d_{2^{j+1}}(f(x))(k)\\
&= \sum_{k=-\infty}^{\infty} \widetilde{g}(2n - k) A^d_{2^{j+1}}(f(x))(k)\,.
\end{aligned}
\tag{2.28}
$$

Therefore, the detail signal at resolution 2^j can be obtained by passing the approximated signal at resolution 2^{j+1} to the filter $\widetilde{g}(n)$ and then downsampling the filtered signal by 2.

Figure 2.4 shows the scheme to decompose signal at resolution 2^{j+1} into approximated signal at resolution 2^j and detail signal at resolution 2^j. This is the process to project a vector in $\mathbf{V}_{2^{j+1}}$ to an approximated vector in $\mathbf{V}_{2^j}$ and a detail signal in $\mathbf{O}_{2^j}$. Figure 2.5 further shows the scheme to decompose the signal in the highest resolution (2^0) to the wavelet representation defined in Eq. 2.23 to the J-th level.

2.1.5 *Inverse wavelet transform*

The wavelet transform is complete as shown in section 2.1.4. Therefore, theoretically, the approximated signal in $\mathbf{V}_1$ thus can be recovered from the wavelet representation defined in Eq. 2.23. In this section, the inverse wavelet transform that can achieve perfect reconstruction of signals is introduced.

From the relationship among $\mathbf{V}_{2^j}$, $\mathbf{O}_{2^j}$, and $\mathbf{V}_{2^{j+1}}$ stated in Eq. 2.15, we can see that $\mathbf{O}_{2^j}$ is the orthogonal complement of $\mathbf{V}_{2^j}$ in $\mathbf{V}_{2^{j+1}}$. Therefore, the union of orthonormal basis of $\mathbf{V}_{2^j}$ (Theorem 2.1) and $\mathbf{O}_{2^j}$ (Theorem 2.2) can form an set of orthonormal basis of $\mathbf{V}_{2^{j+1}}$:

$$\begin{aligned}&\phi_{2^{j+1}}(x-2^{-(j+1)}n)\\&=2^{-j}\textstyle\sum_{k=-\infty}^{\infty}<\phi_{2^{-j}}(u-2^{-j}k),\phi_{2^{j+1}}(u-2^{-(j+1)n})>\phi_{2^{-j}}(u-2^{-j}k)\\&+2^{-j}\textstyle\sum_{k=-\infty}^{\infty}<\psi_{2^{-j}}(u-2^{-j}k),\phi_{2^{j+1}}(u-2^{-(j+1)n})>\psi_{2^{-j}}(u-2^{-j}k).\end{aligned} \tag{2.29}$$

Therefore, for a square-integratable function $f(x)$,

$$\begin{aligned}&<f(u),\phi_{2^{j+1}}(x-2^{-(j+1)}n)>\\&=2^{-j}\textstyle\sum_{k=-\infty}^{\infty}(<\phi_{2^{-j}}(u-2^{-j}k),\phi_{2^{j+1}}(u-2^{-(j+1)n})>\\&\cdot<f(u),\phi_{2^{-j}}(u-2^{-j}k)>)\\&+2^{-j}\textstyle\sum_{k=-\infty}^{\infty}(<\psi_{2^{-j}}(u-2^{-j}k),\phi_{2^{j+1}}(u-2^{-(j+1)n})>\\&\cdot<f(u),\psi_{2^{-j}}(u-2^{-j}k)>).\end{aligned} \tag{2.30}$$

From Eq. 2.12 and Eq. 2.26, the above equation can be further simplified into:

$$\begin{aligned}&<f(u),\phi_{2^{j+1}}(x-2^{-(j+1)}n)>\\&=2\textstyle\sum_{k=-\infty}^{\infty}<\phi_{2^{-1}}(u),\phi(u-(n-2k))><f(u),\phi_{2^{-j}}(u-2^{-j}k)>\\&+2\textstyle\sum_{k=-\infty}^{\infty}<\psi_{2^{-1}}(u),\phi(u-(n-2k))><f(u),\psi_{2^{-j}}(u-2^{-j}k)>.\end{aligned} \tag{2.31}$$

From the definition of discrete-time filter coefficients in Eq. 2.13 and Eq. 2.27,

$$\begin{aligned}&<f(u),\phi_{2^{j+1}}(x-2^{-(j+1)}n)>\\&=2\textstyle\sum_{k=-\infty}^{\infty}h(n-2k)<f(u),\phi_{2^{-j}}(u-2^{-j}k)>\\&+2\textstyle\sum_{k=-\infty}^{\infty}g(n-2k)<f(u),\psi_{2^{-j}}(u-2^{-j}k)>.\end{aligned} \tag{2.32}$$

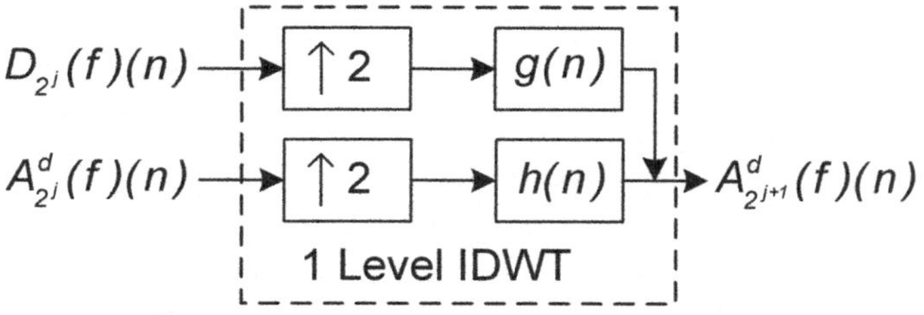

Fig. 2.6 The scheme to reconstruct signal at resolution 2^{j+1} from approximated signal at resolution 2^j and detail signal at resolution 2^j. This scheme is 1 level inverse DWT (IDWT).

Finally, from Eq. 2.11 and Eq. 2.20,

$$\begin{aligned} &A^d_{2^{j+1}}(f)(n) \\ &= 2\sum_{k=-\infty}^{\infty} h(n-2k)A^d_{2^j}(f)(n) + 2\sum_{k=-\infty}^{\infty} g(n-2k)D_{2^j}(f)(n). \end{aligned} \tag{2.33}$$

A scheme for the reconstruction signal at resolution 2^{j+1} from approximated signal at resolution 2^j and detail signal at resolution 2^j thus can be derived similar to the scheme of DWT in Fig. 2.4. Figure 2.6 shows this one-level inverse DWT synthesis filter bank.

Figure 2.7 shows the complete scheme from decomposing a signal in resolution 2^{j+1} into signals in resolution 2^j and reconstructing it. This is the scheme of DWT and IDWT. Please note that in most cases, the filter coefficients in DWT and IDWT are multiplied by $\sqrt{2}$ such that the block of amplified by 2 in IDWT can be eliminated.

Now, we have derived the two-channel DWT analysis filter bank ($\widetilde{h}$ and $\widetilde{g}$) and synthesis filter bank (h and g), which are associated with the scaling function ϕ. The DWT filter is one kind of Quadrature Mirror Filter (QMF), but the coefficients are designed via the properties of ϕ, instead of the frequency response constraints in general DSP filter design. The above deduction is for the orthonormal DWT filter bank. However, it can be proven that there only exists one linear orthonormal DWT filter bank (Haar filter bank) which has only two taps. For designing good linear DWT filter banks, the constraint of Eq. (2.16) can be released, and they are called bi-orthogonal DWT filter banks.

In some cases, the analysis filters are notated as h and g, and the synthesis filters are notated as $\widetilde{h}$ and $\widetilde{g}$.

If the wavelet representation from resolution 1 to resolution 2^J is on

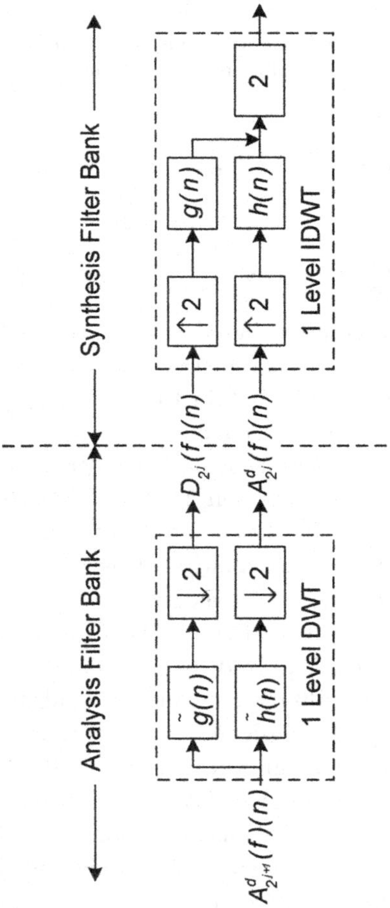

Fig. 2.7 The complete scheme from decomposing a signal in resolution 2^{j+1} into signals in resolution 2^j and reconstructing it.

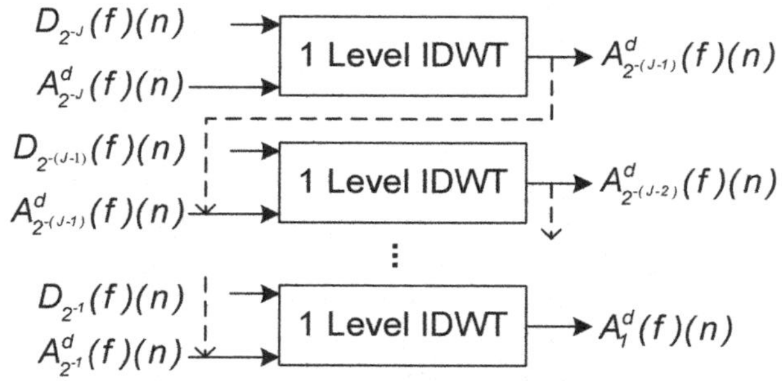

Fig. 2.8 The scheme to of multi-level IDWT.

hand, the signal in the highest resolution, $A_1^d(f)$, can be reconstructed by multi-level IDWT. Figure 2.8 shows the multi-level IDWT scheme which is obtained by cascading *1 Level DWT* modules in Fig. 2.4.

2.1.6 *2-D wavelet transform*

The DWT and IDWT derived in Section 2.1.3 and Section 2.1.5 can be easily extend into 2-D case for image and video processing. Figure 2.9 shows the scheme of single level 2-D DWT and IDWT. The first alphabet in the term LL, LH, HL, and HH means the row direction, and the second alphabet means the column direction. The alphabet "L"means that this signal is an approximated (low-pass) signal, and "H"means that this signal is a detail (high-pass) signal. The subscript "n"means the signal is in resolution 2^{-n}.

Figure 2.10 shows the scheme of two-level 2-D DWT. This scheme is a extension of the multi-level 1-D DWT depicted in Fig. 2.10. The input image can be regarded as the LL-band signal at resolution 2^0. One form of wavelet representation, which is referred to dyadic decomposition or Mallat decomposition in 2-D case thus is:

$$(LL_J, \{LH_j, HL_j, HH_j | 1 \leq j \leq J\}). \tag{2.34}$$

The LH band signal is a low-pass signal in the row direction and a high-pass signal in the column direction. Therefore, the LH signal contains mostly the horizontal edges. Similarly, the HL band signal and the HH band signal contain mostly vertical edges and diagonal edges, respectively.

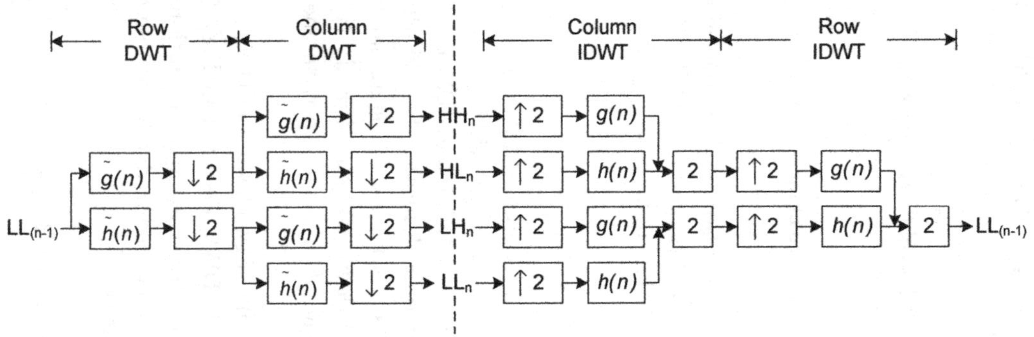

Fig. 2.9 The scheme of single level 2-D DWT and IDWT. The LL_n means the approximated signal (low-pass signal) in both row direction and column direction in resolution 2^{-n}, and LH_n means the signal which is low-pass in the row direction and high-pass in the column direction in resolution 2^{-n}, and so on.

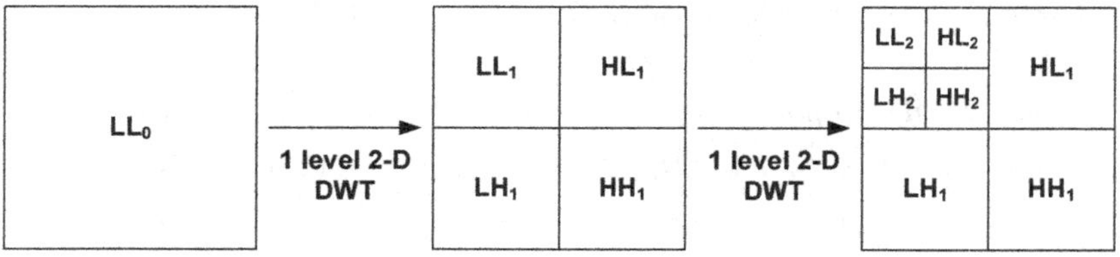

Fig. 2.10 An illustration of performing 2-level 2-D DWT on an image.

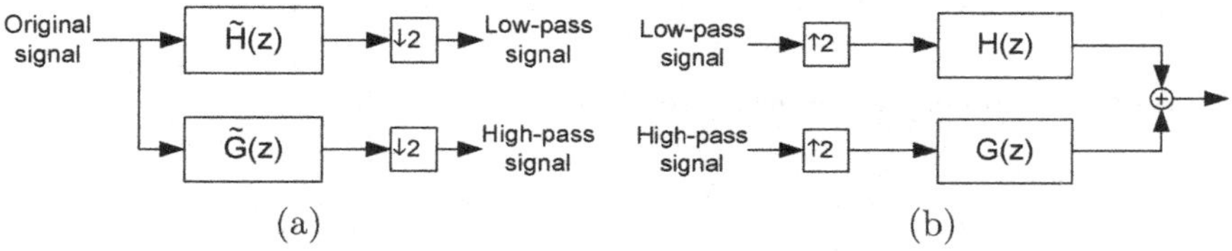

Fig. 2.11 Two-channel filter bank for DWT and IDWT. (a) Analysis filter bank for forward DWT. (b) Synthesis filter bank for inverse DWT.

2.2 Polyphase decomposition

The direct mapping of analysis (DWT) and synthesis (Inverse DWT, IDWT) filter banks is shown in Fig. 2.11, where $\widetilde{H}(z)$ and $\widetilde{G}(z)$ are the z-transform functions of analysis low-pass and high-pass filters, respectively. For perfect reconstruction, the synthesis low-pass and high-pass filters can be defined as

$$\begin{aligned} \widetilde{H}(z) &= G(-z) \\ \widetilde{G}(z) &= -H(-z). \end{aligned} \tag{2.35}$$

However, this direct mapping results in 50% computational waste. As can be seen in Fig. 2.11, in the DWT process, the computed signals will be down-sampled by 2. The hardware utilization thus can not exceed 50%. In the IDWT process, half signal in the input of synthesis filters must be zero because of the up-sample operation.

To achieve no computational waste, polyphase decomposition [36] is usually adopted, which moves the downsampling/upsampling operations to the front/back of the analysis/synthesis filter banks.

There are two possible decomposition types as follows:

$$\begin{aligned}
&Type-I \quad decomposition:\\
&\quad H(z) = H_e(z^2) + z^{-1}H_o(z^2), \qquad G(z) = G_e(z^2) + z^{-1}G_o(z^2)\\
&\quad \widetilde{H}(z) = \widetilde{H}_e(z^2) + z^{-1}\widetilde{H}_o(z^2), \qquad \widetilde{G}(z) = \widetilde{G}_e(z^2) + z^{-1}\widetilde{G}_o(z^2).
\end{aligned} \tag{2.36}$$

$$\begin{aligned}
&Type-II \quad decomposition:\\
&\quad H(z) = H_e(z^2) + zH_o(z^2), \qquad G(z) = G_e(z^2) + zG_o(z^2)\\
&\quad \widetilde{H}(z) = \widetilde{H}_e(z^2) + z\widetilde{H}_o(z^2), \qquad \widetilde{G}(z) = \widetilde{G}_e(z^2) + z\widetilde{G}_o(z^2).
\end{aligned} \tag{2.37}$$

As an example, the following relationships are defined:

$$\begin{aligned}
X(z) &= X_e(z^2) + z^{-1}X_o(z^2)\\
\widetilde{H}(z) &= \widetilde{H}_e(z^2) + z\widetilde{H}_o(z^2)\\
\widetilde{G}(z) &= \widetilde{G}_e(z^2) + z\widetilde{G}_o(z^2)\\
H(z) &= H_e(z^2) + z^{-1}H_o(z^2)\\
G(z) &= G_e(z^2) + z^{-1}G_o(z^2).
\end{aligned} \tag{2.38}$$

The DWT and IDWT schemes thus can be modified according to the relationships stated in Eq. 2.38.

Figure 2.12 shows the analysis filter bank after poly-phase decomposition. After applying the relationships defined in Eq. 2.38 on the scheme in Fig. 2.11(a), the scheme (a) in Fig. 2.12 can be obtained. The scheme (b) can be further obtained by applying the Noble Identity to interchange the order of down-sampling and filtering in scheme (a). Finally, the scheme (c) can be obtained by rearrangement of signals in the scheme (b). Please note that the down-sample operation is performed before filtering. Therefore, the DWT processing core becomes a two-input two-output system and can achieve 100% utilization.

Similarly, Fig. 2.13 shows the synthesis filter bank after poly-phase decomposition. The scheme (a) in Fig. 2.13 can be obtained by applying the relationships defined in Eq. 2.38 on the scheme in Fig. 2.11(b). The scheme (b) can be obtained by applying the other type of the Noble Identity to interchange the order of up-sampling and filtering in scheme (a). Finally, the scheme (c) can be obtained. The up-sample operation is performed after filtering. Therefore, the IDWT processing core becomes a two-input two-output system and can achieve 100% utilization.

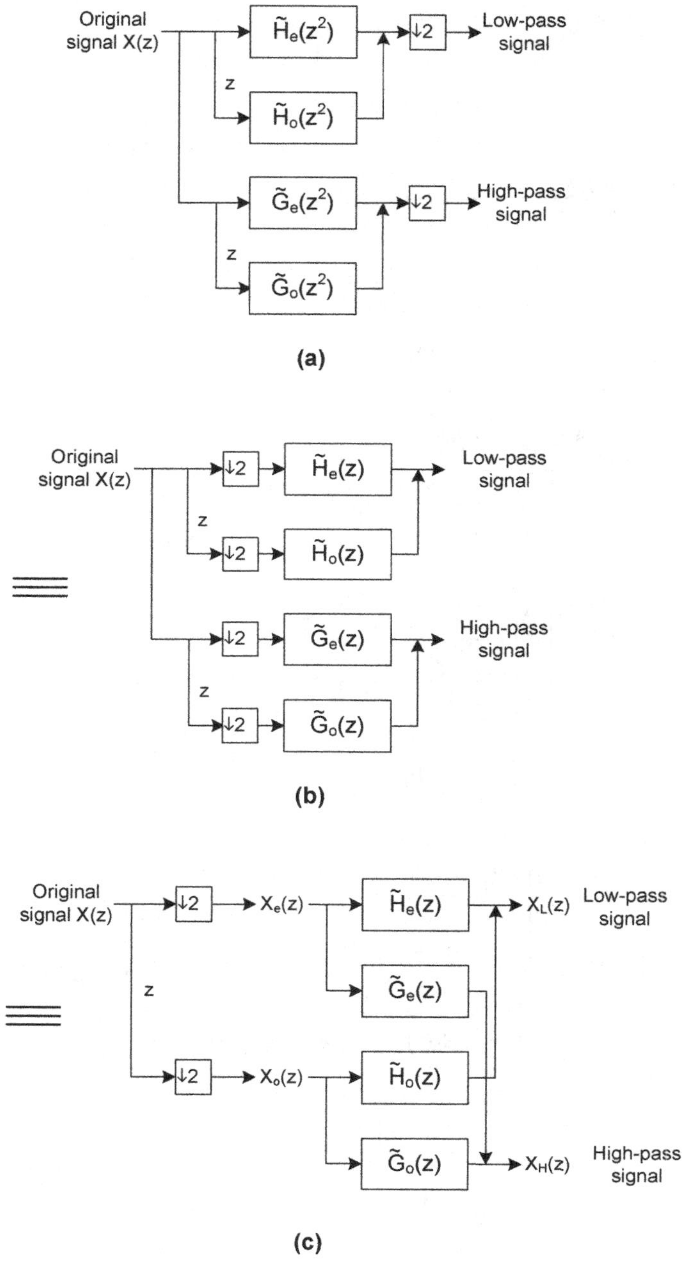

Fig. 2.12 The analysis filter bank after poly-phase decomposition.

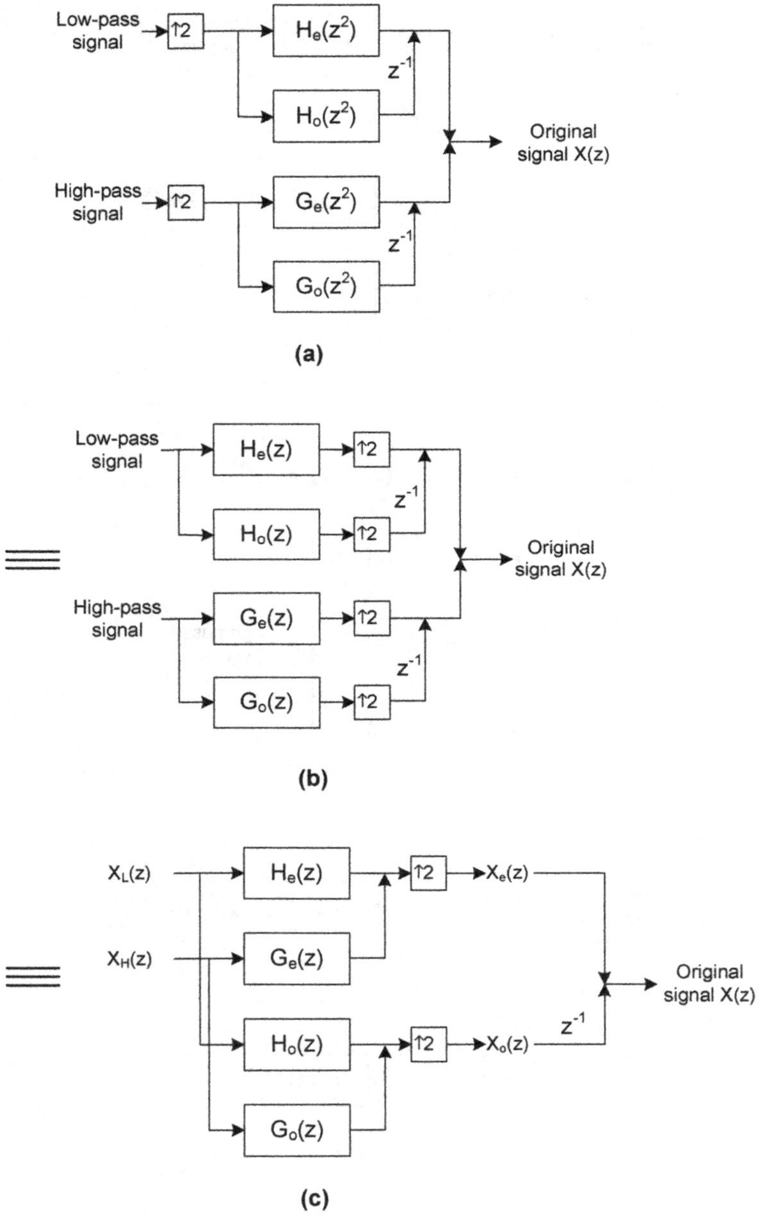

Fig. 2.13 The corresponding synthesis filter bank after poly-phase decomposition.

That is,

$$\begin{bmatrix} X_L(z) \\ X_H(z) \end{bmatrix} = \begin{bmatrix} \widetilde{H}_e(z) & \widetilde{H}_o(z) \\ \widetilde{G}_e(z) & \widetilde{G}_o(z) \end{bmatrix} \begin{bmatrix} X_e(z) \\ X_o(z) \end{bmatrix} \tag{2.39}$$

$$\begin{bmatrix} X_e(z) \\ X_o(z) \end{bmatrix} = \begin{bmatrix} H_e(z) & G_e(z) \\ H_o(z) & G_o(z) \end{bmatrix} \begin{bmatrix} X_L(z) \\ X_H(z) \end{bmatrix}. \tag{2.40}$$

The final scheme for DWT and IDWT with polyphase decomposition is summarized in Fig. 2.14.

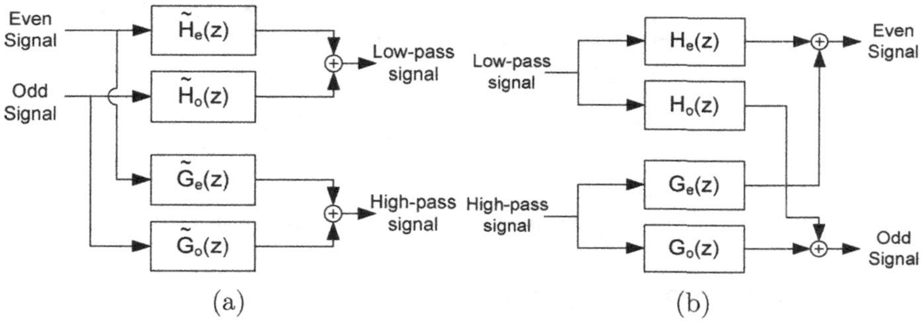

Fig. 2.14 Polyphase decomposition of two-channel filter banks. (a) Analysis filter bank. (b) Synthesis filter bank.

2.3 Lifting Scheme

The lifting scheme is a method for constructing wavelets by spatial approach [37]. The lifting scheme provides many advantages, such as fewer arithmetic operations, in-place implementation, and easy management of boundary extension. According to [38], any DWT filter bank of perfect reconstruction can be decomposed into a finite sequence of lifting stages. This decomposition corresponds to a factorization for the polyphase matrix of the target filter bank into a sequence of alternating upper and lower triangular matrices (prediction and update stages) and a constant diagonal matrix (normalization stage) by using the Euclidean Algorithm. In this section, the lifting scheme is derived according to [38].

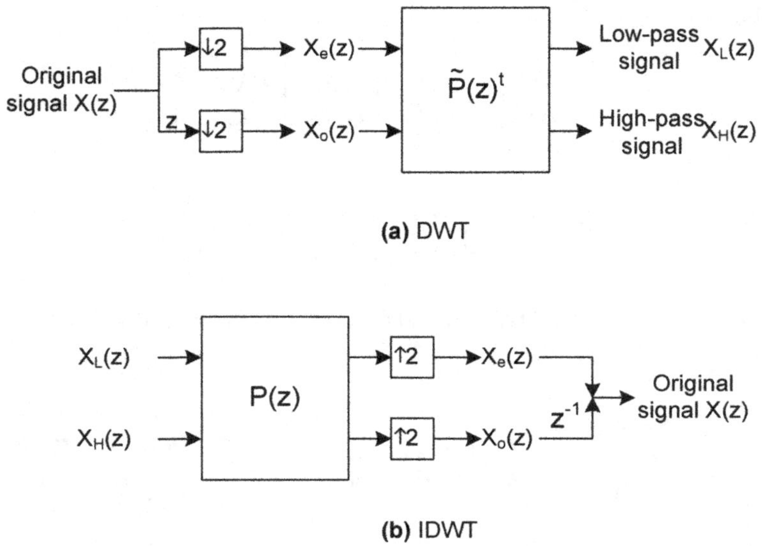

Fig. 2.15 Polyphase representation of DWT with equivalent matrices.

2.3.1 *Lifting steps for wavelet transform*

Define the following relationships:

$$P(z) = \begin{bmatrix} H_e(z) & G_e(z) \\ H_o(z) & G_o(z) \end{bmatrix}. \tag{2.41}$$

Similarly,

$$\widetilde{P}(z) = \begin{bmatrix} \widetilde{H}_e(z) & \widetilde{G}_e(z) \\ \widetilde{H}_o(z) & \widetilde{G}_o(z) \end{bmatrix}. \tag{2.42}$$

From Eq. 2.39–2.42, the polyphase representation of DWT (analysis filter bank) and IDWT (synthesis filter bank) in Fig. 2.14 can be simplified as the scheme in Fig. 2.15. From the prefect reconstruction property of DWT, the following relationship must be satisfied:

$$P(z)\widetilde{P}(z)^t = \mathbf{I} \tag{2.43}$$

where $\mathbf{I}$ is the 2×2 identity matrix.

One possible solution to Eq. 2.43 is:

$$\begin{aligned}\widetilde{H}_e(z) &= G_o(z) \\ \widetilde{H}_o(z) &= -G_e(z) \\ \widetilde{G}_e(z) &= -H_o(z) \\ \widetilde{G}_o(z) &= H_e(z).\end{aligned} \tag{2.44}$$

This further implies:

$$\begin{aligned}\widetilde{G}(z) &= z^{-1}H(-z) \\ \widetilde{H}(z) &= -z^{-1}G(-z).\end{aligned} \tag{2.45}$$

With FIR DWT filters, $P(z)$ and $\widetilde{P}(z)$ are Laurent Polynomials. Equation 2.43 implies that $det\{P(z)\}$ and its inverse are both Laurent Polynomials. This is possible only when $det\{P(z)\}$ is a monomial, that is, $det\{P(z)\} = Cz^l$. When deriving the lifting factorization, $det\{P(z)\}$ is assumed to be 1. If the determinant is not 1, $G(z)$ can be divided by the determinant value to normalize $P(z)$ to be 1.

$$det\{P(z)\} = 1. \tag{2.46}$$

A filter pair (h, g) is said to be *complementary* if and only if $P(z) = 1$. Please note that if (h, g) is complementary, so is $(\widetilde{h}, \widetilde{g})$.

We can define $P^{new}(z)$:

$$P^{new}(z) = P(z)U(z) = P(z)\begin{bmatrix} 1 & s(z) \\ 0 & 1 \end{bmatrix}, \tag{2.47}$$

where $s(z)$ is a Laurent Polynomial.

Because $det\{U(z)\} = 1$, $P^{new}(z)$ is thus still complementary. With this $P^{new}(z)$, $G(z)$ is transformed into $G(z) + H(z)s(z^2)$.

Theorem 2.3 *Lifting*

Let (h, g) be complementary. Then (h, g^{new}) is also complementary.

$$G^{new}(z) = G(z) + H(z)s(z^2) \tag{2.48}$$

where $s(z)$ is a Laurent Polynomial. Conversely, any filter of this form is complementary to h.

The dual polyphase matrix of $P^{new}(z)$, $\widetilde{P}^{new}(z)$ is:

$$\widetilde{P}^{new}(z) = \begin{bmatrix} 1 & -s(z) \\ 0 & 1 \end{bmatrix}\widetilde{P}(z). \tag{2.49}$$

The process of transforming $P(z)$ into $P^{new}(z)$ according to Theorem 2.3 is called a *lifting step*. Figure 2.16(a) shows the schematic representation of applying one lifting step on DWT and IDWT.

Similarly, if $P^{new}(z)$ is defined in another way:

$$P^{new}(z) = P(z)L(z) = P(z)\begin{bmatrix} 1 & 0 \\ t(z) & 1 \end{bmatrix}, \tag{2.50}$$

where $t(z)$ is a Laurent Polynomial.

Again, $P^{new}(z)$ is thus still complementary. With this $P^{new}(z)$, $H(z)$ is transformed into $H(z) + G(z)t(z^2)$.

Theorem 2.4 *Dual lifting*

Let (h, g) be complementary. Then (h^{new}, g) is also complementary.

$$H^{new}(z) = H(z) + G(z)t(z^2) \tag{2.51}$$

where $t(z)$ is a Laurent Polynomial. Conversely, any filter of this form is complementary to g.

The dual polyphase matrix of $P^{new}(z)$, $\widetilde{P}^{new}(z)$ is:

$$\widetilde{P}^{new}(z) = \begin{bmatrix} 1 & 0 \\ -t(z) & 1 \end{bmatrix} \widetilde{P}(z). \tag{2.52}$$

The process of transforming $P(z)$ into $P^{new}(z)$ according to Theorem 2.4 is called a *dual lifting step*. Figure 2.16(b) shows the schematic representation of applying one lifting step on DWT and IDWT.

2.3.2 *The Euclidean algorithm*

In this section, the Euclidean Algorithm for Laurent Polynomials is introduced. Combining with the lifting step and dual lifting step introduced in Theorem 2.3 and 2.4, the lifting factorization algorithm can be derived.

Theorem 2.5 *Euclidean Algorithm for Laurent Polynomials.*

For a Laurent Polynomial $a(z)$, let $\mid a(z) \mid$ be the order of $a(z)$.Define the modulus operator % in Laurent Polynomial:

$$\begin{aligned} a(z) &= b(z)q(z) + r(z)\ , \mid r(z) \mid < \mid b(z) \mid \\ r(z) &= a(z)\%b(z) \\ q(z) &= a(z)/b(z). \end{aligned} \tag{2.53}$$

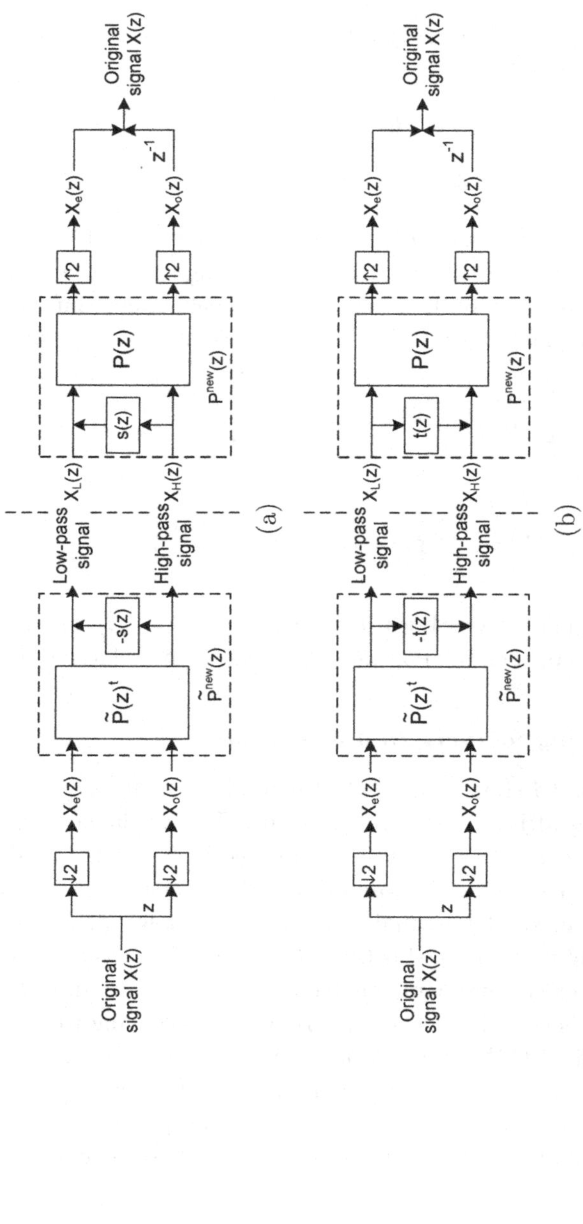

Fig. 2.16 The scheme of DWT and the corresponding IDWT. (a) Lifting scheme. (b) Dual lifting scheme.

Take two Laurent Polynomials $a(z)$ and $b(z) \neq 0$ with $\mid a(z) \mid \geq \mid b(z) \mid$. Let $a_0(z) = a(z)$ and $b_0(z) = b(z)$. The greatest common divider (gcd) of $a(z)$ and $b(z)$ can be obtained from the following iteration process from $i = 0$:

$$\begin{aligned} a_{i+1}(z) &= b_i(z) \\ b_{i+1}(z) &= a_i(z)\%b_i(z). \end{aligned} \tag{2.54}$$

$q_i(z)$ is further defined such that:

$$q_{i+1}(z) = a_i(z)/b_i(z). \tag{2.55}$$

Theorem 2.5 implies that $\mid b_{i+1}(z) \mid < \mid b_i(z) \mid$ for all i. Therefore, there exists an m so that $\mid b_m(z) \mid = 0$. This iterative algorithm then finishes for $n = m + 1$ where $b_n(z) = 0$. The number of iteration steps thus is bounded by $n \leq \mid b(z) \mid +1$. Therefore, the following relationship must exist:

$$\begin{bmatrix} a_n(z) \\ 0 \end{bmatrix} = \prod_{i=n}^{1} \begin{bmatrix} 0 & 1 \\ 1 & -q_i(z) \end{bmatrix} \begin{bmatrix} a(z) \\ b(z) \end{bmatrix}. \tag{2.56}$$

Conversely,

$$\begin{bmatrix} a(z) \\ b(z) \end{bmatrix} = \prod_{i=1}^{n} \begin{bmatrix} q_i(z) & 1 \\ 1 & 0 \end{bmatrix} \begin{bmatrix} a_n(z) \\ 0 \end{bmatrix}. \tag{2.57}$$

Therefore, $a_n(z)$ divides both $a(z)$ and $b(z)$. If $a_n(z)$ is a monomial, that is, $\mid a_n(z) \mid = 0$, then $a(z)$ and $b(z)$ are said to be relatively prime.

2.3.3 *The lifting factorization algorithm*

Theorem 2.3 and 2.4 show that a set of new wavelet filters can be synthesized by applying lifting or dual lifting steps. The Euclidean algorithm is further introduced in section 2.3.2. In this section, we further show that any wavelet filter can be decomposed into lifting steps by use of Euclidean Algorithm for Laurent Polynomials. For more examples, please see [38].

The first thing to be noticed is that $H_e(z)$ and $H_o(z)$ must be relatively prime. If there exists one common factor among $H_e(z)$ and $H_o(z)$, this common factor also divides $det\{P(z)\}$. However, according to the assumption in Eq. 2.46, $det\{P(z)\}$ must be 1. We can thus run the Euclidean algorithm in Theorem 2.5 and the resulted *gcd* will be monomial. According to the definition of quotient in Eq. 2.53, the quotient is not unique. Therefore, we can always choose the quotients $q_i(z)$, such that the resulted

gcd is a constant K. Therefore, from Eq. 2.57,

$$\begin{bmatrix} H_e(z) \\ H_o(z) \end{bmatrix} = \prod_{i=1}^{n} \begin{bmatrix} q_i(z) & 1 \\ 1 & 0 \end{bmatrix} \begin{bmatrix} K \\ 0 \end{bmatrix}. \tag{2.58}$$

Please note that in the case that $\mid H_e(z) \mid > \mid H_o(z) \mid$, $q_1(z)$ will be zero. In the case n is odd, we can interchange $H_e(z)$ with $H_o(z)$ by multiplying $H(z)$ with z and $G(z)$ with z^{-1}. This action will not change $det\{P(z)\}$ and make n even. Therefore, we can always assume that n is even. Give a filter $H(z)$, we can always find a complementary filter $G^0(z)$ such that

$$P^0(z) = \begin{bmatrix} H_e(z) & G_e^0(z) \\ H_o(z) & G_o^0(z) \end{bmatrix} = \prod_{i=1}^{n} \begin{bmatrix} q_i(z) & 1 \\ 1 & 0 \end{bmatrix} \begin{bmatrix} K & 0 \\ 0 & 1/K \end{bmatrix}. \tag{2.59}$$

The final diagonal matrix can force the determinant of $P^0(z)$ to be 1. The matrix representing for one iteration in Euclidean algorithm can be expressed in other forms:

$$\begin{bmatrix} q_i(z) & 1 \\ 1 & 0 \end{bmatrix} = \begin{bmatrix} 1 & q_i(z) \\ 0 & 1 \end{bmatrix} \begin{bmatrix} 0 & 1 \\ 1 & 0 \end{bmatrix} = \begin{bmatrix} 0 & 1 \\ 1 & 0 \end{bmatrix} \begin{bmatrix} 1 & 0 \\ q_i(z) & 1 \end{bmatrix}. \tag{2.60}$$

Combining Eqs. 2.59 and 2.60, the following relationship can be derived:

$$\begin{aligned} P^0(z) &= \prod_{i=1}^{n/2} \left(\begin{bmatrix} q_{2i-1}(z) & 1 \\ 1 & 0 \end{bmatrix} \begin{bmatrix} q_{2i}(z) & 1 \\ 1 & 0 \end{bmatrix} \right) \begin{bmatrix} K & 0 \\ 0 & 1/K \end{bmatrix} \\ &= \prod_{i=1}^{n/2} \left(\begin{bmatrix} 1 & q_{2i-1}(z) \\ 0 & 1 \end{bmatrix} \begin{bmatrix} 0 & 1 \\ 1 & 0 \end{bmatrix} \begin{bmatrix} 0 & 1 \\ 1 & 0 \end{bmatrix} \begin{bmatrix} 1 & 0 \\ q_{2i}(z) & 1 \end{bmatrix} \right) \begin{bmatrix} K & 0 \\ 0 & 1/K \end{bmatrix} \\ &= \prod_{i=1}^{n/2} \left(\begin{bmatrix} 1 & q_{2i-1}(z) \\ 0 & 1 \end{bmatrix} \begin{bmatrix} 1 & 0 \\ q_{2i}(z) & 1 \end{bmatrix} \right) \begin{bmatrix} K & 0 \\ 0 & 1/K \end{bmatrix}. \end{aligned} \tag{2.61}$$

From Theorem 2.3, given a complementary set (h, g), any filter g^{new} that makes (h, g^{new}) complementary must be able to be obtained by applying a lifting step on g. Therefore,

$$P(z) = \begin{bmatrix} H_e(z) & G_e(z) \\ H_o(z) & G_o(z) \end{bmatrix} = P^0(z) \begin{bmatrix} 1 & s(z) \\ 0 & 1 \end{bmatrix}. \tag{2.62}$$

A set of complementary filter pair (h, g^0) can be obtained from Euclidean algorithm in Theorem 2.5, and the results are in Eq. 2.59. Theorem 2.3 further shows that g must be able to be obtained from g^0 by a lifting step. Finally, the lifting factorization algorithm can be derived.

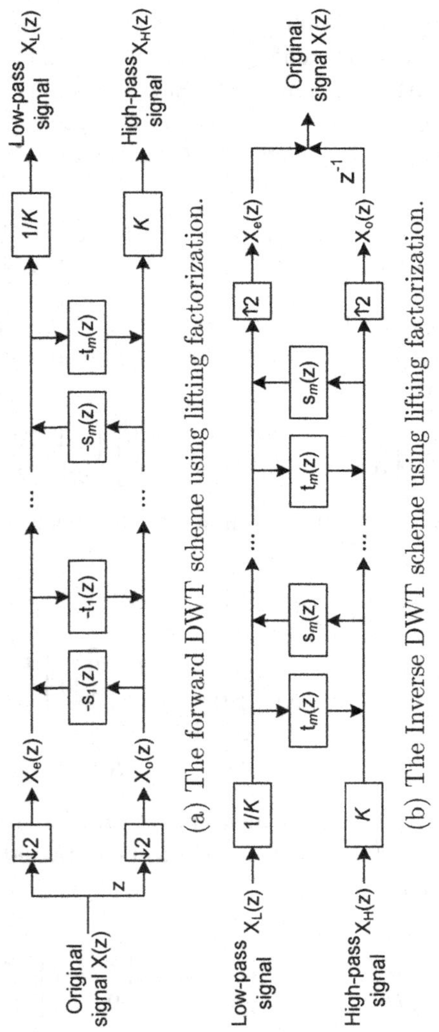

(a) The forward DWT scheme using lifting factorization.

(b) The Inverse DWT scheme using lifting factorization.

Fig. 2.17 The schemes of DWT and IDWT using lifting factorization.

Theorem 2.6 *Lifting factorization algorithm*

Let (h, g) be complementary. Then there exist Laurent Polynomials $s_i(z)$ and $t_i(z)$ for $1 \leq i \leq m$ and a non-zero constant K so that

$$P(z) = \begin{bmatrix} H_e(z) & G_e(z) \\ H_o(z) & G_o(z) \end{bmatrix} = \prod_{i=1}^{m} \left(\begin{bmatrix} 1 & s_i(z) \\ 0 & 1 \end{bmatrix} \begin{bmatrix} 1 & 0 \\ t_i(z) & 1 \end{bmatrix} \right) \begin{bmatrix} K & 0 \\ 0 & 1/K \end{bmatrix}. \quad (2.63)$$

As discussed, m is bounded by $n/2 + 1$. From the Eq. 2.49, the dual polyphase matrix is given by

$$\widetilde{P}(z) = \begin{bmatrix} \widetilde{H}_e(z) & \widetilde{G}_e(z) \\ \widetilde{H}_o(z) & \widetilde{G}_o(z) \end{bmatrix} = \prod_{i=1}^{m} \left(\begin{bmatrix} 1 & 0 \\ -s_i(z) & 1 \end{bmatrix} \begin{bmatrix} 1 & -t_i(z) \\ 0 & 1 \end{bmatrix} \right) \begin{bmatrix} 1/K & 0 \\ 0 & K \end{bmatrix}. \quad (2.64)$$

Figure 2.17 shows the schemes of DWT and IDWT using lifting factorization. When implementation, instead of taking the DWT filter band as two separate filters, the lifting factorization algorithm exploits the properties of perfect reconstruct filter banks. Therefore, the lifting factorization can reduce arithmetic operations compared to the convolution expression by exploring the redundancy between the low-pass and high-pass filters. Although the arithmetic gain of the lifting scheme over convolution-based structures may possibly reach a factor of four [39], the non-uniqueness of lifting factorizations diversifies the design space of lifting-based DWT.

For easy understanding, two examples of factorizing are given.

(1) **Haar wavelets**

Haar wavelets comprise simple wavelet filters with $H(z) = 1 + z^{-1}$ and $g(z) = -\frac{1}{2} + \frac{1}{2}z^{-1}$. The corresponding IDWT filters are $\widetilde{H}(z) = \frac{1}{2} + \frac{1}{2}z^{-1}$ and $\widetilde{G}(z) = -1 + z^{-1}$. By inspection,

$$P(z) = \begin{bmatrix} 1 & -1/2 \\ 1 & 1/2 \end{bmatrix} = \begin{bmatrix} 1 & 0 \\ 1 & 1 \end{bmatrix} \begin{bmatrix} 1 & -1/2 \\ 0 & 1 \end{bmatrix}. \quad (2.65)$$

Therefore, the dual polyphase matrix is:

$$\widetilde{P}(z)^t = P(z)^{-1} = \begin{bmatrix} 1 & 1/2 \\ 0 & 1 \end{bmatrix} \begin{bmatrix} 1 & 0 \\ -1 & 1 \end{bmatrix}. \quad (2.66)$$

Figure 2.18 shows the DWT and IDWT scheme of lifting-based haar filter. It can be directly derived from Eqs. 2.65 and 2.66.

(2) $(9, 7)$ **filter**

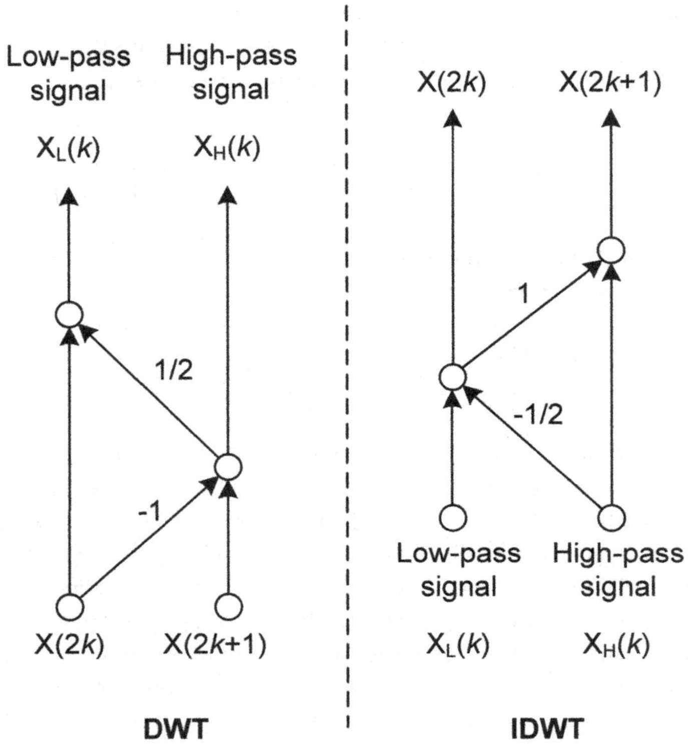

Fig. 2.18 The haar wavelet scheme of DWT and IDWT based on lifting factorization.

The $(9,7)$ filter is a popular filter that has been adopted in JPEG 2000 standard for lossy image compression. The analysis filter $\widetilde{h}$ has 9 coefficients while the synthesis filter h has 7 coefficients for smoother scaling function. The analysis filter can be expressed as:

$$\begin{aligned} \widetilde{H}_e(z) &= h_4(z^2 + z^{-2}) + h_2(z + z^{-1}) + h_0 \\ \widetilde{H}_o(z) &= h_3(z^2 + z^{-1}) + h_1(z + 1). \end{aligned} \tag{2.67}$$

From Euclidean algorithm:

$$\begin{aligned}
a_0(z) &= h_4(z^2 + z^{-2}) + h_2(z + z^{-1}) + h_0 \\
b_0(z) &= h_3(z^2 + z^{-1}) + h_1(z + 1) \\
q_1(z) &= h_4/h_3(1 + z^{-1}) \\
&= \alpha(1 + z^{-1}) \\
\\
a_1(z) &= h_3(z^2 + z^{-1}) + h_1(z + 1) \\
b_1(z) &= (h_2 - h_4 - h_1h_4/h_3)(z + z^{-1}) + (h_0 - 2h_1h_4/h_3) \\
&= r_1(z + z^{-1}) + r_0 \\
q_2(z) &= h_3/r_1(1 + z) \\
&= \beta(1 + z) \\
\\
a_2(z) &= r_1(z + z^{-1}) + r_0 \\
b_2(z) &= (h_1 - h_3 - h_3r_0/r_1)(1 + z) \\
&= s_0(1 + z) \\
q_3(z) &= r_1/s_0(1 + z^{-1}) \\
&= \gamma(1 + z^{-1}) \\
\\
a_3(z) &= s_0(1 + z) \\
b_3(z) &= r_0 - 2r_1 \\
&= \zeta \\
q_4(z) &= s_0/\zeta \\
&= \delta \\
\\
a_4(z) &= \zeta \\
b_4(z) &= 0.
\end{aligned} \tag{2.68}$$

So the polyphase matrix of analysis filters can be decomposed as:

$$\widetilde{P}(z) = \begin{bmatrix} 1 & \alpha(1+z^{-1}) \\ 0 & 1 \end{bmatrix} \begin{bmatrix} 1 & 0 \\ \beta(1+z) & 1 \end{bmatrix} \begin{bmatrix} 1 & \gamma(1+z^{-1}) \\ 0 & 1 \end{bmatrix} \begin{bmatrix} 1 & 0 \\ \delta(1+z) & 1 \end{bmatrix} \begin{bmatrix} \zeta & 0 \\ 0 & 1/\zeta \end{bmatrix}. \tag{2.69}$$

Please note that due to the non-uniqueness of quotient of Laurent Polynomials, many other factorizations exist. The adopted one in [38] is symmetric: every quotient is a multiple of $(z + 1)$, and this makes the multipliers can be halved.

Figure 2.19 shows the DWT scheme of lifting-based $(9, 7)$ filter. It can be directly derived from Eq. 2.69. Please note that the multipliers

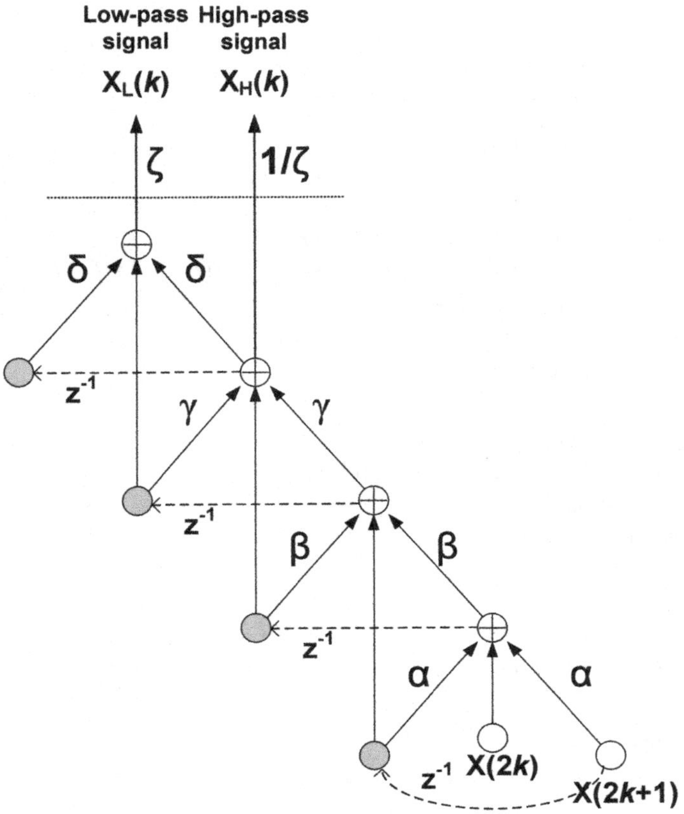

Fig. 2.19 DWT scheme for lifting-based architecture of (9,7) filter.

with the same coefficients can be shared. For example, the two multipliers that multiply signal by α in Fig. 2.19 can become one filter by adding $X(2k+1)$ and $X(2k-1)$ before being multiplied by α.

2.4 B-spline formulation

As mentioned in Section 2.1, the DWT is constructed from CWT and maintains the good time-frequency decomposition characteristic. However, the DWT low-pass and high-pass filters have poor frequency responses because of large transition bandwidth and heavy aliasing effect. Figure 2.20 shows the magnitude response of the popular JPEG 2000 lossy (9,7) filter bank and lossless (5,3) filter bank. The transition bandwidth is quite large, and the aliasing effect of low-pass and high-pass filters is also very significant. It is hard to find out the advantages of DWT in the viewpoints of digital filters and signal processing.

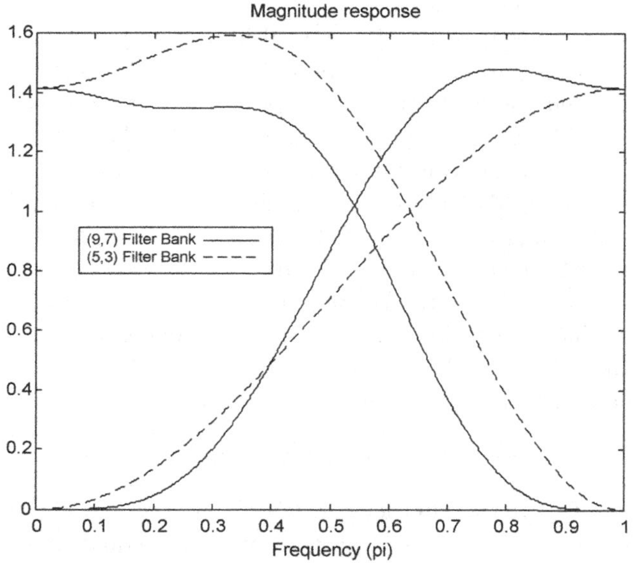

Fig. 2.20 Magnitude response of JPEG 2000 lossy (9,7) filter bank and lossless (5,3) filter bank. The aliasing effect between low-pass and high-pass filters is very significant, and the transition bandwidth is very large.

In [40], the wavelet theory is revisited, which leads to some new insights on wavelets. According to [40], the low-pass filter, $H(z) = \sum_{i=0}^{P_H-1} h_i z^{-i}$, and the high-pass filter, $G(z) = \sum_{i=0}^{P_G-1} g_i z^{-i}$, of any DWT can be factorized as

$$\begin{aligned} H(z) &= \underline{(1+z^{-1})^{\gamma_H}} \cdot \underline{Q(z)} \cdot \underline{h_0} \\ G(z) &= \underline{(1-z^{-1})^{\gamma_G}} \cdot \underline{R(z)} \cdot \underline{g_0} \end{aligned} \tag{2.70}$$

where the first, second, and third terms of the right-hand side can be called the B-spline part, distributed part, and normalization part, respectively. Based on this B-spline factorization, the output of high-pass filter can be viewed as the γ_G-th order difference of the smoothed input signals. For example, the high-pass signals will become all zeros, if the input signal is a $(\gamma_G - 1)$-th order polynomial function.

There are two differences between Eq. (2.70) and the expression of [40]. The first one is that $1 \pm z^{-1}$ is treated as the B-spline part, instead of $\frac{1+z^{-1}}{2}$. And the second one is the normalization part which is extracted here for further implementation issues.

The B-spline part is responsible for all important properties of DWT, such as order of approximation, reproduction of polynomials, vanishing moments, and multiscale differentiation property. The distributed part is used to derive efficient finite-impose-response (FIR) DWT filters. Without the distributed part, the inverse filter bank will contain infinite-impose-response (IIR) filters that are more difficult to implement than FIR filters for image related algorithms, except the simplest 2-tap Haar filter. For this purpose, the order of the distributed part is usually designed as small as possible when the order of the B-spline part is given. For the Daubechies DWT filters which are optimal in the sense that they have a minimum size support with a given number of vanishing moments [35], the filter lengths are constrained with the given vanishing moments, γ_H and γ_G, as follows:

$$F_H + F_G \geq 2(\gamma_H + \gamma_G)$$

where F_H and F_G are the filter lengths of the low-pass and high-pass DWT filters, respectively. Daubechies wavelets satisfy the equal sign. Thus, the filter lengths F_Q and F_R of the distributed part $Q(z)$ and $R(z)$ are constrained by

$$F_Q + F_R \geq (\gamma_H + \gamma_G).$$

As for the normalization part, it is very similar to the normalization stage in the lifting scheme.

2.5 Classification of 1-D DWT Algorithms

A DWT filter bank is derived from a CWT associated with a scaling function. Using the relations between CWT coefficients, the DWT filter coefficients can be derived. The expression of DWT coefficients is exactly a complete two-channel filter bank. The convolution-based expression is the direct one from the filter bank expression, and polyphase decomposition is usually adopted for 100% hardware utilization.

The lifting scheme is an efficient expression of any two-channel filter bank that guarantees perfect reconstruction (PR). It can provide many advantages, including less computational complexity and in-place implementation. It can also be used to construct good DWT filter banks.

A new representation of DWT, called B-spline factorization, can easily show the advantages of using DWT for signal analysis. Moreover, the B-spline part is the intrinsic property of DWT, and make DWT different from other kinds of two-channel filter bank.

The three different mathematical formulations of DWT/IDWT are summarized in Fig. 2.21. Instead only for DWT, the convolution-based expression can be applied to any two-channel filter bank. The lifting-based expression can be used to implement any perfect reconstruction two-channel filter bank. The B-spline-based expression is dedicated for DWT properties.

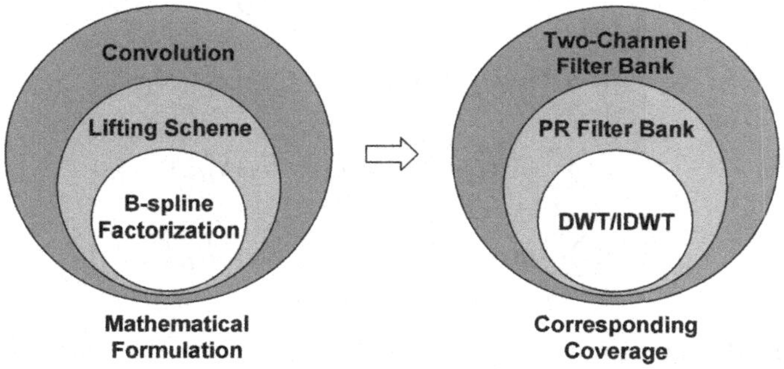

Fig. 2.21 Categories of mathematical formulations for DWT/IDWT and the corresponding coverage.

2.6 Algorithms of 2-D DWT

There are two kinds of filter banks for the one-level 2-D DWT: non-separable and separable. The non-separable 2-D DWT filters are intrinsically of 2-D coefficients. Instead, the separable 2-D DWT filters consist of one 1-D filter in the row direction and one 1-D filter in the column direction. In the following, the separable 2-D DWT is focused. The separable 2-D DWT of the dyadic decomposition type can be formulated recursively as follows:

$$
\begin{aligned}
x_{LL}^{J}(n_1,n_2) &= \sum_{i_1,i_2} h(i_1)h(i_2)x_{LL}^{J-1}(2n_1-i_1,2n_2-i_2) \\
x_{LH}^{J}(n_1,n_2) &= \sum_{i_1,i_2} h(i_1)g(i_2)x_{LL}^{J-1}(2n_1-i_1,2n_2-i_2) \\
x_{HL}^{J}(n_1,n_2) &= \sum_{i_1,i_2} g(i_1)h(i_2)x_{LL}^{J-1}(2n_1-i_1,2n_2-i_2) \\
x_{HH}^{J}(n_1,n_2) &= \sum_{i_1,i_2} g(i_1)g(i_2)x_{LL}^{J-1}(2n_1-i_1,2n_2-i_2) \qquad (2.71)
\end{aligned}
$$

where J is the DWT decomposition level, and x_{LL}^{0} is the input image. Correspondingly, the 2-D IDWT can be formulated as:

$$
\begin{aligned}
x_{LL}^{J-1}(n_1,n_2) &= \sum_{i_1,i_2} \tilde{h}(n_1-2i_1)\tilde{h}(n_2-2i_2)x_{LL}^{J}(i_1,i_2) \\
&+ \sum_{i_1,i_2} \tilde{h}(n_1-2i_1)\tilde{g}(n_2-2i_2)x_{LH}^{J}(i_1,i_2) \\
&+ \sum_{i_1,i_2} \tilde{g}(n_1-2i_1)\tilde{h}(n_2-2i_2)x_{HL}^{J}(i_1,i_2) \\
&+ \sum_{i_1,i_2} \tilde{g}(n_1-2i_1)\tilde{g}(n_2-2i_2)x_{HH}^{J}(i_1,i_2). \qquad (2.72)
\end{aligned}
$$

The dyadic decomposition can provide a good time-frequency characteristic like Fig. 2.3, where lower frequency components take longer time period for steadier behavior. Contrarily, the conventional block-based transform, such as discrete cosine transform and discrete Fourier transform, has a blocky time-frequency decomposition characteristic as shown in Fig. 2.22. The block-based transform gives all frequency components the same time period, which is not flexible to express the natural signals.

Figure 2.23 shows the most commonly used dyadic DWT decomposition. The multi-level decomposition is derived by recursively performing one-level decomposition on the LL subband. This dyadic decomposition is suitable to decompose natural images because the lower frequency components are concentrated into a smaller LL subband for efficient manipulation like signal analysis or image compression.

One another kind of decomposition is the complete decomposition as shown in Fig. 2.24. All subbands are further decomposed into four subbands. The complete decomposition becomes similar with the block-based

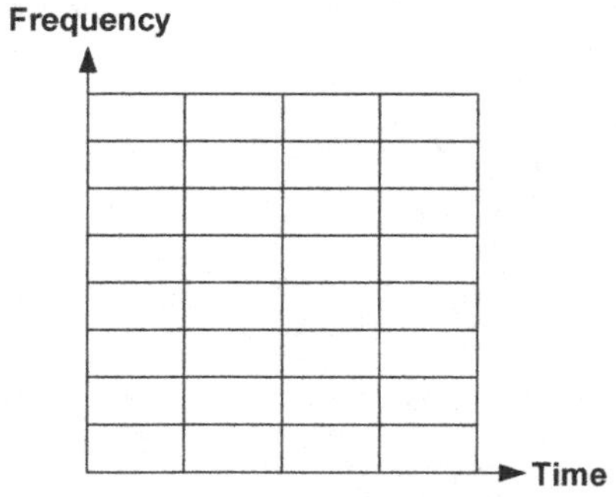

Fig. 2.22 Time-frequency decomposition diagram of block-based transform, such as discrete cosine transform and discrete Fourier transform.

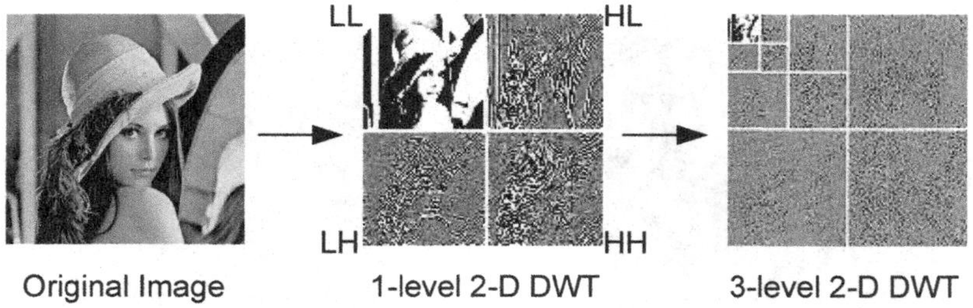

Fig. 2.23 An example of 2-D DWT dyadic decomposition. The multi-level decomposition is to perform one-level decomposition recursively on the LL subband. (LL: Low-pass-Low-pass subband; LH: Low-pass-High-pass subband; HL: High-pass-Low-pass subband; HH: High-pass-High-pass subband;)

transform, but each subband contains the corresponding frequency information of the whole image. Although the complete decomposition is seldom used, the useful wavelet package transform (WPT) is pruned from it. The WPT is to adapt the decomposition of every subband for best manipulation purpose according to the image property. As shown in Fig. 2.25, this image contains much high frequency texture information, so the three high frequency subbands are further decomposed for deriving more details. For images of highly textured property, such as fingerprint and chambray, their high frequency (or high order) components can be explored by decomposing them into more higher frequency subbands, instead of only using the dyadic decomposition.

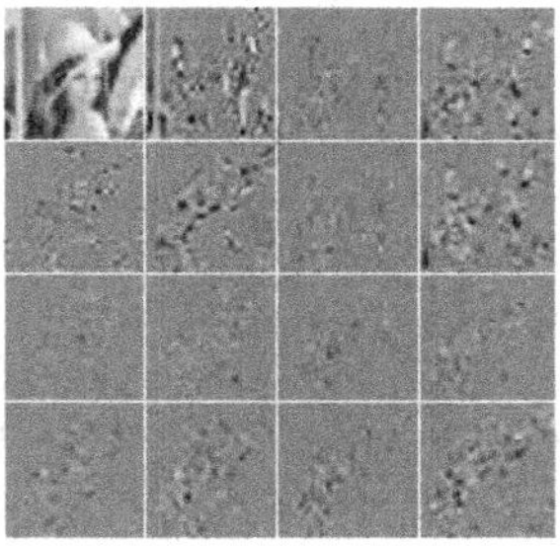

Fig. 2.24 An example of two-level 2-D DWT complete decomposition. Each subband is further decomposed into four subbands.

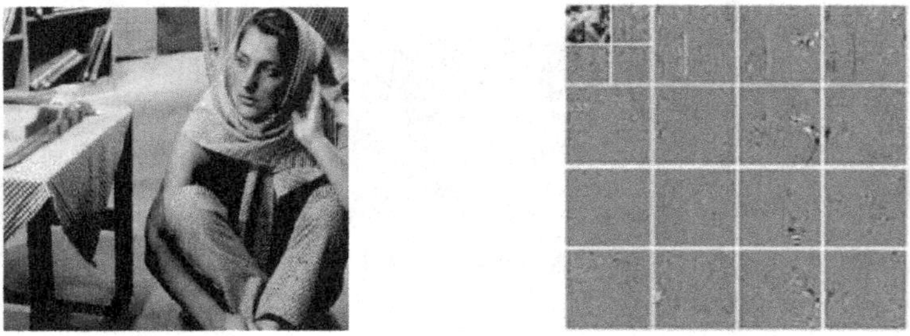

(a) (b)

Fig. 2.25 Wavelet packet transform (WPT). (a) Highly textured image. (b) WPT decomposition for the corresponding frequency characteristic.

The one-level 2-D DWT decomposition is the basic operation of any kind of decompositions. Since the dyadic decomposition is most commonly used, the multi-level decomposition will be considered as a dyadic one for discussion.

2.7 Image Coding Using 2-D DWT

The recently representative image coding algorithms using 2-D DWT are all based on bit-plane coding. Instead of traditional word-level coding, the bit-plane coding considers the DWT coefficients as bit-planes as shown in Fig. 2.26. One coefficient is split into one sign bit and many refinement bits for magnitude from most significant bit (MSB) to least significant bit (LSB).

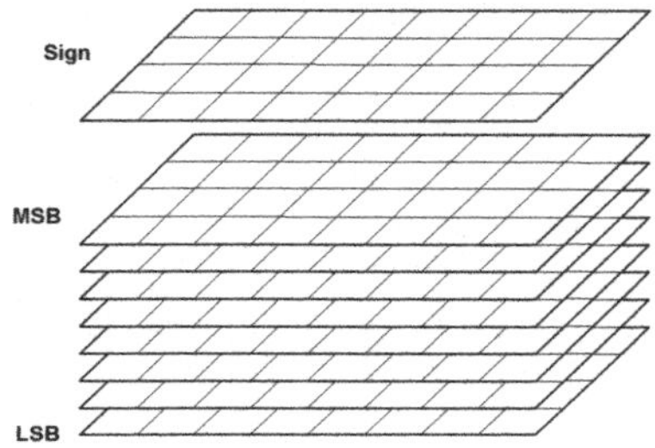

Fig. 2.26 Bit-plane expression of DWT coefficients. The priority of importance is from sign bit, most significant bit (MSB), to least significant bit.

There are two ways to exploit the redundancy of DWT subband coefficients, which are inter- and intra-subband coding schemes. The inter-subband coding is to explore the redundancy among subbands. They usually use a tree structure to represent the relationship between parent and child subband coefficients and utilize the similarity of these trees for high coding performance. The Embedded Zerotree Wavelet (EZW) coding [4] is a breakthrough of DWT-based image coding. After the multi-level DWT decomposition, the EZW constructs the parent-child trees cross subbands as shown in Fig. 2.27. Every tree is scanned in a bitplane-by-bitplane order from MSB to LSB. It is shown that the absolute values of a parent and its children are highly correlated, although their coefficient values are nearly uncorrelated because of the nearly orthogonal decomposition of DWT. When scanning some bit-plane, the coefficient is insignificant if it is smaller than the corresponding threshold value. If a parent is insignificant at some bit-plane, its children are very possibly insignificant. Thus, the EZW utilizes this property to find out the zerotrees for each bit-plane scan. For every zerotree, only one-bit symbol can represent the whole tree such as to save a lot of bits. Furthermore, the coding method called Set Partitioning in Hierarchical Trees (SPIHT) [5] is to increase the compression capability by use of a well-deigned hierarchical tree structure. Based on the set partitioning strategy and the proposed coding flow, the DWT coefficients can be coded in a more efficient way than EZW.

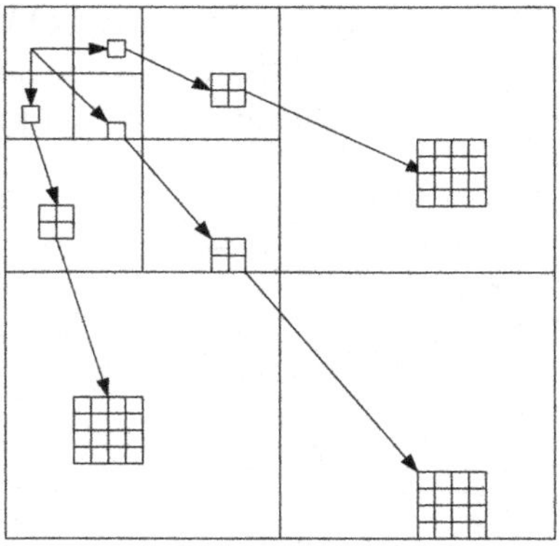

Fig. 2.27 The tree structure of a three-level dyadic DWT decomposition. Except the first level high frequency subbands, every coefficient is a parent that has four children in the corresponding position.

On the other hand, the intra-subband coding scheme utilizes the local redundancy inside each subband, such as the powerful Embedded Block Coding with Optimized Truncation (EBCOT) [6]. The EBCOT algorithm is to separate the subband coefficients into the basic coding units that are called codeblocks. Then the coding algorithm consists of two tiers as shown in Fig. 2.28. In the first tier, each codeblock is encoded into a embedded bitstream separately. In the second tier, the rate-distortion performance is optimized by optimally truncating the less important bitstreams for every codeblock.

The first tier exploits the local redundancy inside every codeblock by context-adaptive coding. The DWT coefficients are also separated into many bit-planes. Each bit-plane is scanned by three passes. In these passes, every sample will be coded into a context which is dependent on the status of the neighboring samples in the context window as shown in Fig. 2.29. In the second tier, the bitstreams derived from each codeblock can be optimally extracted for the minimum mean square error (MSE) under the given bit-rate constraint. The EBCOT algorithm has been adopted in the JPEG 2000 standard [7], which can achieve about 2dB peak-signal-to-noise-ratio (PSNR) gain than JPEG [3]. Besides, the superior scalability is also a new feature compared to the DCT-based block coding.

Moreover, one DWT-based coding algorithm that combines both intra- and inter-subband schemes, called EZBC, has been proposed [8]. The EZBC is to construct zeroblocks inside every subband to utilize the intra-subband

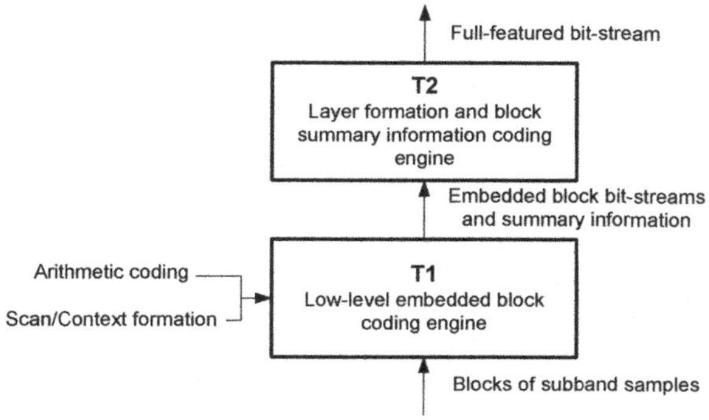

Fig. 2.28 Two-tier coding scheme of JPEG 2000. The first tier is to encode each code-block independently by exploring the local redundancy. The second tier is to optimize the rate-distortion performance by truncating less important bitstreams with a greedy search method.

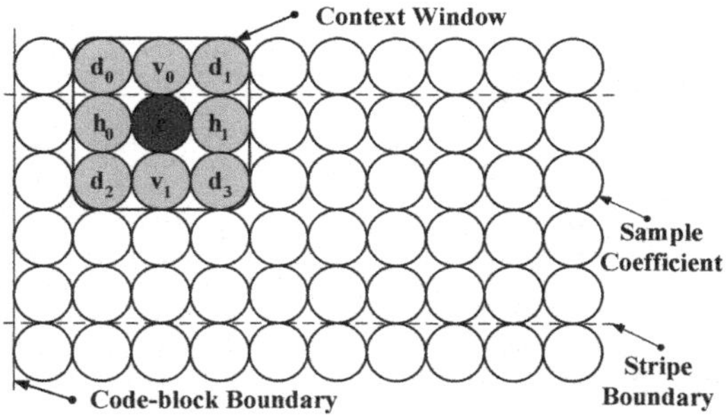

Fig. 2.29 Context formation of EBCOT algorithm. The context of each sample in every bit-plane is derived by exploring the relationship inside the context window. The contexts are further coded by use of arithmetic coding to achieve high coding performance.

redundancy. Every zeroblock is established in a tree structure like the zerotree of EZW. But the zeroblock is constructed by collecting the neighboring coefficients inside a subband. The tree of the corresponding zeroblock is also scanned from root to leaves, and one context is used to represent all children below are all zero. When establishing the contexts, the corresponding context in the upper subband will also be referenced to exploit the inter-subband redundancy. The EZBC can achieve about 0.5dB coding gain more than EBCOT.

Chapter 3

Architectures of One-Dimensional DWT

This chapter provides an overview and performance comparison of processing element designs for 1-D DWT. The convolution-based one is the basic type that requires larger computational complexity. The lifting-based one can reduce the complexity in many cases and requires the fewest registers. The B-spline-based one can provide the smallest logic gate count. The precision issues, including word length and round-off noise, are also discussed.

3.1 Convolution-Based Architectures

The straightforward implementation for DWT and IDWT is to construct the low-pass and high-pass filters independently with fundamental VLSI DSP design techniques, such as folding, unfolding, and pipelining [28]. For 100% hardware utilization, the polyphase decomposition as described in Section 2.2 is usually adopted, and the corresponding architectures are shown in Fig. 2.14. The four separate filters of Fig. 2.14(a) or (b) can be implemented by use of parallel or serial filters.

There have several efficient architectures been proposed for convolution-based DWT [41, 42, 43, 44]. However, the simplest parallel filter architecture is usually used if the throughput is set as two-input/two-output per clock cycle, and the minimal latency and the fewest registers are required. It can be implemented as shown in Fig. 3.1, in which $H_e(z)$ and $H_o(z)$ are combined, and so are $G_e(z)$ and $G_o(z)$. The registers of $H_e(z)$ and $G_e(z)$ are also shared for saving hardware resource, and so are those of $H_o(z)$ and $G_o(z)$. In Fig. 3.1, the critical path is $T_m + (F-1) \cdot T_a$, where T_m is the time taken for a multiplication operation, T_a is the time needed for an addition operation, and $F = max(F_H, F_G)$. The hardware cost is $(F_H + F_G) \cdot C_m + (F_H + F_G - 2) \cdot C_a$, where C_m and C_a are the hardware cost of a multiplier and an adder, respectively. Furthermore, using adder tree to implement these additions can improve the critical path to $T_m + \lceil \log_2 F \rceil \cdot T_a$. As for the number of registers, this architecture requires $F-2$ registers without considering the input nodes, $x(2n)$ and $x(2n-1)$. If the adopted DWT filter is linear, we can reduce the required number of multipliers by one half by use of the symmetric or anti-symmetric structures of linear filters. Moreover, this modification will not change the critical path and the number of registers.

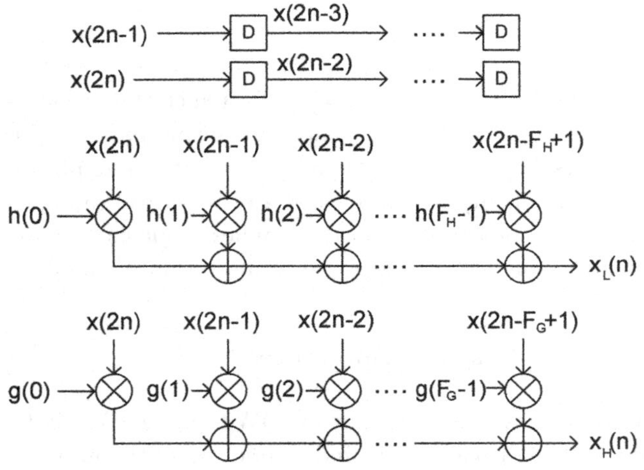

Fig. 3.1 Convolution-based architecture using parallel filters. F_H and F_G are the lengths of low-pass and high-pass filters, respecitively.

Besides the parallel filter, the four filters in Fig. 2.14(a) can also be implemented by use of serial filter architecture as shown in 3.2. The critical path is constrained to only T_m+T_a, but the registers between the four filters cannot be shared as parallel filters.

3.2 Lifting-Based Architectures

The 1-D DWT can be constructed by use of efficient lifting scheme expression. In the following, two kinds of implementations based on lifting scheme will be introduced. The first one is from direct mapping of lifting scheme, and the second one is from an efficient flipping method for lifting stages.

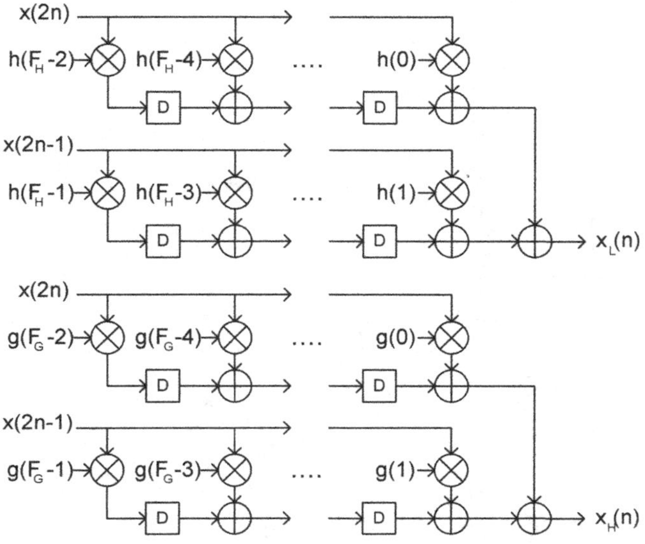

Fig. 3.2 Convolution-based architecture using serial filters. F_H and F_G are assumed to be even only for example.

3.2.1 *Direct implementation of lifting scheme*

Most of the lifting-based architectures in literature are implemented with the lifting factorization directly [45, 46, 47, 48]. The direct mapping from Eq. (2.63) and Eq. (2.64) to lifting-based DWT and IDWT implementation are shown in Fig. 3.3. Although the lifting scheme can provide many advantages, such as fewer arithmetic operations and in-place implementation, the potentially long critical path is a drawback for hardware implementation. In the following, the timing crisis is examined.

The lifting factorization is essentially composed of a series of computing stages that correspond to the upper and lower triangular matrices. The computing unit of upper triangular matrices is shown in Fig. 3.4, and the case of lower triangular matrices is similar. In Fig. 3.4, the computation node performs the summation of all input signals, the register node stores the data in the previous clock cycle, and the input node receives the coming data in the current clock cycle. Thus, a lifting-based architecture is a serial combination of such computing units, and the computation node of the previous computing stage is connected to the right input node of the next stage. The critical path of a lifting-based architecture would be the

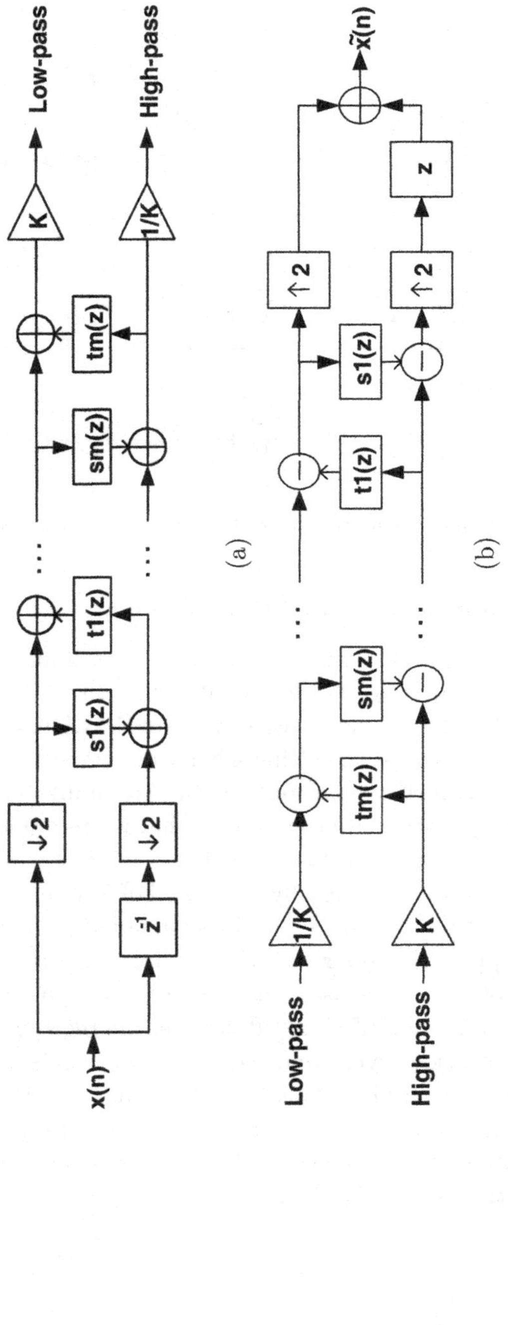

Fig. 3.3 Direct implementation of lifting scheme. (a) Analysis filter bank; (b) Synthesis filter bank.

sum of the timing delay in each computing unit without pipelining. This accumulative timing effect is because the multipliers, $s_{i,0}$ and $t_{i,0}$, are on the connection paths between computing units. Although pipelining can be used to reduce the critical path, the number of additional registers will increase more rapidly as the required critical path becomes shorter.

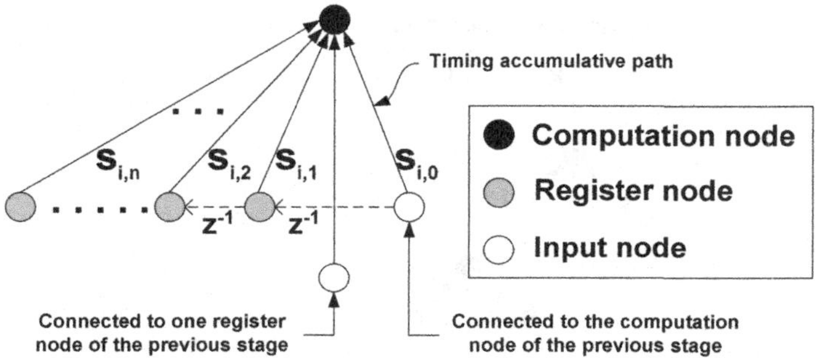

Fig. 3.4 Computing unit of upper triangular matrices.

In order to give a clearer explanation of this crisis, the popular JPEG 2000 lossy (9,7) filter is taken as an example without loss of generality. The (9,7) filter can be decomposed into four lifting stages as follows:

$$P(z) = \begin{bmatrix} 1 & a(1+z^{-1}) \\ 0 & 1 \end{bmatrix} \begin{bmatrix} 1 & 0 \\ b(1+z) & 1 \end{bmatrix} \begin{bmatrix} 1 & c(1+z^{-1}) \\ 0 & 1 \end{bmatrix} \begin{bmatrix} 1 & 0 \\ d(1+z) & 1 \end{bmatrix} \begin{bmatrix} K & 0 \\ 0 & 1/K \end{bmatrix} \tag{3.1}$$

where the coefficients are given as $a = -1.586134342$, $b = -0.052980118$, $c = 0.882911076$, $d = 0.443506852$, and $K = 1.149604398$. The corresponding signal flow graph can be derived as Fig. 3.5. To reduce the number of multipliers, each computing unit should be modified as Fig. 3.6. The normalization step K and $1/K$ can be implemented either independently or together with the quantization if data compression is performed. Thus, only the implementation issue of the lifting stages is discussed here. In comparison with the convolution-based architecture of the (9,7) filter that requires nine multipliers, 14 adders, and seven registers if adder tree and symmetric property are adopted, the lifting-based architecture needs only four multipliers, eight adders, and four registers (K and $1/K$ are not involved). Nonetheless, the critical path of the lifting-based architecture is $4T_m + 8T_a$, whereas the convolution-based one needs only $T_m + 4T_a$. Although pipelining the lifting-based architecture can improve the serious timing problem, this will raise the number of registers rapidly. For instance, the lifting-based architecture for the (9,7) filter can be pipelined into four stages to obtain a critical path $T_m + 2T_a$ with six additional registers, as shown in Fig. 3.7.

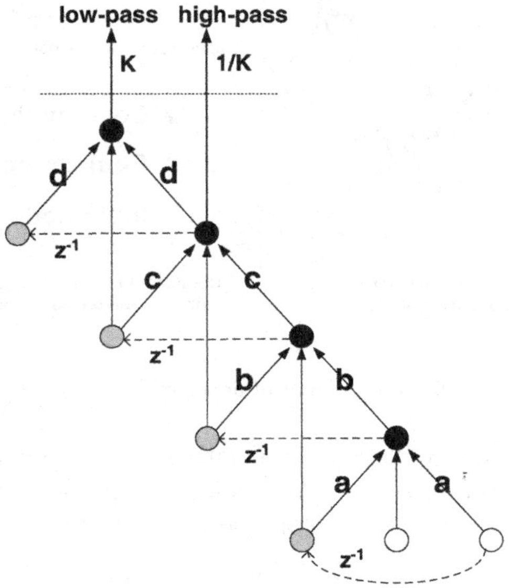

Fig. 3.5 Signal flow graph for lifting-based architecture of (9,7) filter.

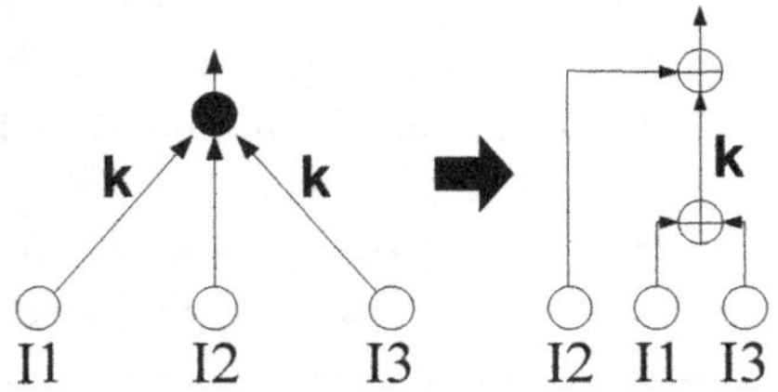

Fig. 3.6 Modified computing unit for Fig. 3.5.

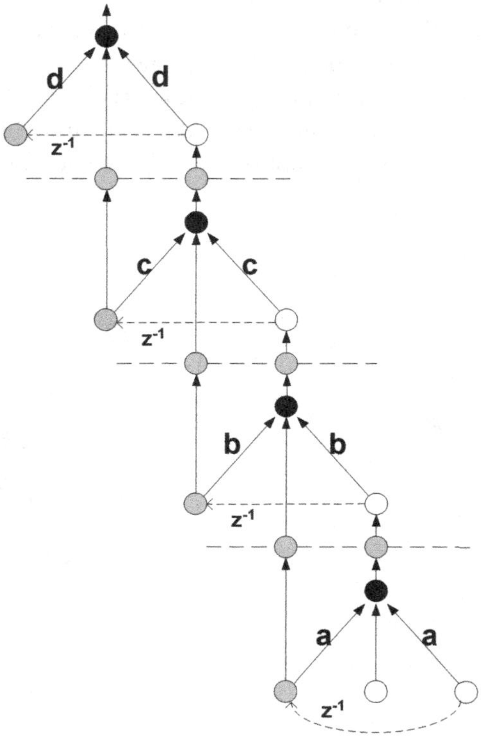

Fig. 3.7 Pipelining four stages for Fig. 3.5.

3.2.2 *Flipping structure*

Since the timing problem is due to the accumulation of timing delays from the input node to the computation node in each computing unit (Fig. 3.4), the flipping structure [49] is proposed to release the accumulation by eliminating the multipliers on the path from the input node to the computation node. This can be achieved by flipping each computing unit with the inverse of the multiplier coefficient. For example, two computing units are possibly connected as Fig. 3.8(a), in which $s(z)$ and $t(z)$ are assumed to be two taps for simplicity. This architecture can be flipped by the inverse coefficients of b and d as shown in Fig. 3.8(b). Flipping is to multiply the inverse coefficient for every edge on the feed-forward cutset which is through the selected multiplier. Then, every computation node can be split into two adders, of which one can process in parallel with other computing units, and the other one is on the accumulative path, as illustrated in Fig. 3.8(c). In addition, the multiplications on the same path can be merged together to reduce the number of multipliers. In this simple example, the critical path is reduced from $2T_m + 3T_a$ to $T_m + 3T_a$, and the reduction rate will increase as the number of serially connected computing units becomes larger.

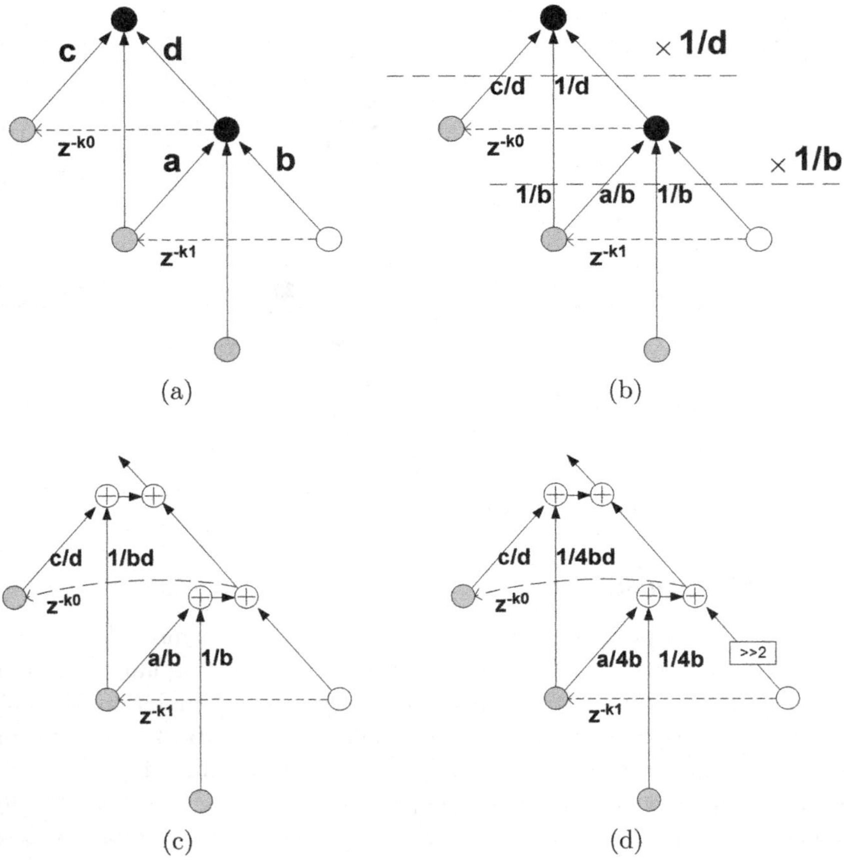

Fig. 3.8 Simple example of flipping structure for lifting-based DWT. (a) Two connected computing units; (b) Flipping computing units with b and d; (c) After splitting computation nodes and merging the multipliers; (d) Flipping with $4b$ and d.

If $s(z)$ and $t(z)$ are more than two taps, the selected flipping coefficients are still from the multipliers between the input and computation nodes. Moreover, the computation nodes can be split into two parts, one is the summation of the multiplication results from register nodes, and the other one is the adder on the accumulative path. The timing accumulation can be greatly reduced by flipping the original lifting-based architectures. Another advantage of flipping structure is that no additional multipliers will be required if the computing units are all flipped. Furthermore, the flipping coefficients should be put into the normalization step to assure that correct low-pass and high-pass coefficients will be obtained.

There are also many alternatives for flipping structures. How many computing units should be flipped is case-by-case and dependent on hardware constraints. This flipping method can also be applied for lifting-based IDWT because the basic computing unit is exactly the same as that of lifting-based DWT.

To compare the performance of these two kinds of lifting-based architectures, three design examples are given in the following, including the JPEG 2000 default DWT (9,7) filter, an integer (9,7) filter, and the (6,10) filter.

3.2.3 *Design example of JPEG 2000 default (9,7) filter*

Since the lifting structure of (9,7) filter is very regular and typical, it is useful to examine its conventional lifting-based architecture and the flipping structure. The lifting-based architecture, as shown in Fig. 3.5, needs only four multipliers, eight adders, and four registers with a critical path of $4T_m + 8T_a$. This critical path can be reduced to $T_m + 2T_a$ by cutting four pipelining stages with six additional registers, as shown in Fig. 3.7. Moreover, 32 registers can be used for fully pipelining such as to minimize the critical path to a multiplier delay.

An efficient flipping structure is designed for the (9,7) filter, as shown in Fig. 3.9, by flipping all computing units. The shifters are designed to make all multiplication coefficients smaller than one such that the outputs of multipliers will not overflow. The critical path of this flipping structure is only $T_m + 5T_a$ without any additional hardware cost over Fig. 3.5. In fact, this flipping structure can be represented by the equation below, with respect to Eq. (3.1) for the lifting-based architecture.

$$P(z) = \begin{bmatrix} \frac{1}{a} & 1+z^{-1} \\ 0 & \frac{1}{a} \end{bmatrix} \begin{bmatrix} \frac{1}{16b} & 0 \\ \frac{1+z}{16} & \frac{1}{16b} \end{bmatrix} \begin{bmatrix} \frac{1}{2c} & \frac{1+z^{-1}}{2} \\ 0 & \frac{1}{2c} \end{bmatrix} \begin{bmatrix} \frac{1}{2d} & 0 \\ \frac{1+z}{2} & \frac{1}{2d} \end{bmatrix} \begin{bmatrix} 64abcdK & 0 \\ 0 & \frac{64abcd}{K} \end{bmatrix} \tag{3.2}$$

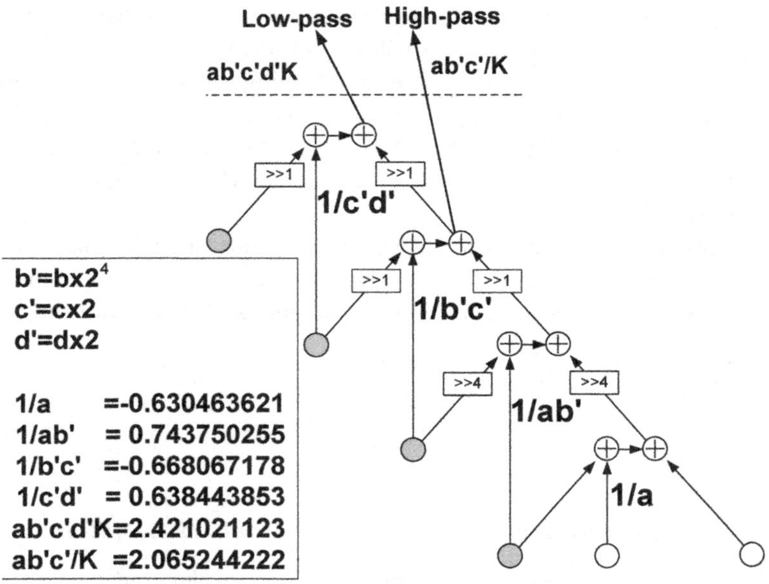

Fig. 3.9 Flipping structure for (9,7) filter.

Furthermore, if three pipelining stages are cut and some arithmetic operations are rearranged as Fig. 3.10(a), the critical path will be reduced to $T_m + T_a$ with three additional registers. The critical path can also be minimized to a multiplier delay by using five pipelining stages, as shown in Fig. 3.10(b), which needs only 11 registers.

To obtain more realistic results, the above-mentioned architectures, including conventional lifting-based architectures, flipping structures, and convolution-based architectures, are compared by use of 12-bit precision multiplier coefficients and 16-bit wordlength registers. The least significant four bits of the internal data are used to preserve the decimal precision.

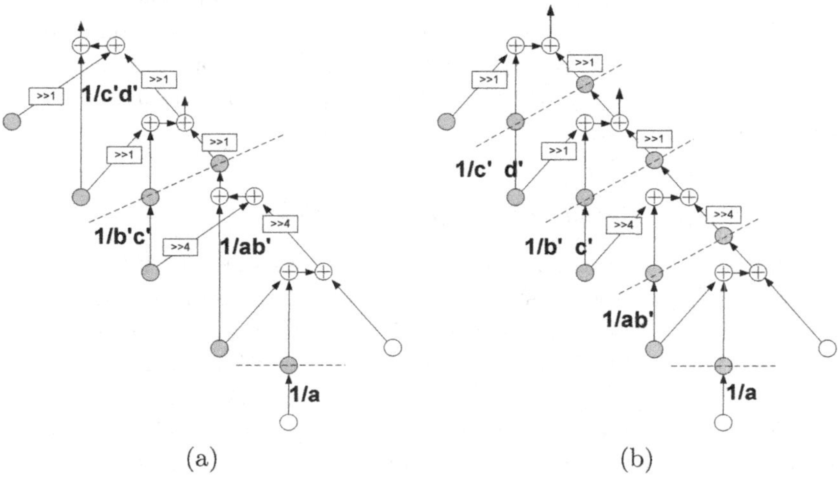

Fig. 3.10 Pipelining the flipping structure of (9,7) filter in Fig. 3.9. (a) Three pipelining stages; (b) Five pipelining stages.

The method of verification is to write Verilog HDL codes first and examine the simulation results. Then Synopsys Design Compiler is used to synthesize the circuits with standard cells from Avant! 0.35-μm cell library. For comparison, the timing constraints for circuit synthesis are set as tight as possible. As a result, the synthesis results for critical paths are very close to the expectation. The experimental results are summarized in Table 3.1, where the case of the pipelined convolution-based architecture is also included. The flipping structures outperform the conventional lifting-based and the convolution-based architectures in every aspect, such as timing, logic gate count, and the number of registers.

Furthermore, in order to examine the timing performance of flipping structures, flipping structures are synthesized under the timing constraints that are the limits of the lifting-based architectures with nearly the same registers. The comparison results are given in Table 3.2, which shows that flipping structures can achieve the timing limits of lifting-based architectures with only about one half of the hardware cost. In the case of no pipelining stages, the maximum of the critical path of the flipping structure, $30.5ns$, is much smaller than the minimum of the critical path of the conventional lifting-based architecture, $55ns$. The gate counts of flipping structures in Table 3.2 are much less than those in Table 3.1 because different adder architectures can be used under different timing constraints. For example, the simplest ripple-carry adders are used under the loose timing constraint in Table 3.2. On the contrary, carry-look-ahead adders are used to meet the tight timing constraint in Table 3.1, which require many more logic gates.

3.2.4 *Design example of integer (9,7) filter*

In addition to the advantages of implementation issues, the lifting scheme can also provide a well-constructed architecture to design wavelet-like filters. At the same time, both [50] and [51] propose a class of integer DWT filters based on the lifting scheme of the (9,7) filter. Moreover, the results of these two classes both can give an excellent integer DWT filter with lifting coefficients, $a = -3/2$, $b = -1/16$, $c = 4/5$, and $d = 15/32$. This integer wavelet filter can achieve nearly the same performance as the original (9,7) filter, but requires much less hardware cost [51]. The multiplication of a, b, and d can be implemented with a few shifters and two adders. However, c needs a floating-point operation. If 12-bit precision of c is considered, three adders and four shifters are sufficient for the implementation of the multiplier c as shown in Fig. 3.11. Therefore, if the conventional lifting-based architecture is used for this integer DWT filter, 13 adders and some shifters are required, and the critical path is $13T_a$.

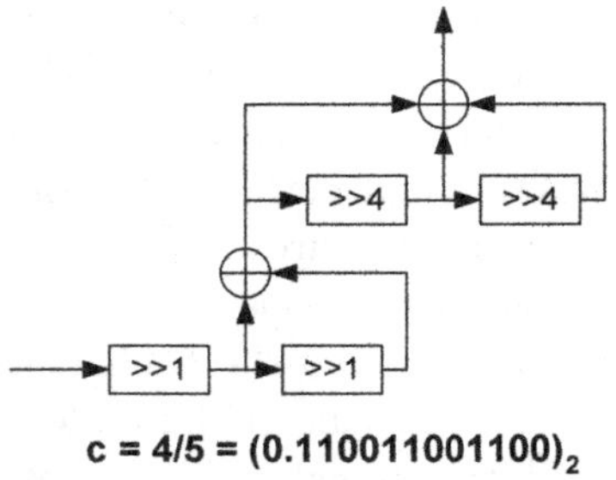

Fig. 3.11 12-bit precision multiplication of 4/5.

However, if the computing unit of c is flipped as Fig. 3.12, 13 adders are required for the hardware implementation with a critical path $7T_a$ after some modification of computation nodes. Furthermore, there is no floating-

Table 3.1 Comparison of hardware architectures for (9,7) filter. Synthesis results are derived by use of Avant! 0.35-μm cell library.

Architecture	Mul.	Add.	Critical Path	Reg.	Timing (ns)	Gate Count
Convolution + no pipeline	9	14	$T_m + 4T_a$	7	19	14.6K
Convolution + 3 stages	9	14	T_m	23	10	13.6K
Lifting + no pipeline	4	8	$4T_m + 8T_a$	4	55	12.4K
Lifting + 4 stages	4	8	$T_m + 2T_a$	10	16	12.9K
Lifting + fully pipeline	4	8	T_m	32	10	12.1K
Flipping + no pipeline	4	8	$T_m + 5T_a$	4	21	10.1K
Flipping + 3 stages	4	8	$T_m + T_a$	7	12	9.7K
Flipping + 5 stages	4	8	T_m	11	10	10.8K

Table 3.2 Comparison of conventional lifting-based architectures and flipping structures with similar registers for (9,7) filter. Synthesis results are derived by use of Avant! 0.35-μm cell library.

Architecture	Reg.	Timing (ns)	Gate Count
Lifting + no pipeline	4	55.0	12.4K
Flipping + no pipeline	4	30.5	6.6K
Lifting + 4 stages	10	16.0	12.9K
Flipping + 5 stages	11	13.9	7.0K

point operation in Fig. 3.12 such that the precision of internal data can also be reduced. This design example shows that flipping structures can be used not only to reduce the critical path but also to provide other efficient design techniques for lifting-based architectures.

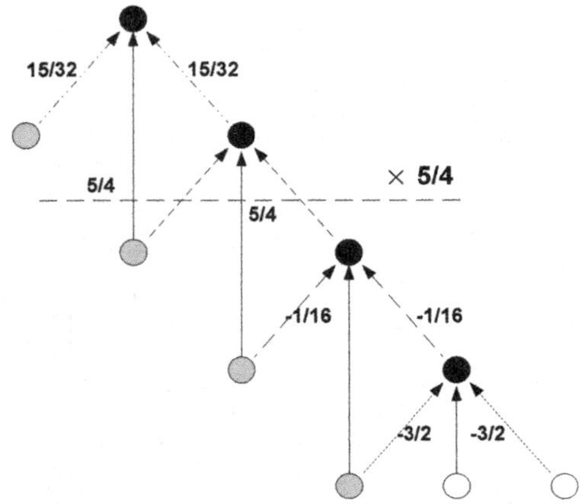

Fig. 3.12 Flipping structure of integer (9,7) filter.

3.2.5 *Design example of linear (6,10) filter*

Besides the above odd symmetric wavelet filters, the even linear (6,10) filter [48] is explored in the following. The polyphase matrix of the (6,10) filter can be decomposed as follows:

$$\begin{bmatrix} G_e(z) & H_e(z) \\ G_o(z) & H_o(z) \end{bmatrix} = \begin{bmatrix} 1 & a \\ 0 & 1 \end{bmatrix} \begin{bmatrix} 1 & 0 \\ b + cz^{-1} & 1 \end{bmatrix} \begin{bmatrix} 1 & e + dz \\ 0 & 1 \end{bmatrix} \begin{bmatrix} 1 & 0 \\ -f + gz^{-1} + fz^{-2} & 1 \end{bmatrix} \begin{bmatrix} K_2 & 0 \\ 0 & K_1 \end{bmatrix} \tag{3.3}$$

where the coefficients are given as $a = -0.369536$, $b = -0.42780$, $c = -0.119532$, $d = -0.090075$, $e = 0.872739$, $g = -0.572909$, $f = 0.224338$, $K_1 = 0.874919$, and $K_2 = 1.142963$ [48]. Thus, the lifting-based architecture can be shown as Fig. 3.13(a) where seven multipliers, eight adders, and five registers are required if K_1 and K_2 are excluded. However, the convolution-based architecture requires eight multipliers, 14 adders, and eight registers if the symmetric and anti-symmetric properties are adopted. The hardware saving ratio of multipliers between lifting-based and convolution-based architectures is not as high as the case of (9,7) filter. Moreover, the lifting-based architecture would require more multipliers than the convolution-based one if K_1 and K_2 are considered. The main advantage of lifting scheme is the number of adders and registers in this case.

The timing accumulation of Fig. 3.13(a) results in a long critical path, $4T_m + 5T_a$. By pipelining through the dot lines in Fig. 3.13(a), the critical path can be reduced to $T_m + 2T_a$ with four additional registers. Furthermore, the critical path can be minimized to T_m by fully pipelining with 22 additional registers. On the other hand, the critical path of the convolution-based architecture is only $T_m + 4T_a$ and can be reduced to T_m with three pipelining stages by use of 16 additional registers.

The flipping structure can reduce the critical path of Fig. 3.13(a) to $T_m + 5T_a$ as shown in Fig. 3.13(b), in which all lifting stages are flipped. The critical path of Fig. 3.13(b) can be further reduced to $T_m + 2T_a$ by pipelining through the dot lines. The minimum critical path T_m can be achieved with 10 pipelining registers.

The above architectures are all synthesized in the same way of Section 3.2.3 with 16-bit wordlength for internal data and 12-bit precision for multiplier coefficients. Table 3.3 gives the experimental results and shows that the flipping structures have better performance than the lifting-based and convolution-based ones in all aspects.

3.3 B-Spline-Based Architectures

The third kind of DWT implementation is based on the intrinsic B-spline factorization property [52, 53]. In the following, the generic architectures will be introduced first. Then the implementation methods of B-spline part will be discussed. Design examples of (9,7) filter, (6,10) filter, and (10,18) filter, will be presented for implementation details.

3.3.1 *B-spline factorized architectures for DWT and IDWT*

From B-spline factorization Eq. (2.70), a different DWT architecture can be constructed. For 100% hardware utilization, the polyphase decomposition is adopted first. After the Type-I or Type-II polyphase decomposition, the general B-spline factorized architecture can be expressed as Fig. 3.14, where

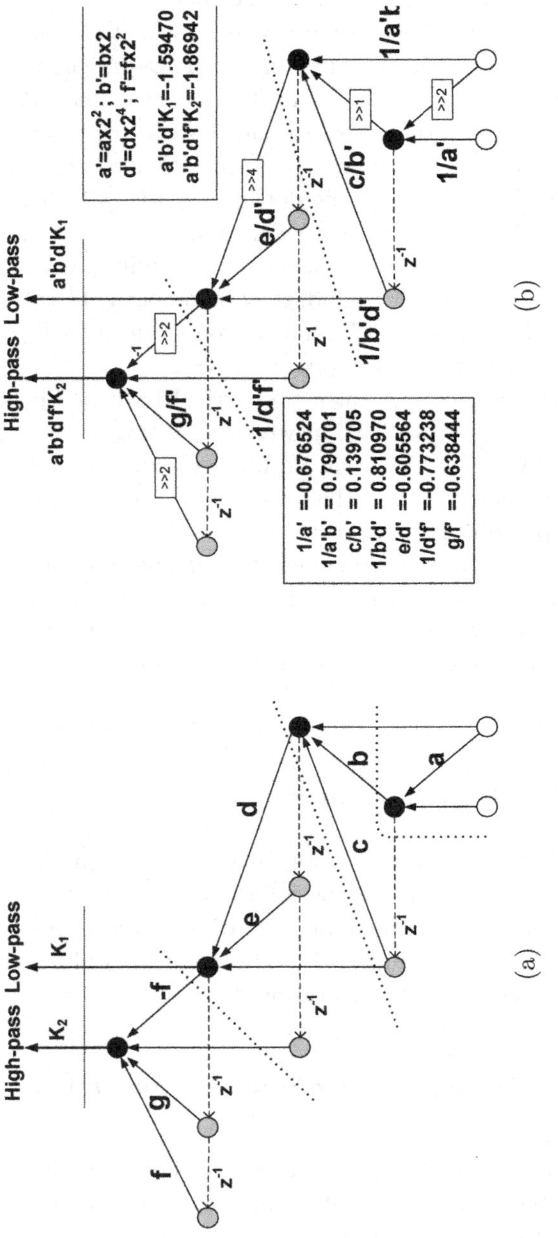

Fig. 3.13 Lifting-based architecture for the (6,10) filter. (a) Conventional lifting; (b) Flipping structure.

Table 3.3 Comparison of hardware architectures for (6,10) filter. Synthesis results are derived by use of Avant! 0.35-μm cell library.

Architecture	Mul.	Add.	Critical Path	Reg.	Timing (ns)	Gate Count
Convolution + no pipeline	8	14	$T_m + 4T_a$	8	20.5	15.2K
Convolution + 3 stages	8	14	T_m	24	9.6	15.4K
Lifting + no pipeline	7	8	$4T_m + 5T_a$	5	42.0	13.6K
Lifting + 4 stages	7	8	$T_m + 2T_a$	11	14.8	13.7K
Lifting + fully pipeline	7	8	T_m	27	9.0	14.5K
Flipping + no pipeline	7	8	$T_m + 5T_a$	5	22.8	13.3K
Flipping + 3 stages	7	8	$T_m + 2T_a$	9	14.3	13.0K
Flipping + 5 stages	7	8	T_m	11	9.8	11.1K

the distributed part, $Q(z)$ and $R(z)$, are polyphase decomposed first, and the left is the B-spline part. The distributed part is the only part that has multipliers, and the four filters ($Q_e(z)$, $Q_o(z)$, $R_e(z)$, and $R_o(z)$) can be implemented by serial or parallel filters. The normalization part, h_0 and g_0, can be implemented independently from the other two parts.

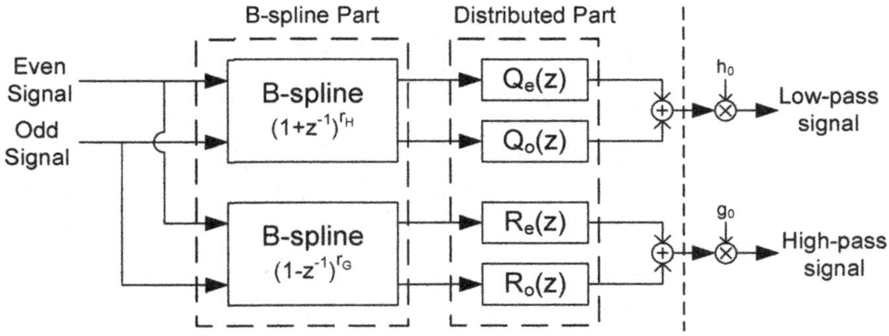

Fig. 3.14 B-spline factorized architecture for DWT.

Using Eq. (2.35) and Eq. (2.70), the B-spline factorization for IDWT can be derived similarly as follows:

$$\widetilde{H}(z) = (1+z^{-1})^{\gamma_{\widetilde{H}}} \cdot \widetilde{Q}(z)$$
$$\widetilde{G}(z) = (1-z^{-1})^{\gamma_{\widetilde{G}}} \cdot \widetilde{R}(z). \tag{3.4}$$

Then substituting this equation into Fig. 2.11(b), the general architecture can be derived by use of polyphase decomposition as shown in Fig. 3.15.

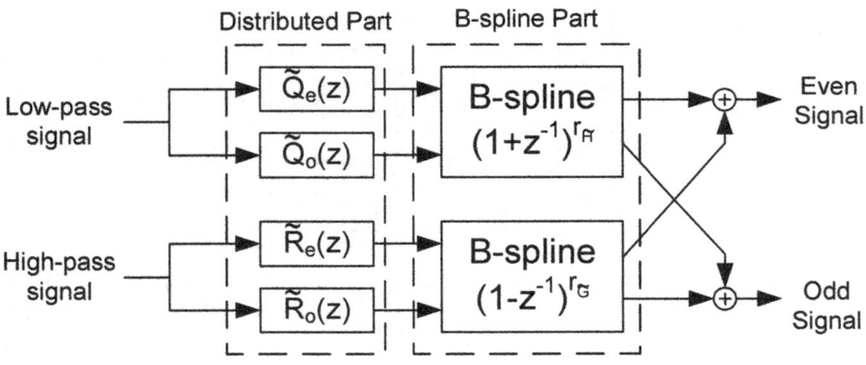

Fig. 3.15 B-spline factorized architecture for IDWT.

Similar to the B-spline-based DWT architectures, the IDWT architecture in Fig. 3.15 comprises of the distributed part and the B-spline part. The normalization part is not extracted because usually no other operations need to be performed before IDWT. The four filters of the distributed part ($\widetilde{Q}_e(z)$, $\widetilde{Q}_o(z)$, $\widetilde{R}_e(z)$, and $\widetilde{R}_o(z)$) can be implemented by use of many DSP VLSI techniques, such as serial filter, parallel filter, pipelining, and retiming. In the following, two implementation methods for the B-spline part will be introduced.

3.3.2 *Implementation methods of B-spline part*

3.3.2.1 *Direct implementation of B-spline part*

The direct implementation of the B-spline part is a straightforward one. The concept is to implement $(1 + z^{-1})$ and $(1 - z^{-1})$ first, and then the B-spline part can be constructed by serially connecting $(1+z^{-1})$ and $(1-z^{-1})$. But two-input-two-output structures of $(1 + z^{-1})$ and $(1 - z^{-1})$ cannot be derived from polyphase decomposition. Instead, they can be implemented by considering the physical connection of signals as shown in Fig. 3.16, where we assume the Type-I decomposition is used so the even signals are prior to odd signals. Thus, the direct implementation requires $2\gamma_H + 2\gamma_G$ (or $2\gamma_{\widetilde{H}} + 2\gamma_{\widetilde{G}}$) adders for a pair of low-pass and high-pass outputs. When connecting the B-spline part to the distributed part, the priority of signals need to be handled carefully.

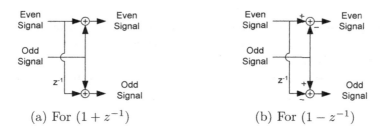

(a) For $(1 + z^{-1})$ (b) For $(1 - z^{-1})$

Fig. 3.16 Direct implementation for the B-spline part (Type-I decomposition). (a) For $(1 + z^{-1})$. (b) For $(1 - z^{-1})$.

Another problem that should be solved is the internal signal wordlength. Since the DC gain of $(1 + z^{-1})$ is 2, the signal magnitude is possible to be double after every $(1 + z^{-1})$ stage, and so is every $(1 - z^{-1})$ stage. However, implementing $(1 \pm z^{-1})/2$ instead will lose too much precision.

The precision and wordlength issues should be handled carefully when the precision criteria is given.

3.3.2.2 *Pascal implementation of B-spline part*

Instead of the direct implementation, the B-spline part can also be constructed by Pascal implementation that can exploit the similarity of the B-spline part to reduce adders. The Pascal implementation expresses the B-spline part ($(1+z^{-1})^{\gamma_H}$ and $(1-z^{-1})^{\gamma_G}$, or $(1+z^{-1})^{\gamma_{\tilde{H}}}$ and $(1-z^{-1})^{\gamma_{\tilde{G}}}$) as the Pascal expansion and saves the repeated computation. For example, $1+6z^{-2}+z^{-4}$ and $4z^{-1}+4z^{-3}$ can be computed first for the implementation of $(1+z^{-1})^4 = 1+4z^{-1}+6z^{-2}+4z^{-3}+z^{-4}$ and $(1-z^{-1})^4 = 1-4z^{-1}+6z^{-2}-4z^{-3}+z^{-4}$. Then the sum of them is $(1+z^{-1})^4$, and the difference is $(1-z^{-1})^4$. Furthermore, the integer multiplications of the B-spline part can be implemented with shifters and adders, instead of multipliers. In this example, the Pascal implementation only requires 12 adders, but the direct implementation will need 16 adders. However, the Pascal implementation of long-tap filters will be too complex to be derived, and the complexity reduction is not guaranteed. The precision and wordlength issues are also more complex than those of the direct implementation.

In the following, three Daubechies biorthogonal filters are studied and implemented by use of B-spline factorized architectures, including the JPEG 2000 default (9,7) filter, the (6,10) filter [48], and the (10,18) filter [54].

The precision and wordlength issues are handled with a simple method for discussion. The signals are scaled down by two after every two $(1 \pm z^{-1})$ stages for precision preservation and preventing from signal overflow. The precision is preserved as more as possible when the internal wordlength is decided.

3.3.3 *Design example of JPEG 2000 default (9,7) DWT filter*

The B-spline factorization of the (9,7) filter can be expressed as:

$$
\begin{aligned}
H(z) &= (1+z^{-1})^4(1+t_1z^{-1}+t_2z^{-2}+t_1z^{-3}+z^{-4})h_0 \\
G(z) &= (1-z^{-1})^4(1+t_3z^{-1}+z^{-2})g_0
\end{aligned}
\tag{3.5}
$$

where $t_1 = -4.630464$, $t_2 = 9.597484$, and $t_3 = 3.369536$. Thus the B-spline factorized architecture of the (9,7) filter will only need three multipliers, excluding the normalization part h_0 and g_0. Here, we use the Pascal implementation for the B-spline part, and the Pascal expression of the (9,7) filter is shown in Fig. 3.17. The B-spline factorized architecture requires 18 adders, of which 12 adders for the B-spline part and six adders for the distributed part, as shown in Fig. 3.18, where Fig. 3.18(a) and (b) represent Type-I and Type-II polyphase decompositions, respectively. The notation for FIR filters is described in Fig. 3.19.

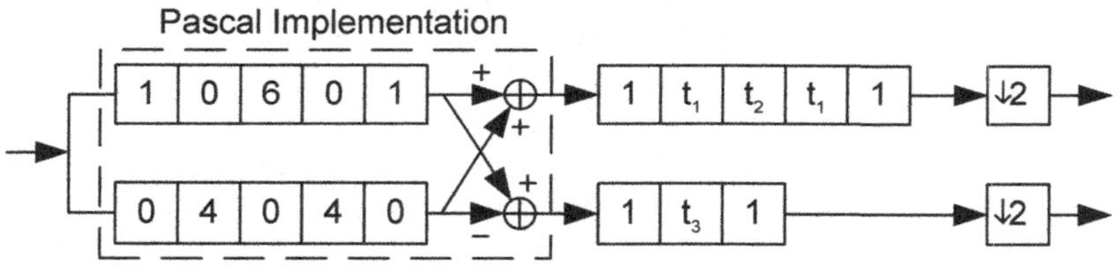

Fig. 3.17 Pascal expression of the B-spline part for (9,7) filter.

The original Type-I architecture requires eight registers, and the critical path is $T_m + 5T_a$. On the other hand, if pipelining is performed through the upside dot line, the critical path can be shortened to $T_m + 2T_a$ with totally 10 registers. However, the critical path of the Type-II architecture is originally $T_m + 2T_a$ with 10 registers.

By extracting the normalization part h_0 and g_0 and utilizing the symmetric property, the convolution-based architecture of the (9,7) filter can be implemented by use of seven multipliers, 14 adders, and seven registers. The critical path is $T_m + 3T_a$ if adder tree is used to connect adders.

The B-spline factorized architectures as well as the convolution-based and lifting-based ones are synthesized into gate-level netlists by Synopsys Design Compiler with standard cells from Artisan 0.25-μm cell library. The comparison and synthesis results are shown in Table 3.4, where the internal bit-widths are all 16-bit, the multipliers are all 16-by-16 multiplications, and the adders are also 16-bit for comparison. The gate counts are given with combinational and non-combinational gate counts separately. The former contributes to the multipliers and adders while the latter is responsible to the registers. For circuit synthesis, the timing constraints are set as tight as possible.

According to Table 3.4, the B-spline-based architectures could require

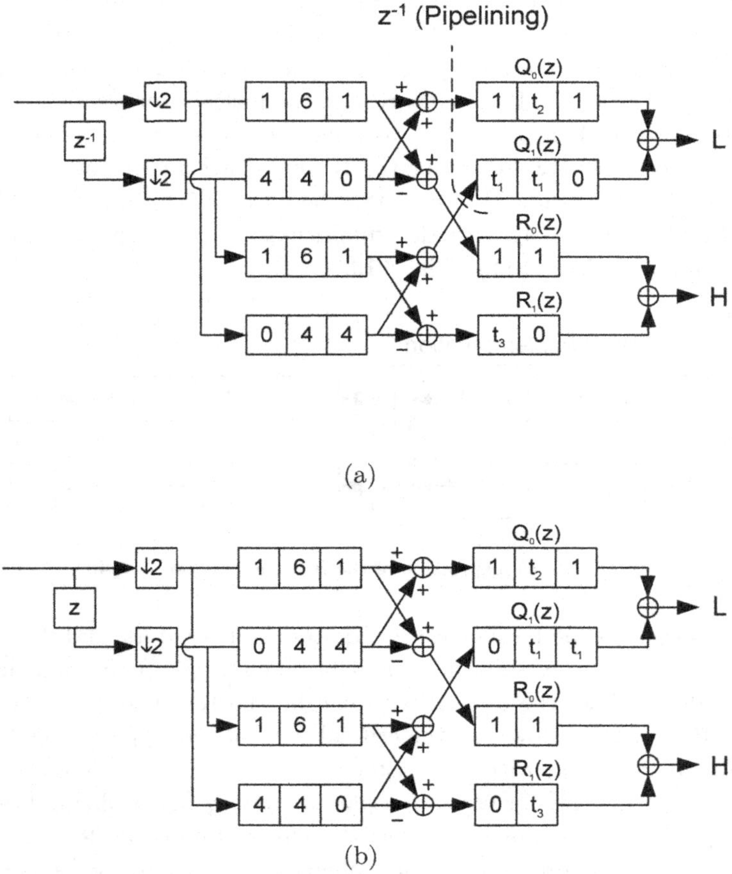

Fig. 3.18 B-spline factorized architectures for (9,7) filter. (a) Type-I polyphase decomposition; (b) Type-II polyphase decomposition.

fewer gate counts under the same timing constraints. Furthermore, the saving of gate counts will be more significant if the multipliers are required to have higher precision.

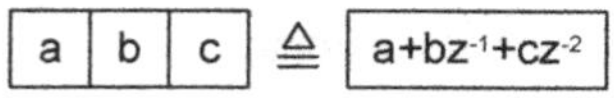

Fig. 3.19 Notation for FIR filters.

3.3.4 *DWT with linear (6,10) filter*

The B-spline factorization of the (6,10) filter can be expressed as:

$$\begin{aligned}H(z) &=(1+z^{-1})^3(1+s_3z^{-1}+z^{-2})h_0 \\ G(z) &=(1-z^{-1})^3(1-z^{-1})^2(1+s_1z^{-1}+s_2z^{-2}+s_1z^{-3}+z^{-4})g_0 \quad (3.6) \\ &=(1-z^{-1})^3(1+r_1z^{-1}+r_2z^{-2}+r_3z^{-3}+r_2z^{-4}+r_1z^{-5}+z^{-6})g_0 \quad (3.7)\end{aligned}$$

where $s_1 = -t_1$, $s_2 = t_2$, $s_3 = -t_3$, $r_1 = 2.630464$, $r_2 = 1.336557$, and $r_3 = -9.934042$. However, the Pascal implementation can only cover $(1 \pm z^{-1})^3$, and there are two solutions for the left part $(1 - z^{-1})^2$ of $G(z)$, Solution-1 and Solution-2, which are corresponding to Eqs. (3.6) and (3.7), respectively. The B-spline-based architectures are shown in Fig. 3.20, where the parts marked with "*"and "##"can be shared. Thus, the Solution-1 of the B-spline factorized architecture requires three multipliers and 20 adders while the Solution-2 needs four multipliers and 18 adders.

The critical path of the Solution-1 architecture could be $T_m + 6T_a$, $T_m + 4T_a$, or $T_m + 2T_a$ by retiming, pipelining, or retiming and pipelining together, respectively. The corresponding numbers of registers are nine, 11, and 13. On the other hand, the Solution-2 architecture can be retimed to obtain a critical path of $T_m + 5T_a$ with totally nine registers.

3.3.4.1 *Comparison*

By extracting the normalization part h_0 and g_0 and utilizing both symmetric and anti-symmetric properties, the convolution-based architecture of the (6,10) filter can be implemented by use of 6 multipliers, 14 adders, and 8 registers. And the critical path is $T_m + 4T_a$ if the adder tree is used.

Similarly, the B-spline-based, convolution-based, and lifting-based architectures have been verified and synthesized. The bit-width is the same as the case of (9,7) filter. The results are listed in Table 3.5. In this case, the lifting-based architecture requires even more multipliers than the convolution-based one because the lifting scheme of even-tap linear DWT filters is not as efficient as that of odd symmetric filters. However, the B-spline-based architecture can still reduce the number of multipliers to

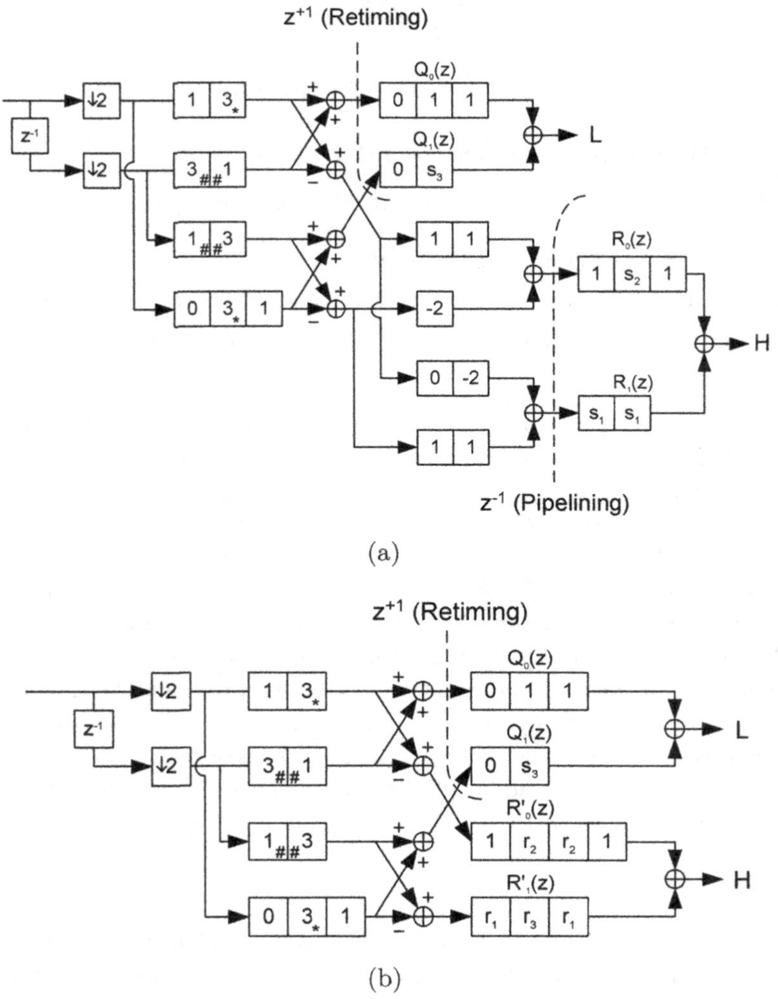

Fig. 3.20 B-spline factorized architectures for the (6,10) filter. (a) Solution-1 with Type-I polyphase decomposition [Eq. (3.6)]; (b) Solution-2 with Type-I polyphase decomposition [Eq. (3.7)].

three. Table 3.5 shows that the B-spline-based architectures can achieve the same timing constraints with fewer gate counts than the other three architectures.

Table 3.4 Comparisons for DWT architectures of the (9,7) filter. Synthesis results are derived by use of Artisan 0.25-μm cell library. (Normalization parts are excluded.)

Architecture	Mul.	Add.	Critical Path	Reg.	Timing (ns)	Combinational Gate Count	Non-combinational Gate Count
Convolution + no pipeline	7	14	$T_m + 3T_a$	7	10.8	17.8K	1.3K
Lifting + no pipeline	4	8	$4T_m + 8T_a$	4	34.0	15.4K	0.8K
Lifting + 4 stages	4	8	$T_m + 2T_a$	10	9.8	15.2K	1.5K
Flipping + no pipeline	4	8	$T_m + 5T_a$	4	14.1	13.3K	0.8K
Flipping + 3 stages	4	8	$T_m + T_a$	7	7.7	12.1K	1.2K
B-spline Type-I	3	18	$T_m + 5T_a$	8	13.6	9.7K	1.3K
B-spline Type-II	3	18	$T_m + 2T_a$	10	10.3	9.4K	1.5K

Table 3.5 Comparisons for DWT architectures of the (6,10) filter. Synthesis results are derived by use of Artisan 0.25-μm cell library. (Normalization parts are excluded.)

Architecture	Mul.	Add.	Critical Path	Reg.	Timing (ns)	Combinational Gate Count	Non-combinational Gate Count
Convolution + no pipeline	6	14	$T_m + 4T_a$	8	12.0	13.7K	1.3K
Lifting + no pipeline	7	8	$4T_m + 5T_a$	5	26.6	12.7K	0.9K
Lifting + 4 stages	7	8	$T_m + 2T_a$	11	9.2	14.2K	1.7K
Flipping + no pipeline	7	8	$T_m + 5T_a$	5	13.6	12.5K	1.0K
Flipping + 3 stages	7	8	$T_m + 2T_a$	9	8.7	12.3K	1.4K
B-spline-1 + retiming	3	20	$T_m + 6T_a$	9	14.1	9.6K	1.3K
B-spline-1 + retiming + pipeline	3	20	$T_m + 4T_a$	11	11.5	8.8K	1.6K
B-spline-1 + pipeline	3	20	$T_m + 2T_a$	13	9.5	8.6K	1.8K
B-spline-2 + retiming	4	18	$T_m + 5T_a$	9	13.1	11.6K	1.4K

Table 3.6 Detailed gate count comparison for the (6,10) filter. Synthesis results are derived by use of Artisan 0.25-μm cell library.

Architecture	Cell Name	Cell Number	Average Gate Count	Total Gate Count
	nbw	7	1477	10339
Lifting + 4 stages	cla	5	483	2415
	bk	3	399	1197
	nbw	3	1071	3213
	cla	1	488	488
B-spline-1 + pipeline	bk	9	291	2619
	rpl	9	208	1872
	rpcs	1	284	284

nbw: non-booth-recorded wallace tree multiplier; **cla**: carry-lookahead adder; **bk**: brent-kung adder; **rpl**: ripple carry adder; **rpcs**: ripple carry select adder.

3.3.4.2 *Detailed gate count comparison*

The B-spline factorized architecture can provide fewer multipliers but introduce more adders. The gate counts of multipliers and adders are compared in more detail to examine the resulting hardware resource reduction. The lifting-based architecture with four pipelining stages and the B-spline Solution-1 architecture with pipelining are chosen, which both have critical path $T_m + 2T_a$.

The detailed comparison of the gate counts is listed in Table 3.6, where the gate counts of different kinds of multipliers and adders are separate. The Synopsys Design Compiler synthesizes all multipliers to non-booth-recorded wallace tree multipliers, which can have trade-offs between the processing speed and the area size. Many kinds of adders are used for circuits synthesis, and the carry-lookahead adders are the fastest but the largest ones.

All multipliers of the lifting-based architecture are on the critical path, so the gate counts of them are quite large and about 1500 gates in average. However, the multipliers of the B-spline factorized architecture are not all on the critical path, so the average gate count is only about 1000 gates. Furthermore, the lifting-based architecture requires four more multipliers than the B-spline factorized one. In the result, the total gate counts of multipliers are about 10000 and 3000 gates, respectively.

On the other hand, only one carry-lookahead adder is used in the B-spline-based architecture while five are used in the lifting-based one. Although more adders are required, most of them are synthesized to the smaller adders in the B-spline-based architecture. The overhead gate count of adders for the B-spline-based architecture is about 1600 gates. By combining the result of multipliers, the net reduction of gate count is about $7000 - 1600 = 5400$. This detailed comparison shows the efficiency of the B-spline-based architecture for reducing gate count.

3.3.5 *Design example of linear (10,18) DWT filter*

The coefficients of the (10,18) analysis filter bank are given in [54]. The analysis low-pass filter is a symmetric 10-tap filter, and the high-pass filter is an anti-symmetric 18-tap filter. The coding efficiency can be better than the well-known (9,7) filter [54, 55]. The B-spline factorization of the analysis filter bank is as follows:

$$\begin{aligned} H(z) =& (1+z^{-1})^5(u_1 z^{-8} + u_2 z^{-7} + z^{-6} + u_2 z^{-5} + u_1 z^{-4}) \cdot h_0 \\ G(z) =& (1-z^{-1})^9(u_3 z^{-8} + u_4 z^{-7} + u_5 z^{-6} + u_6 z^{-5} \\ & + z^{-4} + u_6 z^{-3} + u_5 z^{-2} + u_4 z^{-1} + u_3) \cdot g_0 \end{aligned} \tag{3.8}$$

where $u_1 = 0.1049758$, $u_2 = -0.524577$, $u_3 = 0.0094393$, $u_4 = 0.08498056$, $u_5 = 0.33152476$, $u_6 = 0.74232477$, $h_0 = 0.27485$, and $g_0 = 0.101111$.

For the (10,18) filter bank, the Pascal implementation will be too complex to derive because the degrees of the B-spline parts are five and nine. Thus, we use the direct implementation for the B-spline part. The B-spline-based architecture for the (10,18) filter is as shown in Fig. 3.21, where six multipliers and 40 adders are used if the normalization part is excluded. If retiming z^{+2} is performed, the critical path will become $T_m + 11T_a$ with totally 23 registers. In concept, the critical path can be reduced to $\frac{T_m+11T_a}{2}$ by pipelining with four additional registers.

The following considers the convolution-based architecture of the (10,18) filter is implemented by the parallel filters. If the linear property and the adder tree are adopted, 12 multipliers, 26 adders, and 16 registers are required while the critical path is $T_m + 5T_a$. As the case of (6,10) filter, the lifting scheme of the (10,18) cannot be linear and cannot reduce the hardware complexity. Thus, the lifting scheme is excluded from the comparison.

The B-spline-based and convolution-based architectures are synthesized for comparison. The internal bit-width and multiplier precision are the

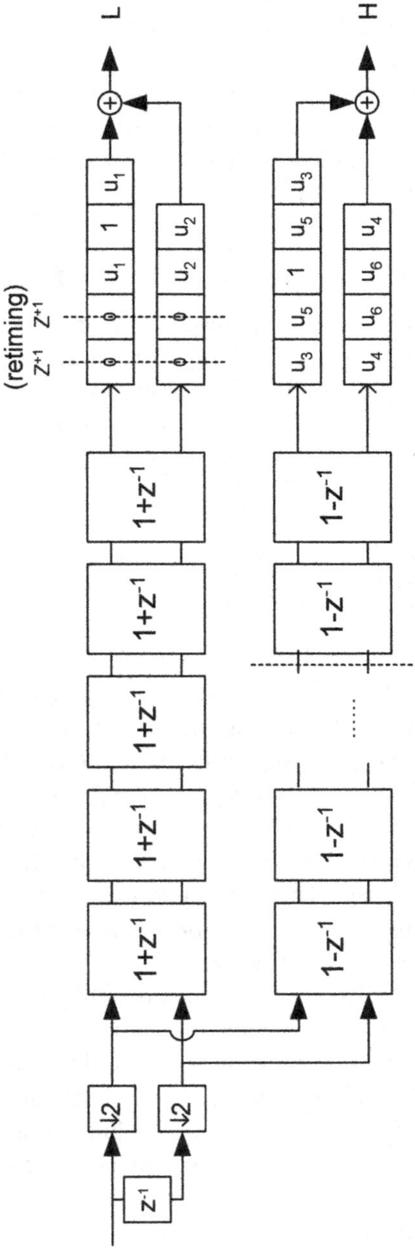

Fig. 3.21 B-spline factorized architecture for the (10,18) filter.

same as the case of (9,7) filter. The results are listed in Table 3.7. The pipelining of the B-spline-based architecture is cut before the last two $1 + z^{-1}$ stages as shown in Fig. 3.21 for Artisan 0.25-μm cell library. The B-spline-based architectures require only about two-thirds of the gate count of the convolution-based one.

3.3.6 *Design example of linear (10,18) IDWT filter*

By use of polyphase decomposition, the convolution-based architecture of the synthesis (10,18) filter can be constructed as Fig. 3.22, where h_i's and g_i's are the coefficients of $H(z)$ and $G(z)$, respectively. $\widetilde{H}_e(z)$ and $\widetilde{H}_o(z)$ are mirror-images of each other, and so are $\widetilde{G}_e(z)$ and $\widetilde{G}_o(z)$. Thus, the number of multipliers can be reduced by using mirror-images, but it would require more registers. Two possible architectures are discussed in the following. The architecture I is to implement the four filters as parallel filters directly such as to minimize the number of registers. The required numbers of multipliers, adders, and registers are 26, 26, and 14, respectively. (h_0 and g_0 can be shared because they are parallel filters.) The architecture II is to minimize the number of multipliers by use of mirror-images. The required numbers of multipliers, adders, and registers are 14, 26, and 24, respectively. The critical path of these two architectures are both $T_m + 4T_a$.

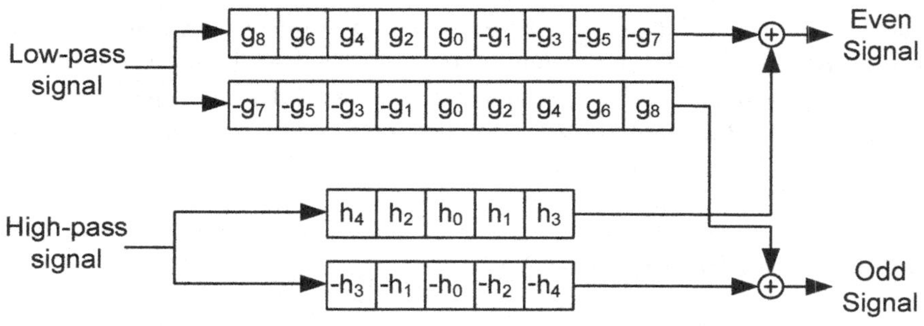

Fig. 3.22 Convolution-based architecture for IDWT with the (10,18) filter.

The B-spline factorization of the synthesis filter bank is as follows:

$$\widetilde{H}(z) = \frac{(1+z^{-1})^9}{8}(v_1 z^{-8} + v_2 z^{-7} + v_3 z^{-6} + v_4 z^{-5} + v_5 z^{-4} + v_4 z^{-3} + v_3 z^{-2} + v_2 z^{-1} + v_1)$$

$$\widetilde{G}(z) = \frac{(1-z^{-1})^5}{4}(v_6 z^{-8} + v_7 z^{-7} + v_8 z^{-6} + v_7 z^{-5} + v_6 z^{-4}) \tag{3.9}$$

where $v_1 = 0.0076535$, $v_2 = -0.0687398$, $v_3 = 0.2681664$, $v_4 = -0.6004576$, $v_5 = 0.808888$, $v_6 = -0.1154104$, $v_7 = -0.57672$, and $v_8 = -1.0994$.
The B-spline-based architecture of the synthesis (10,18) filter bank is shown in Fig. 3.23. The four filters of the distributed part are all symmetric such that the number of multipliers can be reduced into a half. The denominators (eight and four) of the Eq. (3.9) are introduced only for the precision issues. These two denominators are implemented by shifting right the signals between the $(1 + z^{-1})$ and $(1 - z^{-1})$ stages, which are not shown in Fig. 3.23 for simplicity.

There are two possible implementations for these filters: serial or parallel filters. If the four filters are implemented as serial filters, the critical path will be $T_m + 11T_a$. Because the registers cannot be shared among these filters, the required number of registers is 24. On the other hand, the critical path will be $T_m + 13T_a$, and the registers can be shared and the number is reduced to 20 if parallel filters are adopted. In Fig. 3.23, retiming can be performed to $\widetilde{R}_e(z)$ and $\widetilde{R}_o(z)$ to decrease the number of registers. Pipelining can also be used to shorten the critical path. In concept, the pipeline can be cut at the half of the critical path with four additional pipelining registers.

The comparison and synthesis results are shown in Table 3.8, where the internal wordlengths are all 16-bit, the multipliers are all 16-by-16 multiplications, and the adders are also 16-bit for comparison. For Artisan 0.25-μm cell library, we choose the pipelining points for the B-spline-based architectures as shown in Fig. 3.23 to minimize the critical path. According to Table 3.8, the B-spline-based architectures could require fewer gate counts under the same timing constraints.

3.4 General Performance Analysis

In the following, the performance of the three categories of DWT architectures is analyzed, including convolution-, lifting-, and B-spline-based. The

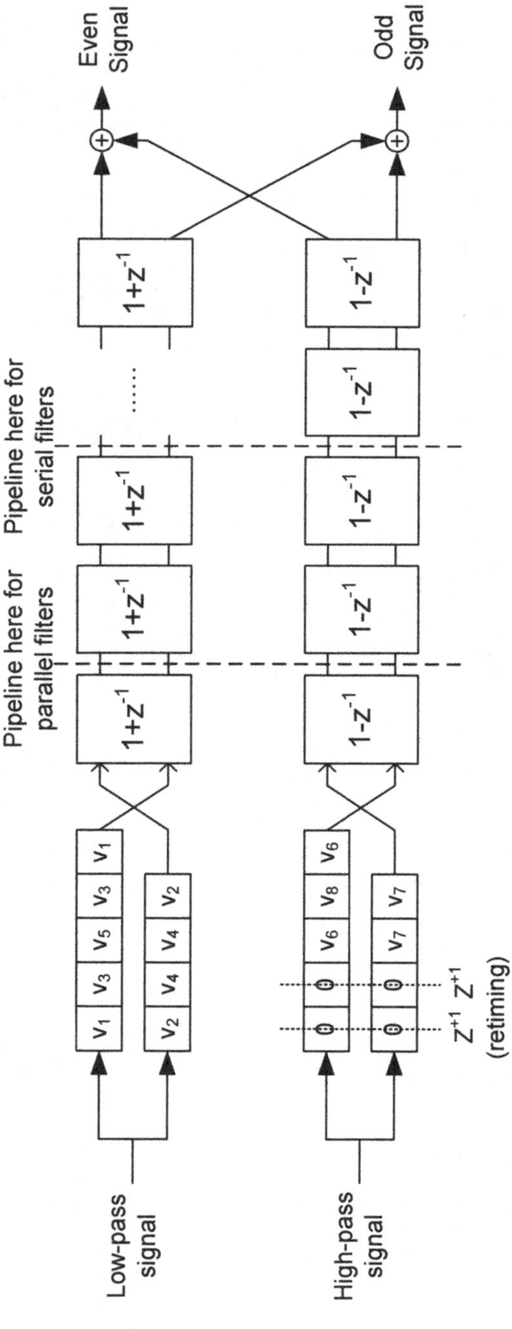

Fig. 3.23 B-spline-based architecture for IDWT with the (10,18) filter.

Table 3.7 Comparisons for DWT architectures of the (10,18) filter. Synthesis results are derived by use of Artisan 0.25-μm cell library. (Normalization parts are excluded.)

Architecture	Mul.	Add.	Critical Path	Reg.	Timing (ns)	Combinational Gate Count	Non-combinational Gate Count
Convolution	12	26	$T_m + 5T_a$	16	13.5	27.2K	2.4K
B-spline + retiming (z^{+2})	6	40	$T_m + 11T_a$	23	21.8	19.2K	2.6K
B-spline + retiming (z^{+1}) + pipeline	6	40	$(T_m + 2T_a)/2$	27	12.7	20.1K	3.1K

Table 3.8 Comparisons for IDWT architectures of the (10,18) filter. Synthesis results are derived by use of Artisan 0.25-μm cell library.

Architecture	Mul.	Add.	Critical Path	Reg.	Timing (ns)	Combinational Gate Count	Non-combinational Gate Count
Convolution Arc. I	26	26	$T_m + 4T_a$	14	12.5	51.0K	2.2K
Convolution Arc. II	14	26	$T_m + 4T_a$	24	12.2	32.8K	2.9K
B-spline-serial + retiming	8	40	$T_m + 11T_a$	24	19.5	19.5K	2.6K
B-spline-serial + retiming + pipeline	8	40	$(T_m + 11T_a)/2$	28	12.3	22.0K	3.1K
B-spline-parallel + retiming	8	40	$T_m + 13T_a$	20	22.5	21.1K	2.4K
B-spline-parallel + retiming + pipeline	8	40	$(T_m + 13T_a)/2$	24	13.4	22.0K	2.9K

result of IDWT is similar to the DWT. Furthermore, the DWT filters are assumed as Daubechies wavelets which are optimal in the sense that they have a minimum size support with a given number of vanishing moments [35]. In other words, all DWT filter lengths are constrained with the given vanishing moments, γ_H and γ_G, as follows:

$$F_H + F_G \geq 2(\gamma_H + \gamma_G) \tag{3.10}$$

where F_H and F_G are the filter lengths of the low-pass and high-pass DWT filters, respectively. Daubechies wavelets satisfy the equal sign. In practical applications, Daubechies wavelets are usually adopted because there is no reason to use a longer filter of the same vanishing moment. Besides the general case, the linear filters are discussed as well. From the length condition in [56], one can derive

$$F_H + F_G = 4k \tag{3.11}$$

where k is a positive integer. Thus, F_H and F_G can only be both odd or even. The odd-tap linear low-pass and high-pass filters are both symmetric. The even-tap linear low-pass filters are symmetric, but the even-tap high-pass filters are anti-symmetric.

3.4.1 *Multipliers and adders*

In the general case, the convolution-based architecture requires $(F_H + F_G)$ multipliers and $(F_H + F_G - 2)$ adders. For the odd-tap linear filter, the four filters in Fig. 2.14(a) are all symmetric such that totally $(\frac{F_H+F_G}{2} + 1)$ multipliers and $(F_H + F_G - 2)$ adders are required. For the even-tap filter, $H_e(z)$ and $H_o(z)$ are mirror images of each other, so are $G_e(z)$ and $G_o(z)$. Thus, only $\frac{F_H+F_G}{2}$ multipliers and $(F_H + F_G - 2)$ adders are needed.

For comparison, the following analysis of lifting scheme will contain the normalization step. According to [38], the complexity of lifting scheme can be approximated with the assumption that all lifting steps are of degree one, except the final stage. Then the normalization step requires two multipliers, and so does each of $\lceil \frac{F_G+1}{2} \rceil$ lifting steps. The final lifting step needs $(\lceil \frac{F_H+1}{2} \rceil - \lceil \frac{F_G+1}{2} \rceil + 1 = \frac{F_H-F_G}{2} + 1)$ multipliers. In total, lifting scheme requires $(\lceil \frac{F_H+1}{2} \rceil + \lceil \frac{F_G+1}{2} \rceil + 3)$ multipliers in the general case. For odd-tap linear filters, each lifting step can be also linear because $H_e(z)$ and $H_o(z)$ are both symmetric. Thus, each of $\frac{F_G+1}{2}$ lifting steps requires only one multiplier, and the final lifting step needs $(\frac{F_H-F_G+2}{4})$ multipliers. So, totally $(\frac{F_H+F_G}{4} + 1)$ multipliers are required. For even-tap linear filters, the lifting step cannot be factorized into linear phase because the $H_e(z)$ is only the mirror image of $H_o(z)$. The number of required multipliers is the same as that of the general case. As for adders, each of $\lceil \frac{F_G+1}{2} \rceil$ lifting steps requires two, and the final one requires $(\lceil \frac{F_H+1}{2} \rceil - \lceil \frac{F_G+1}{2} \rceil + 1)$ adders. For all cases, the number of adders is $(\lceil \frac{F_H+1}{2} \rceil + \lceil \frac{F_G+1}{2} \rceil + 1)$.

The normalization part is also not extracted for the B-spline-based architectures here. Based on the definition of Daubechies wavelets, the below equation can be derived:

$$\begin{aligned} & F_H + F_G = (\gamma_H + F_Q) + (\gamma_G + F_R) = 2(\gamma_H + \gamma_G) \\ \Longrightarrow \quad & F_Q + F_R = \gamma_H + \gamma_G = \frac{F_H + F_G}{2} = 2k \end{aligned} \tag{3.12}$$

where F_Q and F_R are the lengths of $Q(z)$ and $R(z)$, respectively. For the general case, the B-spline-based architecture requires $(F_Q + F_R = \frac{F_H+F_G}{2})$ multipliers. For the linear filters, $Q(z)$ and $R(z)$ are also linear because of the linearity of the B-spline part. Thus, they can be implemented with the symmetric property, and the number of required multipliers is $(\lceil \frac{F_Q+1}{2} \rceil + \lceil \frac{F_R+1}{2} \rceil)$ that can be simplified to $(\frac{F_H+F_G}{4} + 1)$ or $(\frac{F_H+F_G}{4} + 2)$ according to (3.12). Assume the direct implementation is used for the B-spline part. Then the number of required adders is $(F_Q - 1 + F_R - 1 + 2(\gamma_H + \gamma_G) = \frac{3}{2}(F_H + F_G) - 2)$.

The above deduced results are summarized in Table 3.9. Relatively to the convolution-based architectures, the B-spline-based ones can reduce the multipliers by about a half in all cases. The lifting-based ones can reduce about a half of multipliers for the general case and the odd-tap linear filters. For the even-tap linear filters, the lifting-based architectures fail to reduce multipliers and even require more multipliers than the convolution-based ones. However, the B-spline-based ones need about 1.5 times of adders than the convolution-based ones while the lifting-based ones need only about one half of adders of the latter. But the complexity of adders is always much less than that of multipliers.

3.4.2 *Critical path and registers*

The above analysis can be used to evaluate the performance of both hardware and software implementations. For hardware implementation, the critical path and the register number are very important. However, they are hard to estimate exactly because pipelining can be used to reduce the critical path with additional registers. Here we approximate them without pipelining and ignore the difference of $O(1)$ based on the assumption that $F = \max(F_H, F_G)$ is very large.

If the convolution-based architectures are implemented with parallel filters, there will be about F registers and the critical path is about $T_m + \log_2 F \cdot T_a$ by use of the adder tree. The critical path can be reduced to $T_m + 2T_a$ if serial filters are implemented instead, but the number of registers will become $(F_H + F_G)$.

The conventional lifting-based architectures implement the lifting factorization directly and would introduce a long critical path $\frac{F}{2}(T_m + 2T_a)$ with $\frac{F}{2}$ registers because there are about $\frac{F}{2}$ lifting stages. The flipping structure can reduce the critical path to $T_m + \frac{F}{2}T_a$ without any additional register.

The B-spline-based architectures require $(F_H + F_G)$ registers of which $(F_Q + F_R)$ ones are in the distributed part and $(\gamma_H + \gamma_G)$ ones are in the B-spline part. If the distributed part is implemented with parallel filters, the critical path will be $T_m + (\frac{F}{2} + \log_2 F)T_a$ of which $\frac{F}{2}T_a$ comes from the B-spline part and the other term comes from the distributed part. The critical path can be reduced to $T_m + \frac{F}{2}T_a$ if serial filters are implemented instead. The approximation is listed in Table 3.10. The flipping structure and the convolution-based architectures with serial filters are the most efficient in terms of the register number and the critical path, respectively.

3.4.3 *Summary*

The B-spline-based architecture requires the fewest multipliers but the most adders, such that it can provide the smallest die area because adders are usually much smaller than multipliers. The lifting-based one fails to reduce the multipliers for the even-tap linear filters, but always requires the fewest adders. It also can use the fewest registers with a proper critical path if the flipping structure is used. The above analysis shows the trade-off among hardware complexity, critical path, and the number of registers.

3.5 Wordlength Analysis in Single-Level 1-D DWT

In hardware implementation, the circuitry like adders, multipliers, and registers cannot support infinite wordlength (bitwidth). If the adopted wordlength of arithmetic circuits is wider, the calculated results can be more accurate. However, larger hardware area usually accompanies with

Table 3.9 Performance comparisons of 1-D DWT architectures for Daubechies wavelets in three cases: general case, odd linear filters, and even linear filters.

Category	Convolution-based		Lifting-based		B-spline-based	
Function	Mul.	Add.	Mul.	Add.	Mul.	Add.
General Case	$F_H + F_G$		$\lceil \frac{F_H+1}{2} \rceil + \lceil \frac{F_G+1}{2} \rceil + 3$		$\frac{F_H+F_G}{2}$	
Odd Linear	$\frac{F_H+F_G}{2} + 1$	$F_H + F_G - 2$	$\frac{F_H+F_G}{4} + 1$	$\lceil \frac{F_H+1}{2} \rceil + \lceil \frac{F_G+1}{2} \rceil + 1$	$\frac{F_H+F_G}{4} + 1, 2$	$\frac{3}{2}(F_H + F_G) - 2$
Even Linear	$\frac{F_H+F_G}{2}$		$\lceil \frac{F_H+1}{2} \rceil + \lceil \frac{F_G+1}{2} \rceil + 3$		$\frac{F_H+F_G}{4} + 1, 2$	

Table 3.10 Approximation of the register number and the critical path for 1-D DWT architectures without pipelining.

Category	Convolution-based		Lifting-based		B-spline-based	
Implementation Method	Parallel Filter	Serial Filter	Conventional	Flipping	Parallel Filter	Serial Filter
Register Number	F	$F_H + F_G$	$F/2$	$F/2$	$F_H + F_G$	$F_H + F_G$
Critical Path	$T_m + (log_2 F)T_a$	$T_m + 2T_a$	$F/2(T_m + 2T_a)$	$T_m + (F/2)T_a$	$T_m + (F/2 + log_2 F)T_a$	$T_m + (F/2)T_a$

wider wordlength. Therefore, the wordlength should be designed such that it can just meet the desired signal quality level.

In this section, the methods to estimate the finite wordlength effects are introduced. To make a floating-point number become a fixed-point word, a round-off operation has to be made. This round-off operation will induce round-off error in signals whose value is a function of adopted wordlength. Having this function and the desired signal quality level on hand, the required wordlength can be determined.

There are two phenomena to be analyzed in designing wordlength of a DWT filter. One is about the integral part, and the other is about the fractional part of a fixed-point word.

The first phenomenon is the dynamic range growing effect. During the arithmetic operation of DWT, there may be a growing in signal dynamic range. If overflow occurs, the quality of the reconstructed signal will be severely degraded.

The second phenomenon is the round-off errors. Round-off errors are induced by the round-off after the floating-point multiplication. The round-off-errors will break the original relationship of perfect reconstruction between DWT and IDWT. Therefore, the wordlength has to be carefully designed such that the signal quality can still be satisfactory.

Both dynamic range growing effect and round-off error are analyzed in this section. The dynamic range analysis and round-off error analysis of registers in 1-D DWT architecture are shown as examples. It is because the registers in 1-D DWT have a great influence on the hardware power/area of 2-D DWT. This can be seen in Section 3.5.2. However, the discussed methodology can be suitable for all data paths in 1-D DWT. For example, adders, multipliers, and the like. The round-off error analysis of 1-D DWT is presented in Section 3.5.2, and the dynamic range analysis is presented in Section 3.5.1. Only single-level DWT will be analyzed. In Section 4.5, a more general case of multi-level 2-D DWT/IDWT will be analyzed. The mothodology proposed in [57] is introduced, and other related work can be seen in [28][58].

3.5.1 *Dynamic range analysis for single-level 1-D DWT*

In Section 3.5.1.1, some basics of dynamic range analysis is introduced. The dynamic range analysis in single-level 1-D DWT is presented in Section 3.5.1.2. Figure 3.24 shows the architecture of lifting-based (9,7) filter, and the intrinsic registers labeled *R1, R2, R3,* and *R4* will be analyzed as an example. Those registers are named as intrinsic registers since they are originally defined in the lifting-based algorithm. Intrinsic registers are not registers for pipelining usage.

3.5.1.1 *Dynamic range analysis for the output of cascaded FIR filters*

Suppose an input sequence $x(n)$ is fed into a FIR filter $H(z) = \sum_{i=-L}^{T} h(i)z^{-i}$, the output $y(n)$ can be expressed as:

$$y(n) = \sum_{i=-L}^{T} h(i)x(n-i). \tag{3.13}$$

Assuming $-S \leq x(n) \leq S, S > 0$, the maximum possible dynamic range at filter output will exactly be $S \times \sum_{i=0}^{T+L} |h(i)|$. The filter is said to have a dynamic range gain G:

$$G = \sum_{i=-L}^{T} |h(i)|. \tag{3.14}$$

Consider the case that the input sequence $x(n)$ is fed into two cascaded FIR filters $H_1(z) = \sum_{i=-L_1}^{T_1} h_1(i)z^{-i}$ and $H_2(z) = \sum_{i=-L_2}^{T_2} h_2(i)z^{-i}$. These two filters can be merged into an equivalent FIR filter H_{total} with coefficients $h_{total}(n) = \sum_{i=-L_1}^{T_1} h_1(i)h_2(n-i)$. The total dynamic range gain G_{total} is thus:

$$\begin{aligned} G_{total} &= \sum_{n=-(L_1+L_2)}^{T_1+T_2} |h_{total}(n)| \\ &= \sum_{n=-(L_1+L_2)}^{T_1+T_2} \left| \sum_{i=-L_1}^{T_1} h_1(i)h_2(n-i) \right|. \end{aligned} \tag{3.15}$$

3.5.1.2 *Dynamic range analysis for single level 1-D DWT*

In the hardware architecture of a FIR filter, each node can be represented as linear combination of input signal. Therefore, the relationship from the input of the 1-D DWT at certain level to each word of the intrinsic register can be regarded as an equivalent FIR filter.

For example, if lifting-based (9,7) filter is adopted, there are four words of intrinsic registers as shown in Fig. 3.24. Therefore, there are four equivalent filters inside column DWT hardware. For example, the equivalent filter for the intrinsic register indicated as "2" in Fig. 3.24 is $az^{-2} + z^{-1} + a$. Thus

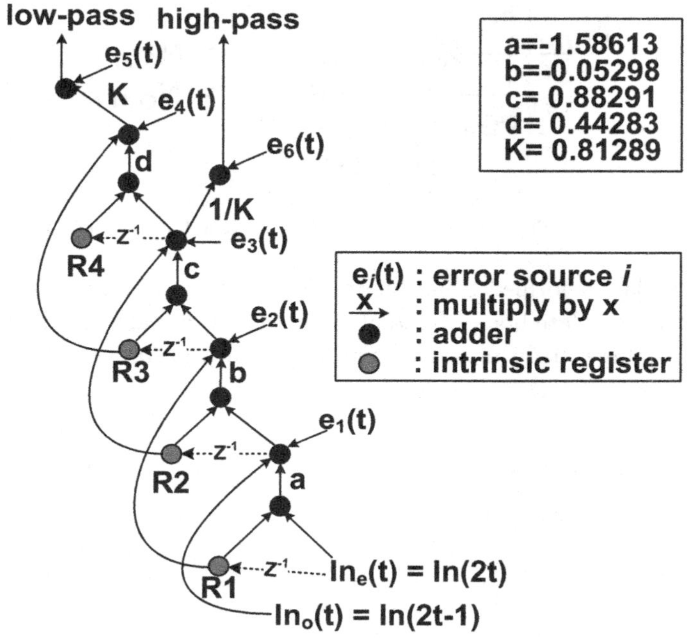

Fig. 3.24 Hardware architecture of lifting-based (9,7) filter.

the corresponding dynamic range gain will be $G_2 = 2|a| + 1 = 4.17226$. By proceeding in this manner, all dynamic range gain from 1-D DWT input to intrinsic registers can be obtained.

At this point, the equivalent dynamic range gain of the nodes in DWT circuits can be calculated. The required additional wordlength can be obtained from the calculated dynamic range gain. Take the intrinsic register "2"in Fig. 3.24 as an example, the dynamic range gain is $G_2 = 4.17226$, and therefore the wordlength of register 2 should be at least 3 bits more than input signal to prevent the overflow.

3.5.2 *Round-off noise analysis basics for single level 1-D DWT*

Once a round-off operation is performed after a floating-point multiplication, an error in signal is introduced. This error is modeled as an additive error source as the $e_1(t)$, $e_2(t)$, $e_3(t)$, $e_4(t)$ in Fig. 3.24. Each error source is a random process where at anytime, the value is uniformly distributed. The

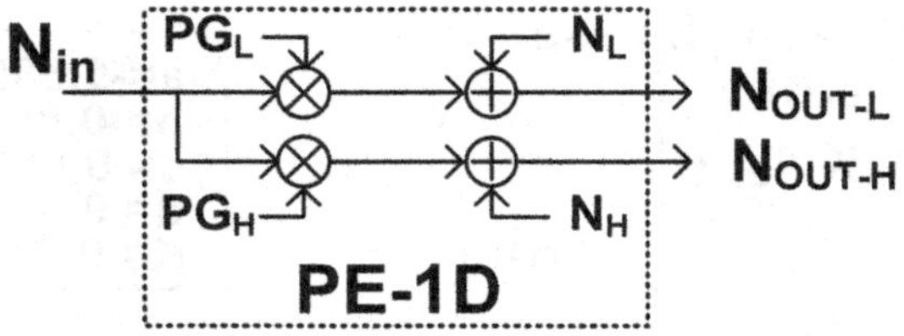

Fig. 3.25 The proposed noise model for single-level 1-D DWT.

random variables formed from different fimes of error source are assumed mutually uncorrelated, and different error sources are also assumed uncorrelated. If there are n fractional bits in all data paths, for error sources $\{e_i(t) : i = 0, 1, 2, ...\}$:

$$E\{e_i(t_1)e_i(t_2)\} = 0, \qquad t_1 \neq t_2 \tag{3.16a}$$

$$E\{e_i(t_1)e_j(t_2)\} = 0 \qquad \forall t_1 t_2, i \neq j \tag{3.16b}$$

$$E\{e_i(t)e_i(t)\} = \sigma^2, \qquad \sigma^2 = \int_{-\frac{1}{2^{n+1}}}^{\frac{1}{2^{n+1}}} 2^n x\, dx = \frac{2^{-2n}}{12} \tag{3.16c}$$

To analyze the noise power at filter output, the noise sources are taken as real signals in the filter architecture. Therefore, the noise in every node can be expressed as linear combination of the noise sources induced directly from round-off operations. The noise power can be evaluated from the expression of noise sources. For example, consider the contribution of noise source $e_3(t)$, $e_4(t)$ in Fig. 3.24 to the low-pass output, the expression of these two noise sources ($e_{LP}(t)$) is:

$$e_{LP}(t) = Kd(e_3(t) + e_3(t-1)) + Ke_4(t) \tag{3.17}$$

In this case, the estimated noise power $E\{e_{LP}^2(t)\}$ can be derived from assumptions in Eq. 3.16:

$$\begin{aligned} E\{e_{LP}^2(t)\} &= E\{(Kd(e_3(t) + e_3(t-1)) + Ke_4(t))^2\} \\ &= K^2d^2E\{e_3^2(t) + e_3^2(t-1)\} + K^2E\{e_4^2(t)\} \\ &= K^2d^2(E\{e_3^2(t)\} + E\{e_3^2(t-1)\}) + K^2E\{e_4^2(t)\} \\ &= (K^2d^2 + K^2)\sigma^2 \end{aligned} \tag{3.18}$$

Thus the noise power induced by 1-D hardware filtering can be calculated by following this way.

If the input signal is not error-free, this error will also be modeled as a noise source with noise power the same as that in input signal. This input noise source, $e_{in}(t)$, also satisfies Eq. 3.16(a) and 3.16(b). If the filter is $H(z) = \sum_{-L}^{T} h(i)z^{-i}$ and the input noise power is N_{in}, the noise power at filter output induced by input noise, N_{out}^{in}, is modeled as:

$$\begin{aligned} N_{out}^{in} &= E\{(\textstyle\sum_{-L}^{T} h(i)e_{in}(t-i))^2\} \\ &= \textstyle\sum_{-L}^{T} h(i)^2 E\{e_{in}^2(t-i)\} \\ &= E\{e_{in}^2(t)\} \times \textstyle\sum_{-L}^{T} h(i)^2 \\ &= N_{in} \times PG\,, \end{aligned} \tag{3.19}$$

where the PG is defined as the filter noise power gain of:

$$PG = \textstyle\sum_{-L}^{T} h(i)^2. \tag{3.20}$$

Please note that in the analysis methodology, the input noise is assumed to be mutually uncorrelated. This assumption is quite useful when calculating multi-level DWT. The low band output of (n-*1*)-th level is the DWT input of n-th level. In calculating the noise power of n-th level output, the round-off effect of (n-*1*)-th level is assumed to be mutually uncorrelated such that the calculation process can be greatly simplified.

In the noise model proposed in [57], the input noise will be amplified by PG during the filtering operation. Figure 3.25 shows the proposed noise model of single level 1-D DWT. As discussed, the fixed-point hardware will introduce round-off error power (N_L, N_H), and the input noise power will be amplified by noise power gains (PG_L, PG_H). The noise power of multi-level 1-D DWT can be obtained by simply cascade the noise model in Fig. 3.25.

Chapter 4

Architectures of Two-Dimensional DWT

This chapter provides an overview for 2-D DWT implementation. RAM-based architectures are focused for their feasibility and efficiency. Section 4.2 summarizes the scan methods of frame memory and discusses the trade-offs between external memory bandwidth and on-chip memory size. The line-based architectures will be introduced in detail in Section 4.3. Lastly, implementation issues of on-chip memory are discussed in Section 4.5.

4.1 Introduction

For 2-D DWT, there have many VLSI architectures been proposed [42, 43, 44, 59, 60]. Nevertheless, only RAM-based architectures are the most practical for real-life designs because of their greater regularity and density of storage [61], compared to systolic or semi-systolic routing. Furthermore, memory issues dominate the hardware cost and complexity of the architectures for 2-D DWT, instead of multipliers that decide the performance of 1-D DWT architectures. Contrary to the block-based DCT, the DWT is basically frame-based. The huge amount of the internal memory size and external access bandwidth is the bottleneck of the implementation for 2-D DWT.

The separable 2-D DWT and IDWT of the dyadic decomposition type can be formulated recursively as Eqs. (2.71) and (2.72), respectively. When the 1-D DWT and IDWT are both implemented into two-input-two-output systems, the methods extending them into 2-D DWT and IDWT are very similar. The following discussion of 2-D DWT architectures is also applicable to 2-D IDWT. The performance of 2-D DWT architectures is mainly determined by frame memory scan method, internal buffer size, and DWT logic gate count. Because the frame memory size is very large, it is usually assumed off-chip. The frame memory access would consume the most power in the 2-D DWT architecture because it consists of large external memory access power and bus interconnect power [61, 62, 23]. Even using embedded frame memory, it is still a very power-hungry factor. Moreover, it may occupy much system memory bandwidth. As for the die area, the contribution of DWT logic is fixed when the adopted 1-D DWT filter and implementation method are determined. The contribution of internal buffer depends on the adopted 2-D DWT architecture and is a trade-off for frame memory access. The die area of internal buffer is related to the required memory size and the implementation method.

4.2 Frame Memory Scan Methods

In this section, 1-level 2-D architectures are focused, which perform 1-level 2-D DWT at a time [63]. There are two ways to extend them to multi-level decompositions. The first one is recursively performing 1-level DWT on the LL subband, which increases the frame memory access by the factor $1 + \frac{1}{4} + ... + (\frac{1}{4})^J = \frac{4}{3}(1 - (\frac{1}{4})^J)$ [59] if J-level decompositions are required. However, the internal buffer size is unchanged. The other one is to extend the 1-level architecture to the multi-level one that performs all levels of DWT decomposition at a time, which will be mentioned for each scan method except the direct scan.

4.2.1 *Direct scan*

The most straightforward implementation of Eq. (2.71) is to perform 1-D DWT in one direction and store the intermediate coefficients in the frame memory, and then to perform 1-D DWT with these intermediate coefficients in the other direction to complete 1-level 2-D DWT. For the other decomposition levels, the LL subband of the current level is treated as the input signals of the next level, and the above steps are then performed recursively. As illustrated in Fig. 4.1(a), this direct architecture requires the least hardware cost and no internal memory due to its simplicity, but it requires much external memory access. For example, if the decomposition level is three, the data flow of the external memory access will be as shown in Fig. 4.1(b). Thus, the bandwidth of external memory access, including

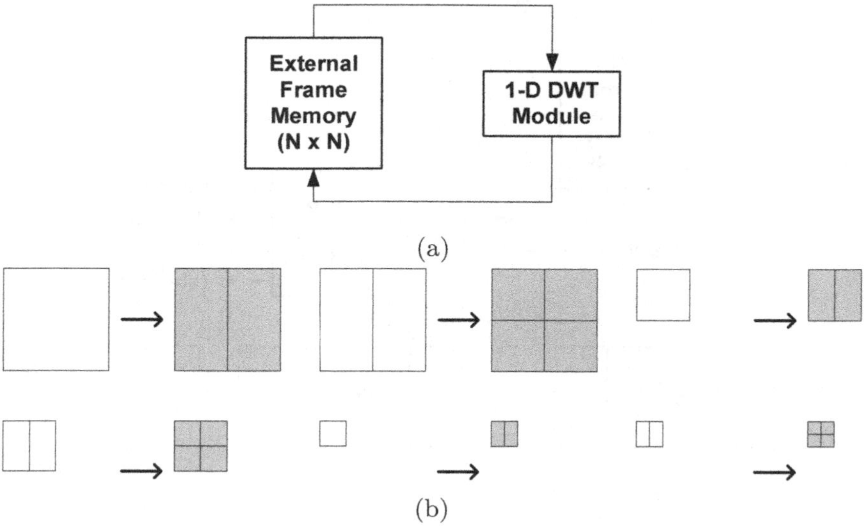

Fig. 4.1 Direct 2-D implementation. (a) System architecture (The number in brackets represents the memory size in terms of words); (b) Data flow of external memory access ($J = 3$; White and grey parts represent external frame memory reads and writes, respectively.)

both reads and writes, can be expressed as

$$4 \times (1 + \frac{1}{4} + \frac{1}{16} + ... + (\frac{1}{4})^{J-1})N^2 \qquad (words/image) \qquad (4.1)$$

where N is the width and height of the image.

4.2.2 *Row-column-column-row scan*

The priorities of row and column directions are identical. Therefore, it is unnecessary to process the row coefficients first for every level decomposition all the time, such as the direct architecture. Instead, the priority can be assumed as row-column for the odd-level decompositions and column-row for the even-level decompositions [64]. Then, the successive two row or column coefficient decompositions can be performed simultaneously.

The DWT module of this RCCR architecture can be implemented by two approaches. One is to fold the two successive decompositions into one 1-D DWT module by RPA scheduling [65] without any line buffer. The other one is to perform the former level decomposition and store the

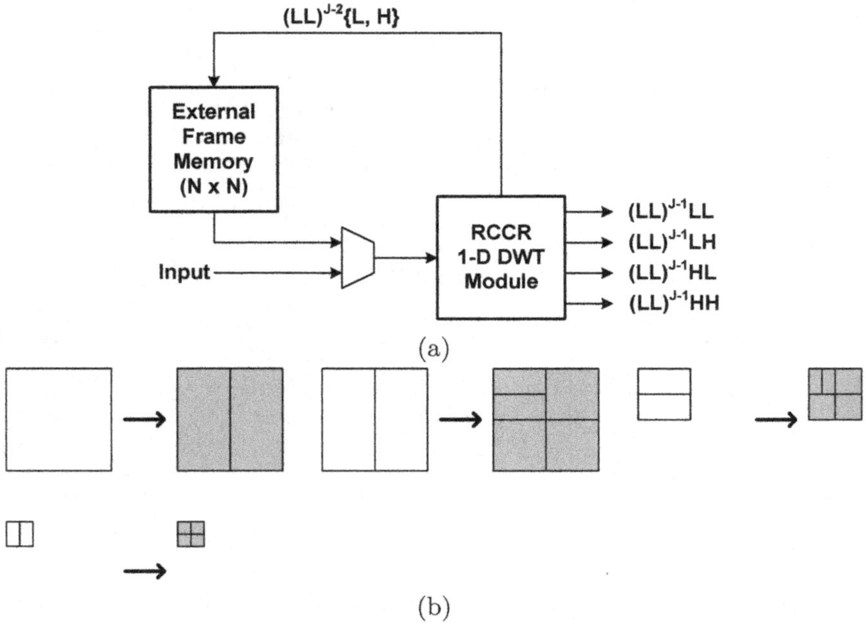

Fig. 4.2 (a) RCCR 2-D architecture; (b) Data flow of external memory access (J = 3)

coefficients in a line buffer of size N/2, and then to perform the latter level decomposition with the stored coefficients. The RCCR architecture is shown in Fig. 4.2(a), and the data flow of external memory access is shown in Fig. 4.2(b). The merging of two successive decompositions in the same direction can decrease the external memory access bandwidth by one half for every level, except the first level decomposition. The external memory access bandwidth can be formulated by:

$$(2 + 2 \times (1 + \frac{1}{4} + \frac{1}{16} + ... + (\frac{1}{4})^{J-1}))N^2 \qquad (words/image)\,, \qquad (4.2)$$

where N is the width and height of the image.

4.2.3 *Line-based scan*

According to the evaluation in [61], external memory access consumes the most power in the 2-D DWT hardware implementation. The line-based

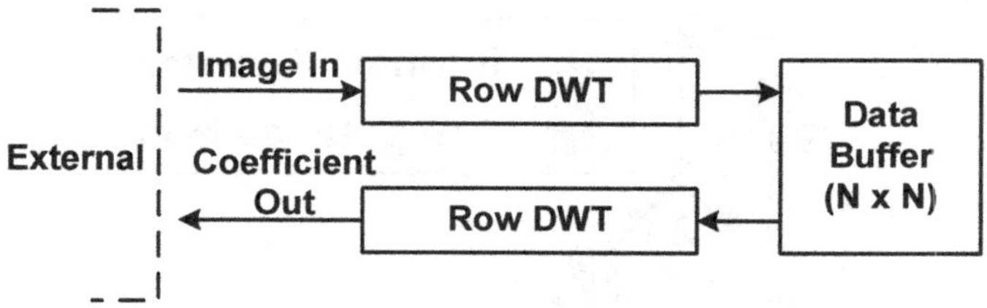

Fig. 4.3 Direct implementation scheme with minimum external bandwidth.

method [66] may be preferred because of the smaller external memory access.

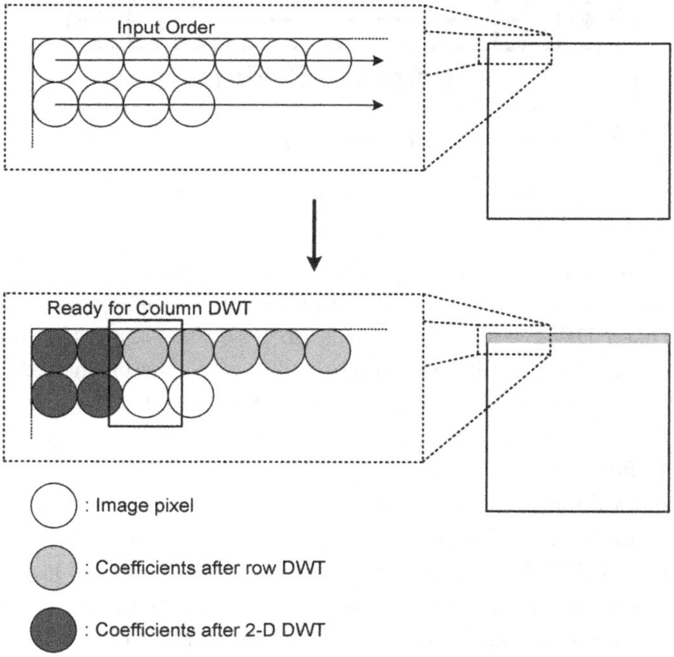

Fig. 4.4 The conceptual line-based scheduling for single level 2-D DWT.

To achieve the minimum bandwidth (one read and one write of image, $2N^2$), an on-chip memory defined as data buffer is required to buffer the coefficients after 1-D DWT (either row-DWT or column-DWT). Figure 4.3 shows this direct implementation scheme with minimum external band-

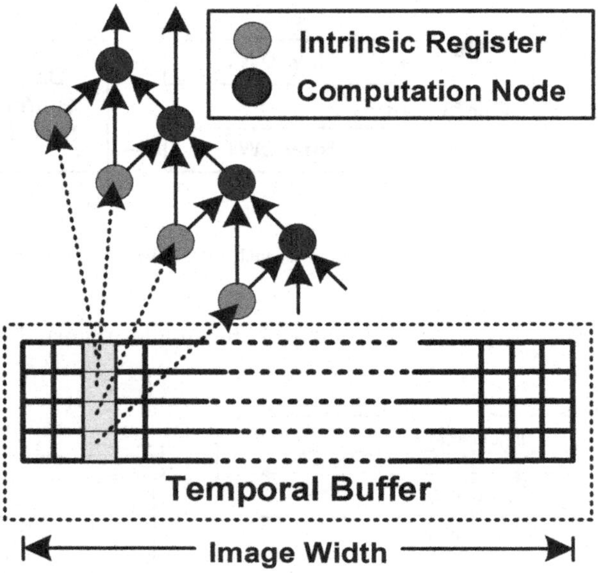

Fig. 4.5 Temporal buffer scheme in lifting-based (9,7) filter.

width. In this scheme, a large on-chip memory is introduced, and this will occupy large chip area and consume a large amount of power.

Line-based DWT scheduling [66] is proposed to shrink this large data buffer. The basic idea of line-based scheduling is to shorten the data-lifetime of temporary coefficients after 1-D DWT. With shorter data-lifetime, the number of temporary coefficients needed to be buffer is smaller, and the required buffer size can be smaller.

Figure 4.4 illustrates the conceptual line-based scheduling of 2-D DWT in row-column order. Assume the image pixels are input in raster scan order, the row DWT can be performed with the input of image pixels. With only one line of coefficients processed by row DWT, the column DWT cannot be started as can be seen in the upper part of Fig. 4.4. When the first row of coefficients processed by row DWT are finished, one column DWT operation can be performed right after a coefficient of the second row is produced by row DWT as shown in the lower part of Fig. 4.4.

With the direct implementation, a coefficient after row DWT should wait for the finish of row DWT of entire image. With the line-based scheduling, however, a coefficient after row DWT should wait for only the finish of row DWT of current row. Theoretically, the buffer size for storing the coefficients after row DWT thus can be reduced from the entire image to only one row. That is, only the grey line in the low part of Fig. 4.4 is required to be buffered.

The temporary register data of column DWT also have to be buffered, and these register data are defined as intrinsic register values. As shown in Fig. 4.4, one column can not be consecutively processed by column DWT module. Therefore, there must exist another buffer to store the register data of column of each row. Figure 4.5 is an example of column DWT of lifting-based (9,7) filter. With lifting-based (9,7) filter, there are four register values each column have to be buffered. The size of this buffer is thus (Image Width $\times$ Number of Intrinsic Registers $\times$ Wordlength of Each Intrinsic Register). In the case of Fig. 4.5 with 16 bits per intrinsic register, a buffer with size of $8N$ ($N \times 4 \times 16$) bytes are required.

Although theoretically only one row of row DWT coefficients has to be buffered, the control complexity will be very high with multi-level DWT, the scheduling proposed in [66] is buffering two rows of coefficients. In the following, scheduling with buffer smaller than two rows is presented under the assumption that the throughput of adopted 1-D DWT module is two-input/two-output per clock cycle [67].

4.2.3.1 *Data flow for data buffer of size* $1.5N$

Since the adopted 1-D DWT module is defined as two-input/two-output per clock cycle, the column DWT module requires that two lines of signals are inputted simultaneously. However, the row DWT module gives the output signals in a line-by-line way. The first line of these two lines of signals which are immediately required by the column DWT module is defined as LINE_1, and the second line is defined as LINE_2. The data flow of these signals should be designed carefully by using the data buffer and its address generator. Contrary to [68] where FIFO is used, the proposed data flow uses feasible two-port RAM, which can provide high regularity and density.

The data flow proposed in [67] is described as follows. As shown in Fig. 4.6, one RAM, called RAM_A, of size N is used for storing the coefficients of LINE_1, and the other one, called RAM_B, of size $0.5N$ is for LINE_2. After the LINE_1 coefficients fill up RAM_A, as Fig. 4.6(a), the data flow can be performed as the following steps. From Fig. 4.6(a) to (d), the LINE_2 coefficients enter RAM_B while the column 1-D DWT module consumes data from both RAM_A and RAM_B. Fig. 4.6(b), (c), and (d) represent that 1/2, 3/4, and all of the LINE_2 coefficients are filled

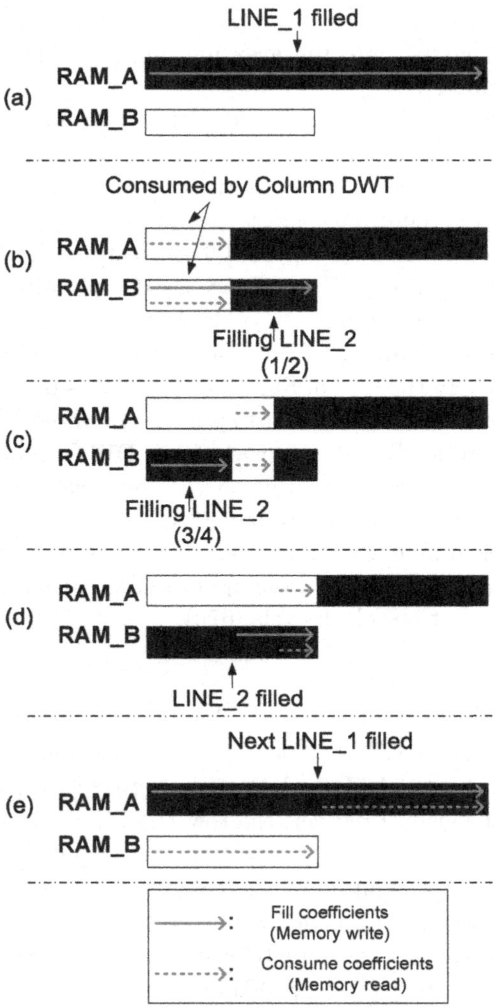

Fig. 4.6 Data flow for data buffer of size $1.5N$ (Black: data filled; White: no data).

into RAM_B, respectively. Then the next LINE_1 coefficients feed RAM_A from Fig. 4.6(d) to (e), and the data flow continues from Fig. 4.6(b) recursively. In summary, the data flow is illustrated by Fig. 4.6 in the order of (a)→(b)→(c)→(d)→(e)→(b)→(c). . . .

This data flow is without conflict because the speed of writing data is double that of reading data for each line buffer. The above steps illustrate only the main idea of the data flow. In fact, RAM_A and RAM_B should both be composed of two two-port RAMs, one for low-pass signals and the other for high-pass signals. Nonetheless, the data flow can work well after this modification.

4.2.4 *Complete data flow for data buffer of size $(1 + (1/2)^k)N$*

The lower bound of the data buffer (one row of coefficients) can be drawn arbitrarily near with the price of control complexity. For this data flow, $2^k + 1$ split RAMs of size $N/2^k$ are required, where k is an arbitrary integer.

At first, the LINE_1 coefficients are filled into 2^k split RAMs. Then the data flow can be recursively performed for every two new lines of coefficients as follows.

The first $1/2^{k-1}$ of the entering LINE_2 coefficients are filled into the left split RAM as the RAM_B from Fig. 4.6(b) to (d). Then the following steps are performed recursively until the next LINE_1 coefficients are filled into 2^k split RAMs. In the beginning, take the two split RAMs, in which the stored data are required by the column 1-D DWT module immediately, as RAM_C and RAM_D while the empty split RAM is called RAM_E, as shown in Fig. 4.7. Then the data can be transferred from Fig. 4.7(a) to (d). Thus, another empty split RAM is obtained as RAM_D, and the entering coefficients are stored in RAM_C and RAM_E. The data flow is summarized in Fig. 4.8.

Although the lower bound can be approached very closely, the additional control circuits and complex address generators may become impractical if k is too large. Moreover, some additional storage devices for controlling data flow would be inevitable, and the size of these storage devices will become larger as k increases. In addition to the data flows mentioned above, no control circuits will be required if a data buffer of size $3N$ is allowable. In [64], six two-port RAMs, three for low-pass signals and three for high-pass signals, and a rotation-like address generator are used to perform the data transfer between the row and column 1-D DWT modules.

4.2.4.1 *1-level line-based architecture*

Unlike the direction-by-direction approach of direct architectures, each level of the DWT decomposition can be performed at a time, and the multi-

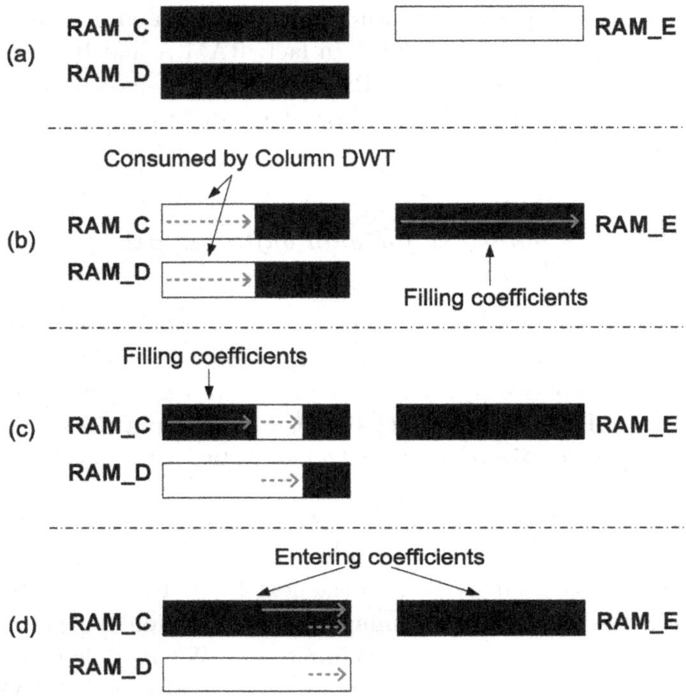

Fig. 4.7 Data transfer among the three working split RAMs for the data buffer of size $(1 + (1/2)^k)N$.

level decompositions can be achieved by using a level-by-level approach. However, this approach may require some internal memory, whose size is proportional to the image width, to store the intermediate DWT coefficients of one direction and to supply the input signals for the DWT decomposition in the other direction [69]. The architecture proposed in [59] is based on this approach as shown in Fig. 4.9(a). The size of the required internal memory, called line buffer, is LN, where $L = L_{raster} + L_{reg}$ represents how many line buffers are used. L_{raster} corresponds to the additional line buffer if the image is inputted in a raster scan fashion. L_{reg} is the number of registers in the adopted 1-D DWT architecture.

Figure 4.9(b) shows the data flow of external memory access, and the

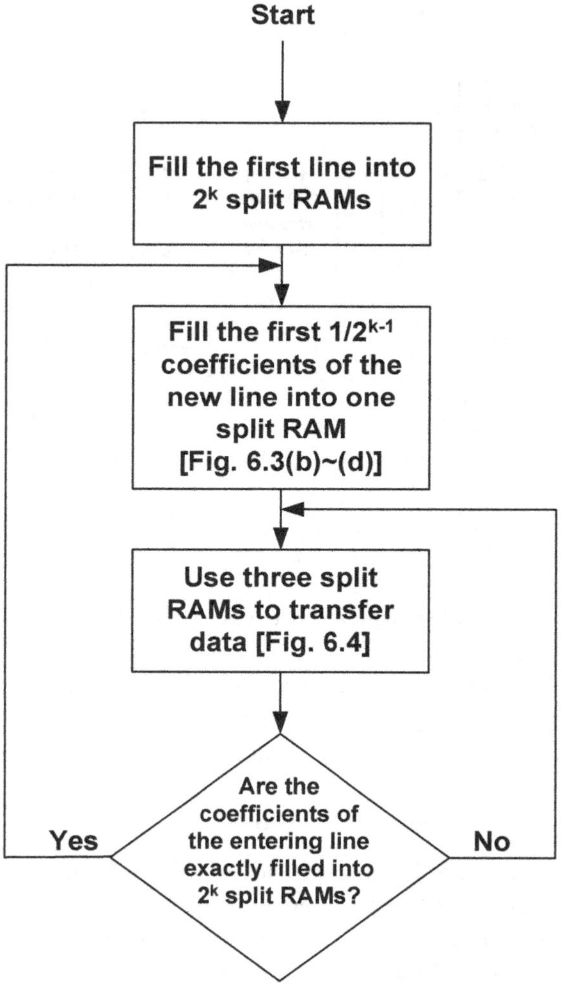

Fig. 4.8 Data flow for data buffer of $(1 + (1/2)^k)N$.

external memory bandwidth can be expressed by:

$$2 \times (1 + \frac{1}{4} + \frac{1}{16} + ... + (\frac{1}{4})^{J-1})N^2 \qquad (words/image). \qquad (4.3)$$

The external memory bandwidth of this 1-level line-based architecture is exactly one half of that of the direct architecture. This is due to the utiliza-

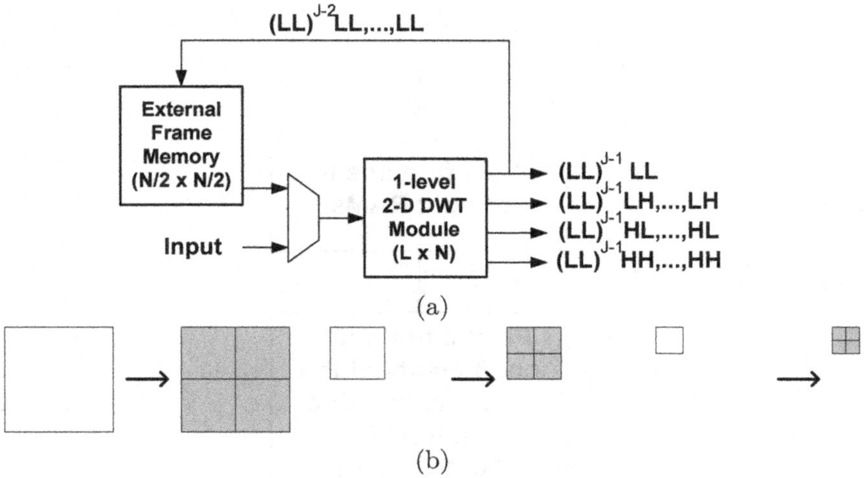

Fig. 4.9 1-level line-based implementation. (a) System architecture; (b) Data flow of external memory access ($J = 3$).

tion of internal line buffers which store exactly one half of the intermediate DWT coefficients.

Furthermore, unlike the direct architecture that uses the whole frame buffer of size N^2 as the intermediate coefficient buffer, the 1-level line-based architecture only uses one quarter of the frame buffer.

4.2.4.2 *Multi-level line-based architecture*

Beyond the level-by-level approach, all of the decomposition levels can be performed simultaneously as the multi-level 2-D architecture in Fig. 4.10(a). However, using cascaded J 1-level line-based architectures to implement directly will result in very low hardware utilization. Generally, the tasks of all decomposition levels will be allocated to a few 1-D DWT modules [43, 44]. Compared to 1-level line-based architecture, the size of required internal line buffers is increased by a factor α to αLN where

$$\alpha = 1 + \frac{1}{2} + \frac{1}{4} + ... + (\frac{1}{2})^{J-1} \tag{4.4}$$

and L is the number of line buffers if this kind of architecture is degenerated into the 1-level line-based architecture.

As described above, the data flow of external memory access is simple and regular as shown in Fig. 4.10(b). Although this multi-level 2-D architecture requires more internal buffer and suitable task assignments for 1-D DWT modules, it can reduce the external memory access bandwidth to the minimum, $2N^2$.

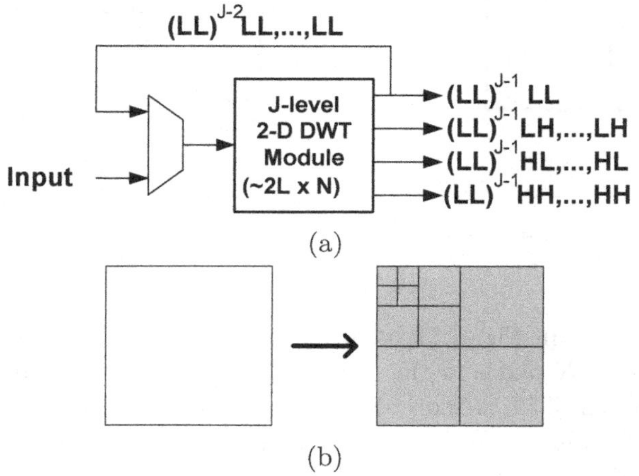

Fig. 4.10 Multi-level line-based implementation. (a) System architecture; (b) Data flow of external memory access ($J = 3$).

4.2.5 *Non-overlapped and overlapped block-based scans*

Block-based methods scan the frame memory block-by-block, and the DWT coefficients are also computed block-by-block. If the blocks are not overlapped with each other, the frame memory reads and writes are both N^2 words for 1-level DWT [70, 47]. For each block, some intermediate data need to be stored for two neighboring blocks as shown in Fig. 4.11(a), where the grey area represents the intermediate data. The blocks are assumed to be scanned in the row direction first. Then the size of the internal buffer is $L_{reg}N + L_{reg}B_y$. For the multi-level architecture, the size of line buffer is also increased by the factor α.

On the other hand, the buffer $L_{reg}N$ can be eliminated if the column-wise intermediate data are not stored. Instead, the required data at the block boundary can be retransmitted from the frame memory. The block-based scheme in [71] is generalized to the overlapped block-based scan

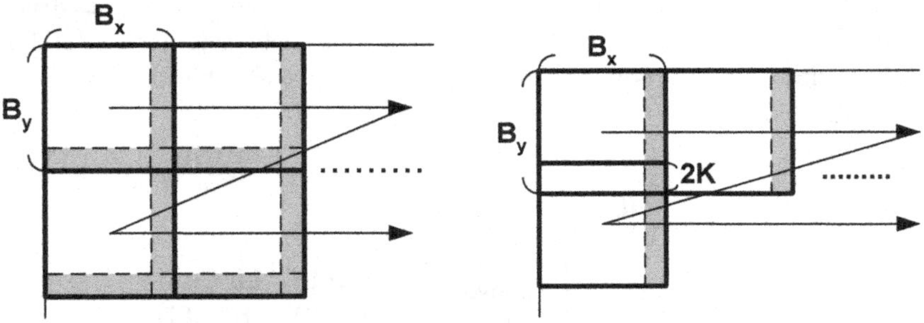

(a) (b)

Fig. 4.11 Block-based scan methods. (a) Non-overlapped block-based scan; (b) Overlapped block-based scan.

method as shown in Fig. 4.11(b), where $K = \lceil \frac{F-1}{2} \rceil$. That is, the blocks are overlapped $2K$ pixels in the column direction. The overlapped area is described in Fig. 4.12 in more detail. The DWT coefficients of the first K and last K columns are not valid. Thus, the overlapped pixels are $2K$ for deriving all DWT coefficients. The retransmission scheme increases the frame memory reads to $N^2 \frac{B_y}{B_y - 2K}$ words while the frame memory writes is still N^2 words. The internal buffer size $L_{reg}B_y$ can be reduced by shrinking the block size, but it would also increase the frame memory read bandwidth. As for the multi-level architecture, the overlapped area will become $2^J K$ that increases exponentially as J, and the frame memory reads become $N^2 \frac{B_y}{B_y - 2^J K}$ words. Thus, the overlapped block-based scan is not feasible for multi-level architectures.

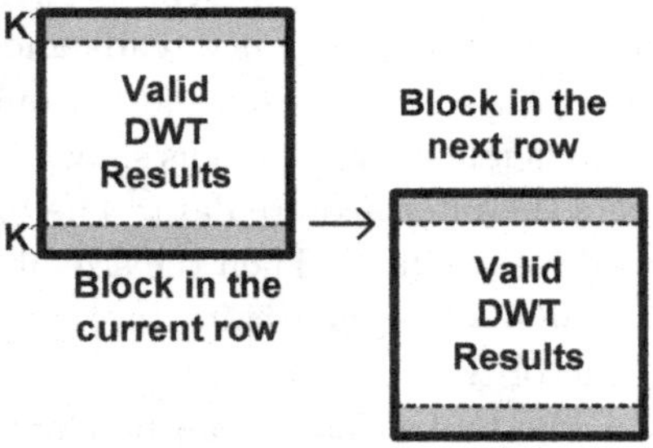

Fig. 4.12 Details of the overlapped blocks.

4.2.6 *Non-overlapped and overlapped stripe-based scans*

The optimal Z-scan method is proposed in [72], which is equivalent to performing the line-based scan in the wide block ($B_x = N$). In concept, the wide blocks can be viewed as stripes. So, this kind of method is categorized as the non-overlapped stripe-based scan as shown in Fig. 4.13(a). The internal buffer size is $L_{reg}(N + S)$, where S is the width of the stripe. The first term is for the intermediate buffer between stripes, and the second term is for the line buffer inside stripes. For the multi-level architecture, the size of line buffer is also increased by the factor α.

Similarly with the block-based scans, the overlapped stripe-based scan method [53] is as shown in Fig. 4.13(b). All parameters are the same as that of the overlapped block-based scan method, except the stripe width S is used instead of B_y. This scan method can avoid the complex control circuits for block-based DWT architectures. It can be implemented by use of a line-based 2-D DWT architecture with the width S and an external memory address generator that provides the address of the scan patterns. One simple control circuit is also required to inform the line-based architecture about the first and last lines of the stripe for boundary extension.

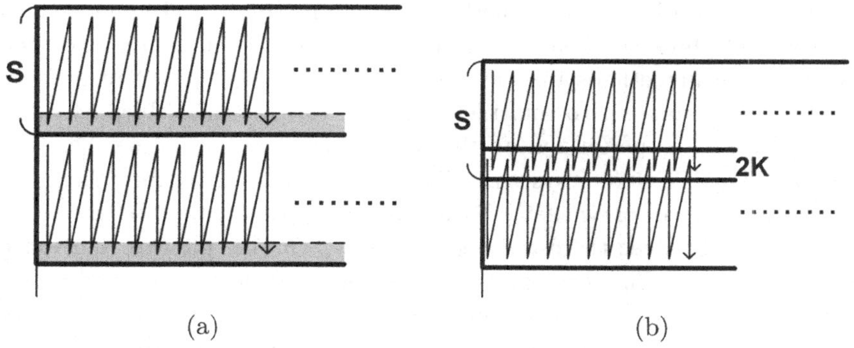

Fig. 4.13 Stripe-based scan methods. (a) Non-overlapped stripe-based scan; (b) Overlapped stripe-based scan.

4.2.7 *Comparison of scan methods for 1-level 2-D DWT architectures*

The comparisons of the six scan methods are listed in Table 4.1. The trade-off between the external memory access and the internal buffer size is presented. The direct scan does not require any internal buffer but suffers nearly double external memory bandwidth than other scan methods. The line-based and two non-overlapped scan methods can minimize the external memory access but require larger internal buffer. Between the two overlapped scan methods, the stripe-based one may be preferred for its simplicity. Especially, the overlapped stripe-based scan method is degenerated to the line-based scan when $S = N$.

For giving more realistic comparisons, the HDTV image quality (1080p 24frames/sec YUV 4:2:0) is considered as the implementation specification for 5-level 2-D DWT with the (9,7) filter. It is assumed that the column DWT module is lifting-based, and $L_{raster} = 0$ and $L_{reg} = 4$ for the internal buffer. The image pixel rate can be calculated as

$$1920 \times 1080 \times 24 \times 1.5 \simeq 74.65 \times 10^6 \quad (words/sec).$$

If the 1-level architecture is used to recursively perform 5-level decomposition, the memory reads and writes need be timed by $1 + \frac{1}{4} + \frac{1}{16} + \frac{1}{64} + \frac{1}{256} = 1.332$. On the other hand, the size of the internal buffer would be increased by $\alpha = 1.9375$ if the multi-level architecture is used.

The comparisons of different scan methods are shown in Table 4.2. Since the two non-overlapped scan methods require more internal buffer in this case, only the line-based one is shown in this table. The direct scan and two overlapped scan methods are considered to perform 1-level DWT recursively because the extension to multi-level architectures is infeasible. Besides, the DWT can be performed on the whole image or only on smaller tiles separately in JPEG 2000 systems. Two cases are considered here, in which no tiles and the tile of size 256×256 are assumed, respectively. In this table, the trade-off between the frame memory access and the internal buffer size is shown clearly. The overlapped scan methods would be preferred in the case of no tiles because the frame memory access can be decreased very much with few overheads of the internal buffer. However, the line-based scan would be better in the case of the tile size 256 because the overheads of the overlapped scan methods become larger.

4.2.8 *Summary*

In this section, the 2-D DWT architectures are classified according to different frame memory scan methods. The performance is evaluated using trade-offs between frame memory access and internal buffer size. The direct implementation requires no internal buffer but suffers the largest frame

Table 4.1 Comparisons of scan methods for 1-level 2-D DWT architectures.

	Direct	Line-Based	Non-Overlapped Block-Based	Overlapped Block-Based	Non-Overlapped Stripe-Based	Overlapped Stripe-Based
Frame Memory Read (words/image)	$2N^2$	N^2	N^2	$\frac{N^2 B_y}{B_y - 2K}$	N^2	$\frac{N^2 S}{S-2K}$
Frame Memory Write (words/image)	$2N^2$	N^2	N^2	N^2	N^2	N^2
Internal Buffer Size (words)	0	LN	$L_{reg}(N + B_y)$	$L_{reg}B_y$	$L_{reg}(N + S)$	$L_{reg}S$
Control Complexity	Low	Medium	High	High	Medium	Medium

Table 4.2 Comparisons of 2-D DWT architectures with 5-level decomposition for HDTV images (assume $L_{raster} = 0$ and $L_{reg} = 4$ for the (9,7) filter).

	Direct	Line-Based		Overlapped Block-/Stripe-Based		
		Recursive 1-Level	Multi-Level	$B_y = S = 16$	$B_y = S = 64$	$B_y = S = 256$
Frame Memory Read (Mwords/s)	198.9	99.4	74.6	198.9	113.7	102.6
Frame Memory Write (Mwords/s)	198.9	99.4	74.6	99.4	99.4	99.4
Internal Buffer Size/No Tile (words)	0	4320	8370	64	256	1024
Internal Buffer Size/Tile Size=256 (words)	0	1024	1984	64	256	-

memory access. The line-based and two non-overlapped scans can minimize the frame memory access by use of large internal buffer. The two overlapped scans can provide various trade-off between these two extremes.

4.3 Line-Based Architecture

In the 2-D DWT architectures, the line-based one requires the largest on-chip memory that induces significant die area. Thus, how to optimize the implementation of line buffers is an important issue for line-based architectures. In this section, some general line-based architectures are introduced and compared. In the next section, the implementation issues of line buffer will be discussed.

4.3.1 *Systolic-parallel and parallel-parallel architectures*

The systolic-parallel [43] and parallel-parallel [44] architectures are multi-level line-based implementation of 2-D DWT by adopting convolution-based 1-D DWT modules. Their basic architecture is shown in Fig. 4.14, which consists of four DWT filter modules and two storage units. The main difference of these two architectures is that systolic-parallel architecture uses serial filters to implement DWT filter modules 1 and 2 of Fig. 4.14, and parallel-parallel one uses parallel filters to implement them. Both DWT filter modules 3 and 4 are implemented by parallel filters. The DWT filter module 1 is responsible to the first decomposition level in the row direction. The DWT filter module 2 is responsible to the following decomposition levels in the row direction. The DWT filter module 3 and 4 perform the DWT decompositions in the column direction.

Each DWT filter module can produce a pair of low-pass and high-pass DWT coefficients in every two cycles. However, the structure of these DWT filter modules is different from Figs. 3.1 and 3.2 that use fixed coefficient multipliers. Instead, the DWT filter module uses programmable coefficients to switch the coefficients between low-pass and high-pass filters. For example, it can be programmed to become the low-pass filter in even cycles and the high-pass filter in odd cycles.

As for the storage units 1 and 2, they are used to store the intermediate data for multi-level DWT decomposition. The storage unit 1 is to store the DWT results from DWT filter modules 1 and 2 and provides the input data to DWT filter modules 3 and 4 in a parallel way. The storage unit 2 is to

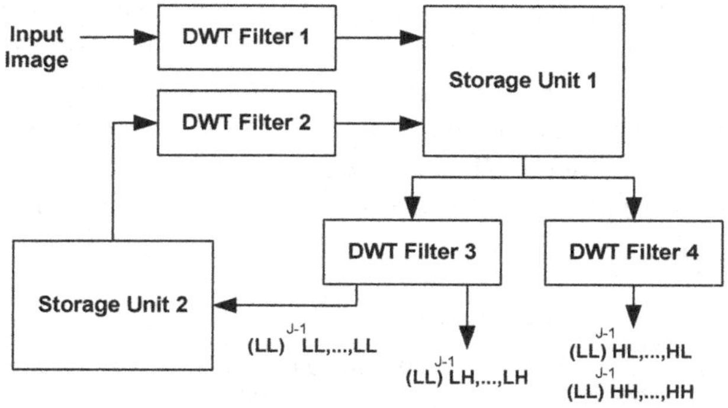

Fig. 4.14 Systolic-parallel or parallel-parallel architecture. DWT filter modules 1 and 2 are implemented by use of serial and parallel filters for the former and latter ones, respectively. DWT filter modules 3 and 4 are implemented by use of parallel filters.

store the LL subbands that are the input data of DWT filter module 4 for following decomposition levels. According to [43] and [44], the storage size of systolic-parallel architecture is $(2F+4)N$ where F is the filter length, and that of parallel-parallel one is $(2F+1)N$ This difference is due to different and detailed storage management.

4.3.2 *Wu's architecture*

As mentioned in Section 4.2.3, the multi-level DWT decompositions can be achieved by performing 1-level DWT recursively on the LL subbands. Wu [59] proposed one 1-level line-based architecture that performs 2-D DWT in a level-by-level way as shown in Fig. 4.9. Compared to the multi-level architectures, this 1-level line-based architecture can reduce about one half of on-chip storage size. In [59], the detailed structure is proposed for convolution-based 1-D DWT as systolic-parallel and parallel-parallel architectures. The row directional DWT is implemented by use of parallel filters, and the on-chip storage size is FN.

4.3.3 *Generic 1-level line-based architecture*

In [67], one generic 1-level line-based architecture is proposed. First, it handles the on-chip storage in a more detailed way to reduce the storage size. Second, the architecture can adopt any kind of DWT filter module that is two-input-two-output per cycle as described in Chapter 3.

As shown in Fig. 4.15, the generic 1-level line-based architecture for 2-D DWT is basically composed of some line buffers and two 1-D DWT modules, one for row-wise decomposition and the other one for column-wise decomposition. These line buffers can be classified into two categories: data buffer and temporal buffer. The decomposition order can be row-column or column-row. Without loss of generality, the row-column order is assumed in the following.

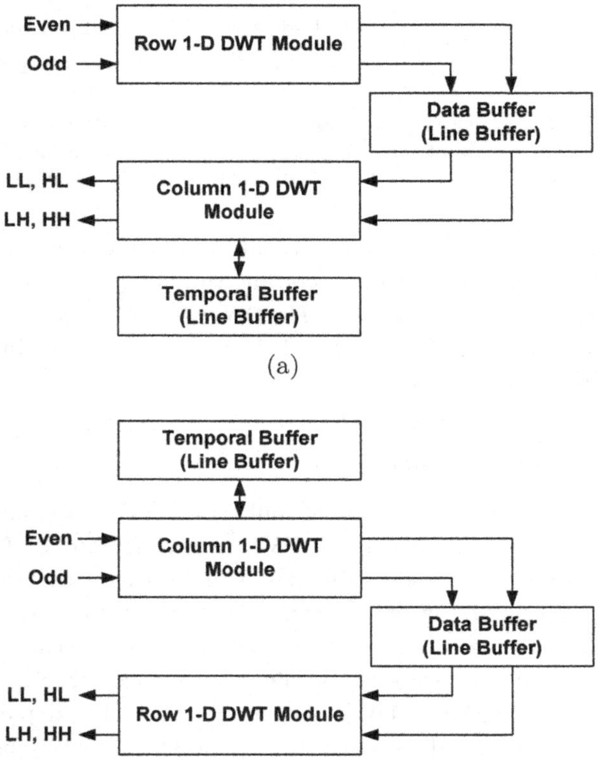

(b)

Fig. 4.15 Generic 1-level line-based architecture. (a) row-column decomposition order; (b) column-row decomposition order.

The data buffer is used to store the intermediate decomposition coefficients after 1-D DWT in the row direction and to provide the input signals of the column 1-D DWT module. Thus, the data buffer results from the raster input order, and it is independent of adopted 1-D DWT architectures and only related to the throughput. On the other hand, the temporal buffer is highly dependent on the adopted 1-D DWT architecture. If the original circuits in the adopted 1-D DWT architecture are as constructed as Fig. 4.16(a), the column 1-D DWT module and the temporal buffer can be modified as Fig. 4.16(b). The temporal buffer is used to store the data that should originally be stored in the registers for the column 1-D DWT module. Because the memory access of temporal buffer is very regular and simple, L_{reg} copies of two-port RAMs of size N can be used to implement it, where L_{reg} is the number of registers in the adopted 1-D DWT module. Moreover, these L_{reg} RAMs can be merged into a single RAM of size $L_{reg}N$ for higher density. The memory address of these temporal buffers can be generated easily by a rotation-like address calculator. According to Table 3.10, the lifting-based 1-D DWT can provide the smallest L_{reg} as well as the smallest temporal buffer. Besides, the B-spline factorized architecture requires large L_{reg}, so it is not suitable to implement the column-DWT module.

As for the data buffer, the lower bound of its size is $1N$ because the data flow always keeps two-input/two-output per clock cycle after the 1-D DWT coefficients of the first row are obtained. However, extremely high complexity will be required with this minimal data buffer size. In [67], two data flows for data buffer of sizes $1.5N$ and $(1 + (1/2)^k)N$ are presented. The control circuits for the former one are quite simple. However, the latter one requires more overhead registers and more complex control circuits as k increases.

If lifting-based 1-D DWT module is adopted, the number of multipliers can be further reduced by two because of the scaling effect of the normalization step in Fig. 4.17, where K is the normalization coefficient. Originally, two multipliers are required for both the row and column 1-D DWT modules. However, the normalization multipliers can be taken out of the two 1-D DWT modules, and instead, two multipliers, K^2 and $1/K^2$, are used to implement the normalization step at the output of the column 1-D DWT module.

4.3.4 *Generic multi-level line-based architecture*

The concepts about data buffer and temporal buffer presented above can be used to construct multi-level architectures with allocating the multi-level

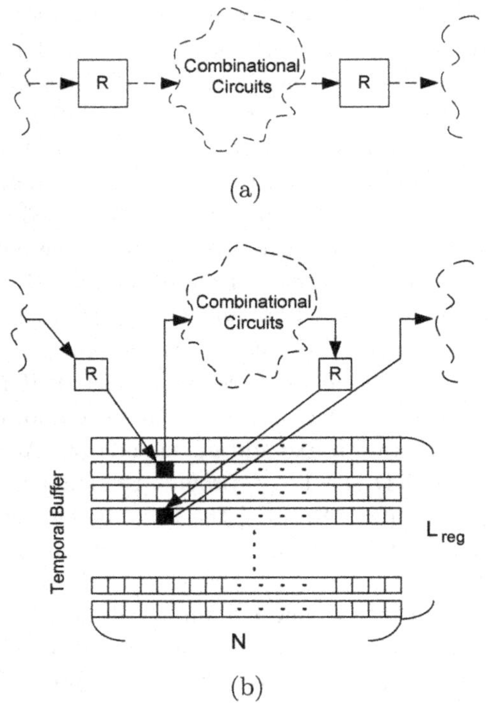

Fig. 4.16 Mapping method for temporal buffer. (a) Original circuits; (b) Modified line-based circuits (R: register).

DWT decomposition tasks to a few 1-D DWT modules. In [67], two generic multi-level line-based architectures are also proposed by using two and three 1-D DWT modules, and the throughputs are one-input/one-output and two-input/two-output per clock cycle, respectively.

4.3.4.1 *Adopting two 1-D DWT modules (2DWTM)*

The generic 1-level architecture can be easily extended to the multi-level architecture by scheduling the multi-level DWT decomposition tasks to the two 1-D DWT modules with recursive pyramid algorithm (RPA) [65], as shown in Fig. 4.18. The RPA schedule for 3-level 2-D DWT is shown as an example in Fig. 4.19, where the numbers represent which level of DWT decomposition should be performed. The throughput of this multi-level architecture is one-input/one-output per clock cycle in average, which is

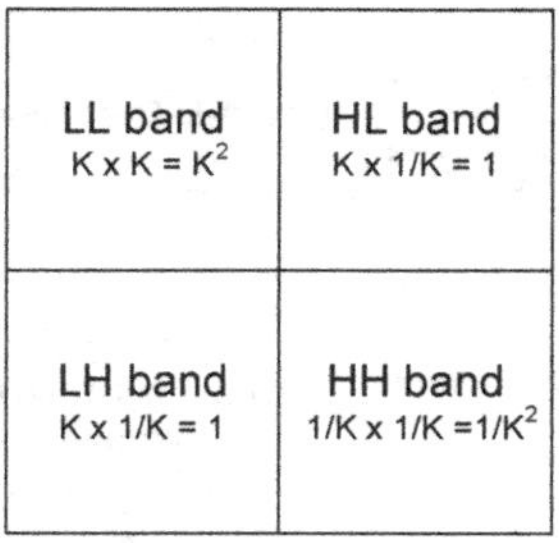

Fig. 4.17 Normalization step of 2-D lifting-based DWT.

one half that of the 1-level architecture. The number of registers in the row DWT module should be increased to J times the original number in order to store the intermediate data of J level DWT decompositions. Because the amount of data in the next level is only one quarter of the current level, the hardware utilization is only:

$$\frac{1}{2} \times (1 + \frac{1}{4} + \frac{1}{16} + ... + (\frac{1}{4})^{J-1}). \tag{4.5}$$

And the limit is 2/3 as J is indefinitely large. The total size of data buffer and temporal buffer becomes

$$(1 + \frac{1}{2} + \frac{1}{4} + ... + (\frac{1}{2})^{J-1})(L_{reg} + L_{raster})N \qquad (words) \tag{4.6}$$

where L_{reg} and L_{raster} are the numbers of line buffers for the temporal buffer and data buffer, respectively, in the original 1-level line-based architecture.

4.3.4.2 *Adopting three 1-D DWT modules (3DWTM)*

The throughput of the 2DWTM architecture is one-input/one-output because of only using two 1-D DWT modules. Moreover, the hardware utilization is not high due to the imbalanced task allocation with RPA scheduling. The problem of the above RPA scheduling is allocating only one half of the hardware resources to perform the first level decomposition in which the arithmetic operations are more than the three-fourths of the total operations.

To increase the hardware utilization, DWT decomposition tasks can be allocated to three 1-D DWT modules of which two are for the first

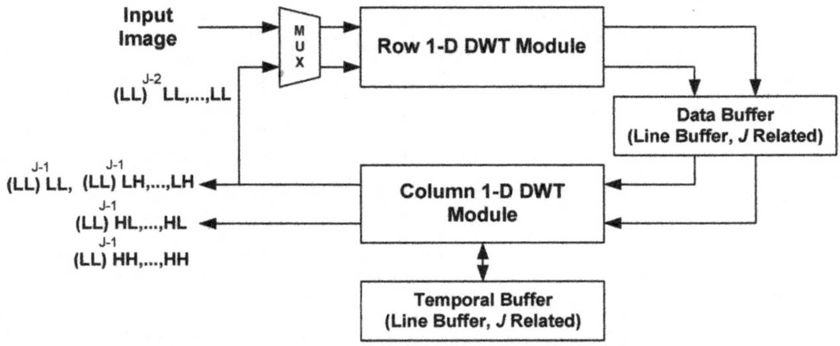

Fig. 4.18 Generic multi-level line-based architecture using two 1-D DWT modules (2DWTM).

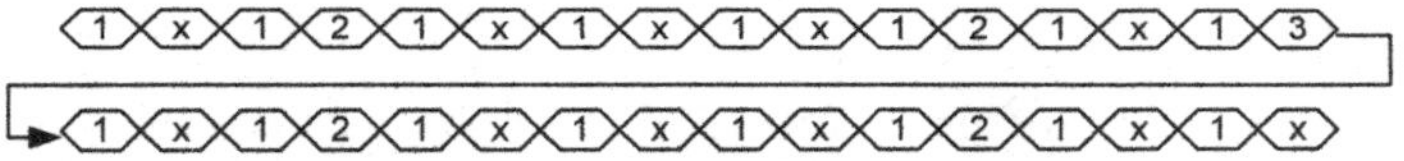

Fig. 4.19 RPA schedule for 3-level 2-D DWT. The numbers represent which level of decomposition is performed, and the "x" means a bubble cycle.

level and one is for all higher levels. Fig. 4.20 shows the proposed multi-level line-based architecture using three 1-D DWT modules (3DWTM). This architecture consists of one proposed 1-level architecture and one two-slow and folded 2DWTM architecture. The two-slow multi-level 2DWTM architecture folds the row and column DWT modules into the same module and serves for DWT decompositions of all levels, except the first level. The throughput can achieve two-input/two-output again, and the hardware utilization is increased to:

$$(2 + \frac{1}{2} \times (1 + \frac{1}{4} + \frac{1}{16} + ... + (\frac{1}{4})^{J-2}))/3 \tag{4.7}$$

and the limit is 8/9 as J is indefinitely large. The total size of data buffer and temporal buffer can be the same as 2DWTM if the data flow is carefully handled. ([67] requires an additional transfer buffer, but it can be eliminated with a proper data flow.) Compared to (4.5), the hardware utilization is increased by about 2/9.

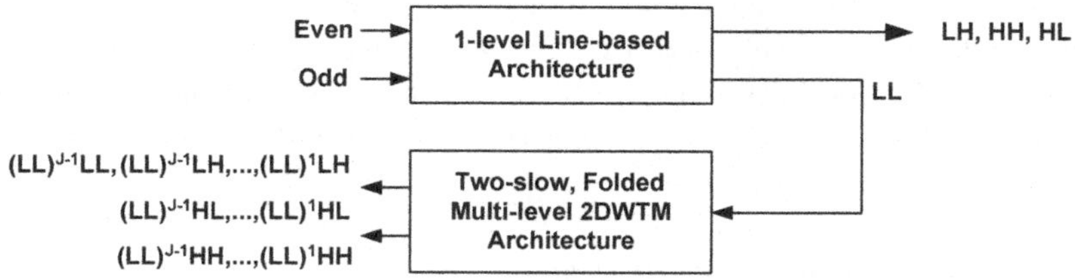

Fig. 4.20 Generic multi-level line-based architecture using three 1-D DWT modules (3DWTM).

4.3.5 *Comparison*

In the following, the above-mentioned architectures are compared in the general case and in the popular case that adopts JPEG 2000 default lossy (9,7) filter. The parameter L_{raster} of the generic architectures is assumed to be 1.5 for comparison because the minimum data buffer size depends on the image size and the memory access delay time.

4.3.5.1 *General case*

The comparison results of systolic-parallel [43], parallel-parallel [44], Wu's [59], and generic architectures [67] are given in Table 4.3, where F represents the filter length, and J is assumed to be infinitely large. In this table, only general convolution-based 1-D DWT modules are considered, so the required numbers of multipliers and adders of these architectures are all proportional to the number of adopted 1-D DWT modules.

Among these architectures, only the generic 1-level line-based and the Wu's architectures are classified into 1-level 2-D DWT architectures, whereas the others belong to multi-level architectures. The hardware utilization of the two 1-level architectures can reach 100%. The product of hardware utilization, computing time, and the number of adopted 1-D DWT modules, should be a constant which is equal to the total decomposition operations. Thus, raising hardware utilization can lower the computing time if the numbers of 1-D DWT modules are the same, as described in [59]. In addition, the generic 1-level line-based architecture outperforms the 1-level 2-D one in the aspect of the number of line buffers due to careful management of the data buffer.

As for the multi-level line-based architectures, the sizes of line buffers in the generic architectures are all smaller than those of the systolic-parallel and parallel-parallel architectures. Moreover, the generic architecture using three 1-D DWT modules can increase the hardware utilization and throughput so as to decrease the computing time to one half of other multi-level architectures.

4.3.5.2 *JPEG 2000 default (9,7) filter*

The popular JPEG 2000 default lossy (9,7) filter is used as the target 1-D DWT module for comparison because of its good time-frequency decomposition. For simplicity, only the multi-level line-based architectures, which adopt the same number of 1-D DWT modules, are considered. The comparison of the generic architecture using two 1-D DWT modules, systolic-parallel architecture, and parallel-parallel architecture is given in Table 4.4. The lifting-based and the convolution-based DWT modules both adopt the symmetric property of this linear filter.

The systolic and parallel filters also can utilize the symmetric property. Although the generic architecture adopting convolution-based module has nearly the same number of multipliers and adders as those of systolic-parallel and parallel-parallel architectures, the details of the implementation of 1-D DWT modules are extremely different. The multipliers of the generic architectures are all fixed coefficients, whereas those of the other two all require programmable coefficients. Thus, the hardware cost of the generic architecture is smaller than those of the other two architectures.

Furthermore, the generic architecture adopting lifting-based 1-D DWT module outperforms other architectures in all aspects. This outstanding performance comes from the adoption of lifting-based modules, which not only decreases the number of multipliers and adders but also greatly reduces the size of the temporal buffer.

4.4 Line Buffer Wordlength Analysis for Line-Based 2-D DWT

The on-chip line buffer dominates the total area and power of line-based 2-D DWT. Therefore, the line buffer wordlength has to be carefully designed to maintain the quality level due to the dynamic range growing and the round-off errors. In this section, a complete analysis methodology that

Table 4.3 Comparison of 2-D architectures for the general case. Assume $J \to \infty$ and the 1-D DWT module is convolution-based. The data buffer of the proposed architectures is assumed to be $1.5N$ only for comparisons, and it can be further reduced to about $1N$. (The unit of line buffer size is word.)

Architecture	Mul.	Add.	Line Buffer Size	Computing Time	Control Complexity	Hardware Utilization	Throughput
Wu's	$4F$	$4F$	FN	$0.67N^2$	Simple	100%	2
Generic 1-level	$4F$	$4F$	$(F-1/2)N$	$0.67N^2$	Simple	100%	2
Systolic-Parallel	$4F$	$4F$	$(2F+4)N$	N^2	Complex	66.7%	1
Parallel-Parallel	$4F$	$4F$	$(2F+1)N$	N^2	Complex	66.7%	1
Generic 2DWTM	$4F$	$4F$	$(2F-1)N$	N^2	Complex	66.7%	1
Generic 3DWTM	$6F$	$6F$	$(2F-1)N$	$0.5N^2$	Complex	88.9%	2

Table 4.4 Comparison of multi-level 2-D architectures for (9,7) filter ($J \to \infty$). The data buffer of the proposed architectures is assumed to be $1.5N$ for comparisons. (The unit of line buffer size is word.)

Architecture	Mul.	Add.	Line Buffer	DWT Module
Systolic-Parallel	20	36	$22N$	Convolution-based
Parallel-Parallel	20	36	$19N$	Convolution-based
Generic 2DWTM	18	28	$17N$	Convolution-based
Generic 2DWTM	10	16	$11N$	Lifting-based

proposed in [57] is introduced to derive the required wordlength of line buffer given the desired quality level of reconstructed image. This analysis is an extension and a generization of the simple analysis presented in Section 3.5. This methodology can guarantee to avoid overflow of coefficients, and the difference between predicted and experimental quality level is within 0.1dB in terms of PSNR.

4.4.1 *Background to wordlength analysis in line-based DWT*

As can be seen in Section 4.3, the line-based implementation [66] can achieve minimum external memory access with the price of relatively large on-chip line buffer. Line-based implementation has become the mainstream of 2-D DWT VLSI implementation.

Figure 4.21 shows a generic scheme for single-level line-based 2-D DWT in column-row order. The scheme for line-based 2-D DWT in row-column order is shown in Fig. 4.15. The line buffer needed in line-based DWT can be decomposed into data buffer and temporal buffer as shown in Fig. 4.21. The data buffer can be reduced into only few words of registers [73]. Therefore, analysis of data buffer can be skipped.

Temporal buffer is used to buffer the intrinsic register values of every column for column DWT as illustrated in Fig. 4.22. Being different from those registers for pipelining usage, the intrinsic registers are originally defined in the 1-D DWT scheme. Therefore, the intrinsic registers of every column have to be buffered. From the above discussion, the temporal buffer contains (*Image Width* × *Number of Intrinsic Registers*) intrinsic register values. This large size makes temporal buffer be the dominant factor of both area and power in 2-D DWT processor. From the implementation results of [74], the line-buffer occupies 49% total area and 75% total power of the entire 2-D DWT processor. This implementation results will also be shown and discussed in Section 4.5. The wordlength of temporal buffer thus has to be carefully designed. However, there are two phenomena that make the wordlength of temporal buffer in multi-level 2-D DWT hard to be determined.

The first phenomenon is the dynamic range growing effect. In multi-level DWT, the coefficients are iteratively filtered for several times. This may lead to variations in signal dynamic range. If overflow occurs, the reconstructed image quality will be severely degraded.

The second phenomenon is the round-off errors which are induced by

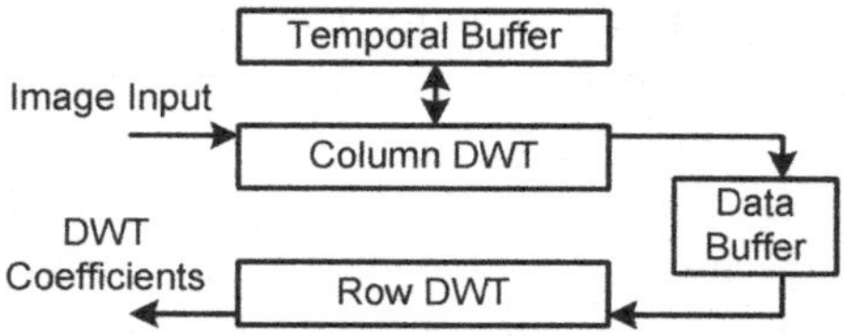

Fig. 4.21 Line-based scheme for single-level column-row 2-D DWT.

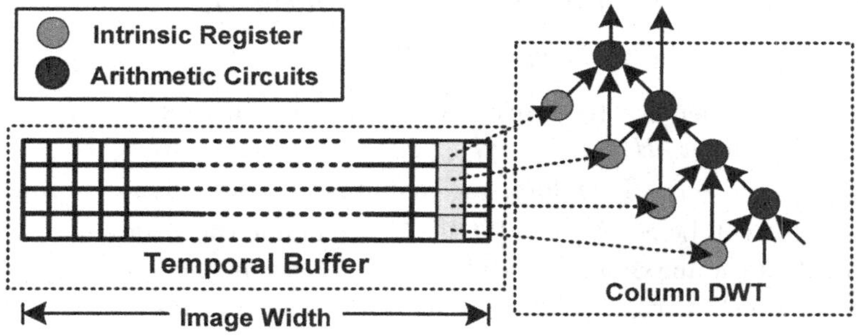

Fig. 4.22 An example of the temporal buffer scheme. There are 4 words of intrinsic register in lifting-based (9,7) filter, and the temporal buffer contains (4×*Image Width*) intrinsic register values.

transferring the floating-point data into data with fixed wordlength. The errors in DWT introduce an upper bound of quality level in image/video system. To control the wordlength such that the reconstructed image can achieve the desired quality level is thus important.

Except the analysis proposed in [57], recently there are some reports presented for wordlength designing [75] [58]. Reference [75] uses an experimental but a theoretical method to determine the wordlength of datapaths. In [58], the round-off errors of only 1-D DWT are analyzed. One error source at each level is assumed. The methodology proposed in [57] analyzed not only round-off errors but dynamic range growing effects of multi-level 2-D DWT. This methodology allows multiple noise sources per decomposition level, and the signal quality is measured in reconstructed image. It is more reasonable.

In this section, the analysis methodology for deriving required line-buffer wordlength in multi-level 2-D DWT proposed in [57] is presented. Wordlength derived with the proposed dynamic range analysis methodology was proved to guarantee the avoidance of overflow. The wordlength required to achieve the desired quality level in reconstructed image can also be derived with the round-off error analysis with a simple distortion model.

The dynamic range analysis methodology and round-off-error analysis methodology are presented in Section 4.4.2 and 4.4.3, respectively. The experimental results in [57] verifying the methodologies are shown in Section 4.4.4. Finally, Section 4.4.5 summaries the wordlength analysis.

4.4.2 *The dynamic range analysis methodology*

4.4.2.1 *Dynamic range analysis of FIR filters*

Suppose a sequence $x(n)$ with dynamic range within $[-S, S]$ is fed into a FIR filter $H(z) = \sum_{i=-L}^{T} h(i)z^{-i}$, the output is $y(n) = \sum_{i=-L}^{T} h(i)x(n-i)$. Therefore, the maximum possible dynamic range at filter output will be $S \times \sum_{i=-L}^{T} |h(i)|$. The dynamic range gain of a system is defined as the maximum possible value of (*output dynamic range/input dynamic range*). For the dynamic range gain G of this filter:

$$G = \sum_{i=-L}^{T} |h(i)|. \tag{4.8}$$

Consider the case of two cascaded FIR filters $H_1(z) = \sum_{i=-L_1}^{T_1}(h_1(i)z^{-i})$ and $H_2(z) = \sum_{i=-L_2}^{T_2} h_2(i)z^{-i}$, these two filters can be merged into an equivalent FIR filter $H_{total}(z)$ with coefficients $h_{total}(n) = \sum_{i=-L_1}^{T_1} h_1(i)h_2(n-i)$. The total dynamic range gain of these two filters G_{total} is:

$$\begin{aligned} G_{total} &= \textstyle\sum_{n=-(L_1+L_2)}^{T_1+T_2} |h_{total}(n)| \\ &= \textstyle\sum_{n=-(L_1+L_2)}^{T_1+T_2} \left|\sum_{i=-L_1}^{T_1} h_1(i)h_2(n-i)\right|. \end{aligned} \tag{4.9}$$

4.4.2.2 *LL-band dynamic range analysis*

The coefficients of LL-band are analyzed because the dynamic range of coefficients of $(n-1)$-th level LL band will affect the dynamic range of intrinsic registers in n-th level. Figure 4.23 shows the Noble identity 1 applied in two-level 1-D DWT. By applying Noble identity, the operations from signal input to each subbands can be equivalent to one filter and one downsampling that will not affect the dynamic range.

For example, if the low-pass filter is $L(z) = \frac{1}{3}z^{-1} + \frac{1}{2} + \frac{1}{3}z$, the dynamic range gain is $|\frac{1}{3}|+|\frac{1}{2}|+|\frac{1}{3}| = \frac{7}{6}$. Taking both column and row directions into

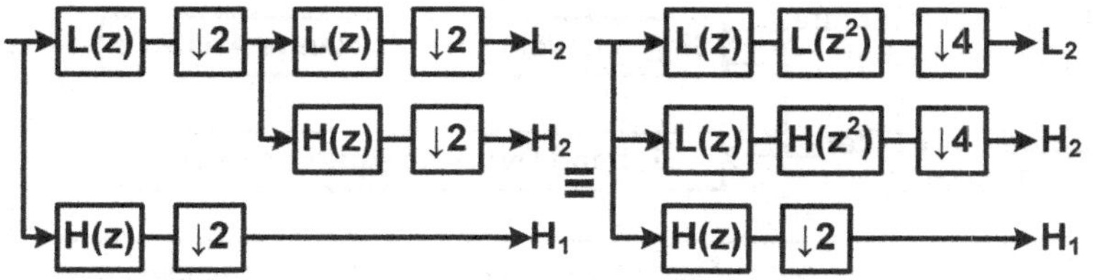

Fig. 4.23 The Noble identity 1 applied in two-level 1-D DWT.

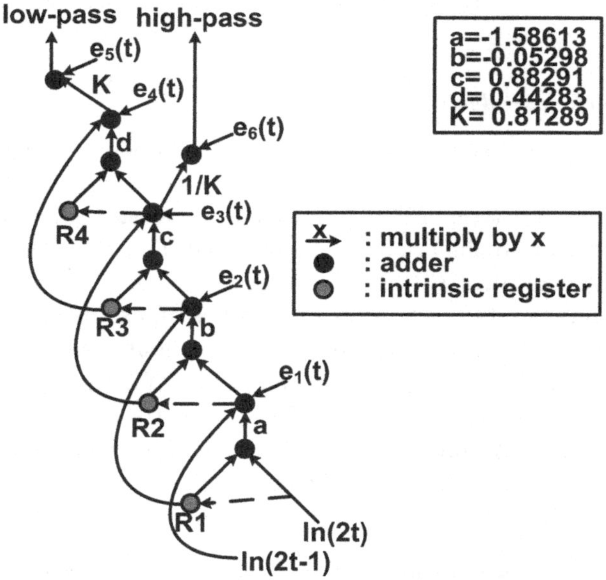

Fig. 4.24 Hardware architecture of lifting-based (9,7) filter.

consideration, the dynamic range gain of first level LL-band is thus $(\frac{7}{6})^2 = \frac{49}{36}$. As for the second level LL-band, the Noble identity 1 has to be applied. The equivalent filter is $L(z)L(z^2) = (\frac{1}{3}z^{-1} + \frac{1}{2} + \frac{1}{3}z)(\frac{1}{3}z^{-2} + \frac{1}{2} + \frac{1}{3}z^2) = \frac{1}{9}z^{-3} + \frac{1}{6}z^{-2} + \frac{5}{18}z^{-1} + \frac{1}{4} + \frac{5}{18}z + \frac{1}{6}z^2 + \frac{1}{9}z^3$, and the corresponding dynamic range gain is $|\frac{1}{9}| + |\frac{1}{6}| + |\frac{5}{18}| + |\frac{1}{4}| + |\frac{5}{18}| + |\frac{1}{6}| + |\frac{1}{9}| = 1.361$. Therefore, the dynamic range gain in the second level LL-band is $1.361^2 = 1.853$. Having the equivalent filter of LL-band at each level, the dynamic range gains of LL-band in all levels can be obtained.

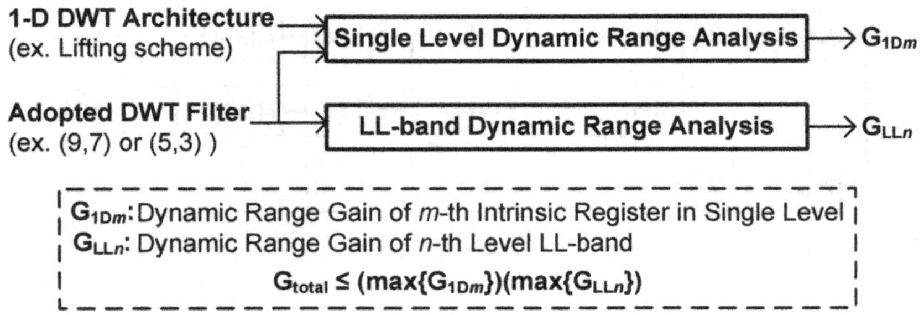

Fig. 4.25 Analysis flow of the dynamic range analysis methodology.

4.4.2.3 *Single level dynamic range analysis*

This part has been described in Section 3.5.1. A brief overview is still given in this section.

Since DWT is a type of FIR filter, intrinsic register values can be represented as linear combinations of input signal, and this relationship can further be an equivalent FIR filter.

Take lifting-based (9,7) filter in Fig. 4.24 as an example, there are four intrinsic registers values. Therefore, there are four equivalent filters for column DWT. For example, the equivalent filter for the intrinsic register "R2"in Fig. 4.24 is $a(z^{-1}+z)+1$. Thus the corresponding filter gain is $2|a|+1 = 4.17226$. All filter gains from input to first-level intrinsic register values in temporal buffer can thus be obtained.

4.4.2.4 *The combined dynamic range analysis methodology*

To analyze the dynamic range gains of the intrinsic register values of all levels is a tedious work. A tight upper bound of dynamic range gain of temporal buffer that can be derived in a much simpler way is thus derived.

Lemma 4.1 *Assume two cascaded FIR filters* $H_1(z) = \sum_{i=-L_1}^{T_1} h_1(i)z^{-i}$ *and* $H_2(z) = \sum_{i=-L_2}^{T_2} h_2(i)z^{-i}$ *have filter gains* G_1 *and* G_2*, respectively. The total filter gain* G_{total} *is smaller than or equal to* G_1G_2.

Proof

From Eq. 3.15:

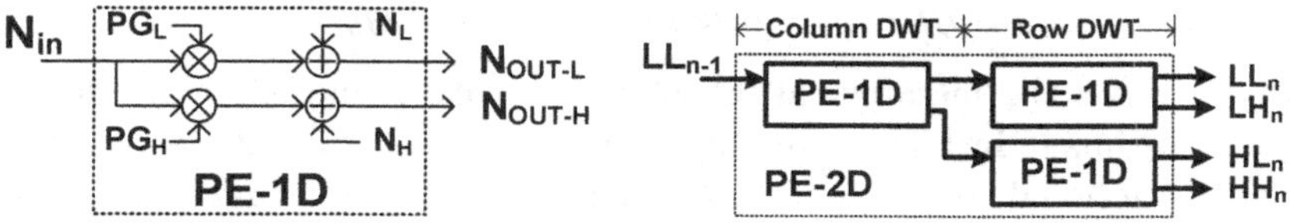

(a) Model for 1-D DWT (b) Model for 2-D DWT

Fig. 4.26 The noise model for single-level DWT.

$$\begin{aligned} G_{total} &= \textstyle\sum_{n=-(L_1+L_2)}^{T_1+T_2} |\sum_{i=-L_1}^{T_1} h_1(i)h_2(n-i)| \\ &\leq \textstyle\sum_{n=-(L_1+L_2)}^{T_1+T_2} \sum_{i=-L_1}^{T_1} |h_1(i)h_2(n-i)| \\ &= (\textstyle\sum_{i=-L_1}^{T_1} |h_1(i)|)(\sum_{j=-L_2}^{T_2} |h_2(j)|) \\ &= G_1G_2. \end{aligned} \tag{4.10}$$

Lemma 4.2 *Let the dynamic range gain from input image to temporal buffer be G_{max}, then $G_{max} \leq (\max_m\{G_{1D_m}\})\times (\max_n\{G_{LL_n}\})$, where G_{1D_m} is the dynamic range gain of the m-th intrinsic register value within single level, and G_{LL_n} is the dynamic range gain from input image to the n-th level LL-band.*

Proof

The relationship from the input to one word in intrinsic register value in n-th level can be taken as the cascade of the relationship from input to $(n-1)$-th level LL-band and the relationship from $(n-1)$-th level LL-band to the intrinsic register value. Assume $G_{total_{m,n}}$ be the filter gain from input to the m-th intrinsic register value in n-th level column DWT. From lemma 4.1:

$$\begin{aligned} G_{max} &= \max_{m,n}\{G_{total_{m,n}}\} \\ &= G_{total_{m1,n1}}(\exists m_1, n_1) \\ &\leq G_{1D_{m1}}G_{LL_{n1}} \\ &\leq (\max_m\{G_{1D_m}\})(\max_n\{G_{LL_n}\}). \end{aligned} \tag{4.11}$$

The analysis flow is shown in Fig. 4.25. G_{LL_n} can be obtained from Section 4.4.2.2, and G_{1D_m} can be obtained from Section 4.4.2.3. With these two values, the upper bound of the dynamic range gain from input image to temporal buffer, G_{max}, can be obtained. Therefore, the wordlength needed to prevent overflow can be obtained.

4.4.3 *The round-off error analysis methodology*

In this section, the hierarchical model to estimate round-off errors in reconstructed image in [57] is presented, and it is a function of the number of bits in fractional part of temporal buffer. The analysis round-off error of 1-D DWT discussed in Section 3.5.2 is also briefly restated in this section.

4.4.3.1 *Model of round-off operations*

As discussed in Section 3.5.2, once a round-off operation is performed, an zero-mean uniformly-distributed and mutually-independent additive error source is introduced, as the $e_1(t)$ to $e_6(t)$ in Fig. 4.24. If there are n fractional bits to represent a coefficient, for error sources $\{e_i(t) : i = 1, 2, ...\}$:

$$E\{e_i(t_1)e_i(t_2)\} = 0, \qquad t_1 \neq t_2 \tag{4.12a}$$

$$E\{e_i(t_1)e_j(t_2)\} = 0 \qquad \forall t_1 t_2, i \neq j \tag{4.12b}$$

$$E\{e_i(t)e_i(t)\} = \sigma^2, \sigma^2 = \int_{-\frac{1}{2^{n+1}}}^{\frac{1}{2^{n+1}}} 2^n x^2 \, dx = \frac{2^{-2n}}{12} \tag{4.12c}$$

4.4.3.2 *Noise power model of single-level 1-D DWT*

To analyze the noise power at 1-D DWT output, the noise sources are taken as real signals in the filter architecture. For example, the contributions of noise source $e_3(t)$ and $e_4(t)$ in Fig. 4.24 to the low-pass output, $(e_{LP}(t))$, are:

$$e_{LP}(t) = Kd(e_3(t) + e_3(t-1)) + Ke_4(t). \tag{4.13}$$

In this case, the estimated noise power $E\{e_{LP}^2(t)\}$ can be derived from the assumptions in Eq. 4.12:

$$\begin{aligned} E\{e_{LP}^2(t)\} &= E\{(Kd(e_3(t) + e_3(t-1)) + Ke_4(t))^2\} \\ &= K^2 d^2 E\{e_3^2(t) + e_3^2(t-1)\} + K^2 E\{e_4^2(t)\} \\ &= (2K^2 d^2 + K^2)\sigma^2. \end{aligned} \tag{4.14}$$

Thus the noise power induced by 1-D DWT can be calculated in this way. If the input signal is with a known noise power, this error will also be modelled as a noise source that satisfies Eqs. 4.12(a) and 4.12(b). If the filter is $H(z) = \sum_{i=-L}^{T} h_i z^{-i}$ and the input noise power is N_{in}, the noise

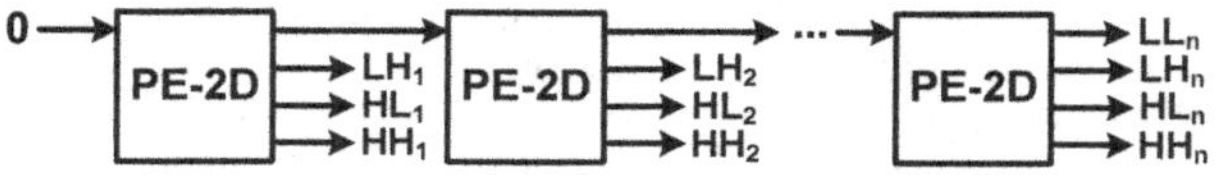

Fig. 4.27 The noise power model of multi-level 2D DWT.

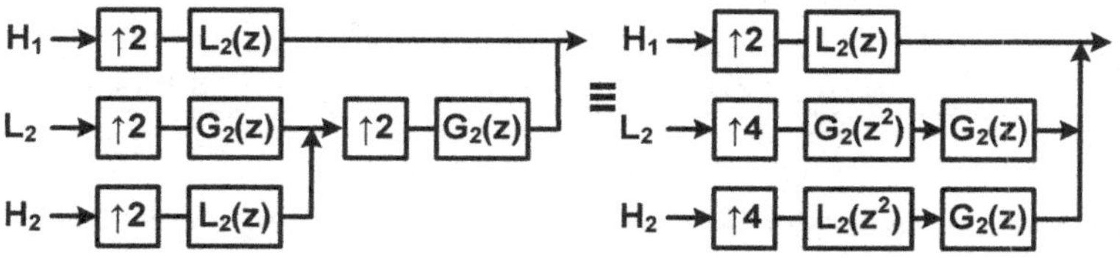

Fig. 4.28 Noble identity 2 applied in two-level 1-D IDWT.

power at filter output induced by input noise, N_{out}^{in}, is:

$$\begin{aligned} N_{out}^{in} &= E\{(\textstyle\sum_{-L}^{T} h_i e_{in}(t-i))^2\} = \textstyle\sum_{-L}^{T} h_i^2 E\{e_{in}^2(t-i)\} \\ &= E\{e_{in}^2(t)\} \times \textstyle\sum_{-L}^{T} h_i^2 = N_{in} \times PG. \end{aligned} \tag{4.15}$$

Where the PG is defined as the power gain of $H(z)$. In the noise model, the input noise will be amplified by PG after the filtering operation.

Figure 4.26a shows this noise model of single level 1-D DWT. As discussed, the fixed-point hardware will introduce round-off error power (N_L, N_H), and the input noise power will be amplified by noise power gains (PG_L, PG_H).

4.4.3.3 *Noise power model of multi-level 2-D DWT*

Figure 4.26b further shows the noise model in single level 2-D DWT. It is a cascade of noise models of 1-D DWT.

The noise model shown in Fig. 4.27 for multi-level 2-D DWT consists of the cascade of the noise models of single level DWT. The input noise power of n-th level is the the LL-band noise power in $(n-1)$-th level. At the first level, the input is the original image, the input noise power is therefore zero.

4.4.3.4 *Noise power analysis in reconstructed image*

In Section 4.4.3.3, the noise powers in all sub-bands are calculated. To estimate the corresponding noise power in reconstructed image, noble identity 2 is utilized. As illustrated in Fig. 4.28, the IDWT can be considered as upsampling, filtering, and addition of each subband. Upsampling by n

Table 4.5 The estimated and the measured dynamic range of reconstructed image with random signals as input image.

	Derived Upper Bound		Experimental Maximum Dynamic Range	
	Value	Required Bits	Value	Required Bits
Lifting-based	731	**10 bits**	549	**10 bits**
Convolution-based	241	**8 bits**	233	**8 bits**

will make the noise power became $\frac{1}{n}$ times, and the equivalent filter can be modelled as a noise power gain as in Section 4.4.3.2.

For example, if an signal with noise power N is upsampled by M then passed to filter $H(z) = \sum_{i=-L}^{T} h(i)z^{-i}$, the noise power at filter output is $\frac{N}{M} \times \sum_{i=-L}^{T} h^2(i)$.

4.4.3.5 *Summary of round-off-error analysis*

In summary, noise power gains (PG_L, PG_H) can be obtained with the DWT filter type. Noise power induced in 1-D DWT (N_L, N_H) can be obtained by analyzing the 1-D hardware architecture. The model of single level 2-D DWT can be obtained by cascading the 1-D noise models. The multi-level 2-D DWT model can be obtained by cascading the single level DWT models. By feeding zero noise power into the multi-level DWT model, the noise power of each subbands can be obtained. Finally, the noise power expression in reconstructed image can be estimated by calculate the power gain of each sub-band using noble identity 2. This noise power expression is a function of the number of fractional bits of data because the value of σ is defined as in Eq. 3.16(c). The noise power in reconstructed image is the mean-square-error of pixels and can directly be mapped into PSNR. Therefore, the required number of fractional bits in temporal buffer can be obtained from the required quality level in image domain.

4.4.4 *Experimental results*

Table 4.5 shows the derived dynamic range upper bound and the experimental maximum dynamic range when random signals are taken as input. Two hardware architectures of DWT, convolutional-based and lifting-based architectures are implemented by Verilog HDL. As can be seen in Table 4.5, the introduced dynamic range upper bound and the experimental maximum

Table 4.6 The estimated and the measured quality of reconstructed image with different number of fractional bits.

Lifting-Based							
Fractional Part	lena	baboon	lake	pepper	Average Experimental Value	**Predicted By Model**	**Difference**
2 bits	52.21	52.27	52.38	52.35	52.30	**52.41**	**0.11**
3 bits	58.36	58.25	58.00	58.26	58.21	**58.43**	**0.21**
4 bits	64.35	64.43	64.31	64.29	64.34	**64.45**	**0.10**
Convolution-Based							
Fractional Part	lena	baboon	lake	pepper	Average Experimental Value	**Predicted By Model**	**Difference**
2 bits	49.43	49.80	49.31	49.55	49.52	**49.66**	**0.14**
3 bits	55.83	55.76	55.80	55.77	55.79	**55.68**	**-0.11**
4 bits	61.75	61.81	61.77	61.79	61.78	**61.70**	**-0.08**

dynamic range yield the same number of required bits in both architectures. Therefore, this upper bound of dynamic range is tight enough in designing the wordlength.

Table 4.6 shows the estimated and the measured quality of reconstructed image with different number of fractional bits in temporal buffer. As can be seen in Table 4.6, the average prediction error of this introduced precision analysis methodology is 0.12 dB, and this prediction error is within the quality variance between different input images. Therefore, the proposed methodology can provide a good reference for designing the number of fractional bits in temporal buffer.

4.4.5 *Summary of wordlength analysis*

Line buffer dominates the area and power in line-based 2-D DWT. In this section, design methodology for the wordlength of line buffer is introduced [57]. The introduced dynamic range analysis methodology can provide a tight upper bound and guarantee to prevent the overflow in line buffer. The round-off error model can predict the image-domain quality level with 0.12 dB difference, and the required fractional wordlength can be obtained from the desired quality level. Both proposed methodologies are simple to be performed.

4.5 On-Chip Memory Implementation Issues

From the VLSI implementation perspective, the dominant factor of hardware cost in 1-D DWT module is the number of multipliers and adders. However, memory issues usually dominate the cost of RAM-based 2-D DWT. Memory access is one of the most important sources of total power, and embedded memory also occupies much area in 2-D DWT [61]. Memory-efficient hardware architecture is therefore an important issue in 2-D DWT VLSI design. In recent years, many 2-D DWT architectures for VLSI implementation are proposed [41, 44, 61, 63, 76].

The multiple-lifting scheme and the corresponding M-scan propsed in [74] are introduced in this section. It is one of memory-efficient VLSI implementations for line-based DWT. Line-based DWT is introduced in Section 4.3. In this section, we will still review it briefly. In conventional 2-D DWT implementation, there are one read and one write of line buffer every cycle, and the line buffer has to be a two-port RAM.

Under the constraint of equal throughput per second, the average memory bandwidth can be reduced to 50% or lower by use of the multiple-lifting scheme. The maximum number of memory access within a clock cycle is also reduced to one access such that the line buffer can be a single-port RAM. The reduction of memory bandwidth in temporal buffer results in the reduction of total power, and the change from two-port RAM to single-port RAM reduces about 50% area of temporal buffer. The reduction of power and area is dependent on the adopted fabrication process. By use of the corresponding M-scan, the data buffer can be eliminated, which avoids the overhead of multiple-lifting scheme.

This Section is structured as follows. Section 4.5.1 gives an overview of memory structure for line-based DWT. Section 4.5.2 and Section 4.5.3 will discuss the multiple-lifting scheme and the corresponding M-scan, respectively. Comparisons of implementation results between multiple-lifting scheme and the conventional line-based scheme with eliminated data buffer will be presented in section 4.5.4.

4.5.1 *Overview*

As discussed in Section 4.4.1, the line buffer needed in line-based DWT can be decomposed into data buffer and temporal buffer. Data buffer is used to buffer the intermediate coefficients after column DWT and temporal buffer is used to buffer the register values inside column DWT core. The temporal buffer may have to buffer the register values in 1-D DWT core at every column. The temporal buffer size is thus the product of image width and the number of registers within the 1-D DWT core.

One memory-efficient VLSI implementation is using a proper Z-scan to eliminate the data buffer [72]. However, because the temporal buffer has to represent registers inside 1-D DWT module, its maximum number of memory access within one cycle is one read and one write so that the temporal buffer has to be a two-port RAM, as the lifting-based architecture in column DWT shown in Fig. 4.29. The computation nodes in Fig. 4.29 are combinational components such as adders, multipliers and nets. The lifting-based (9,7) filter is used for illustration throughout this section.

4.5.2 *Schemes to reduce memory bandwidth*

In this section, two ways to reduce memory bandwidth of line buffer are presented. The multiple-lifting scheme will be discussed in more detail.

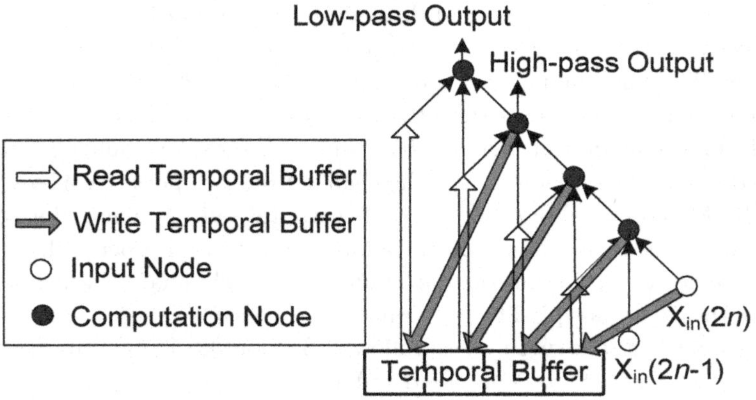

Fig. 4.29 Lifting-based (9,7) filter for line-based column DWT.

There are two important goals of multiple-lifting scheme. The first one is to reduce the average memory bandwidth of temporary buffer and thus reduce the power consumption. The other one is to reduce the maximum number of memory access within one cycle in temporal buffer to one read/write such that the temporal buffer can be a single-port RAM and the memory area can thus be reduced.

The discussion throughout this section will focus on 2-D DWT in column-row order. The comparisons are all under the assumption that the throughput per second is equal in each scheme. All discussed schemes and data scans can be easily modified to be suitable to 2-D DWT in row-column order.

4.5.2.1 *Reducing average memory bandwidth using parallel processing*

One way to reduce the memory bandwidth is to use parallel processing to raise the throughput per clock cycle such that the total number of memory access for the same number of input pixels will be reduced. Under the constraint of the same throughput per second, the clock rate and memory bandwidth of parallel processing thus can be reduced.

Fig. 4.30 shows such a two-parallel processing implementation in which two sets of processing element (PE) are adopted. A set of PE is defined as the combinational circuits including adders and multipliers in 1-D DWT of Fig. 4.29. One action of reading data from temporal buffer can produce two low-pass coefficients and two high-pass coefficients. The clock rate and

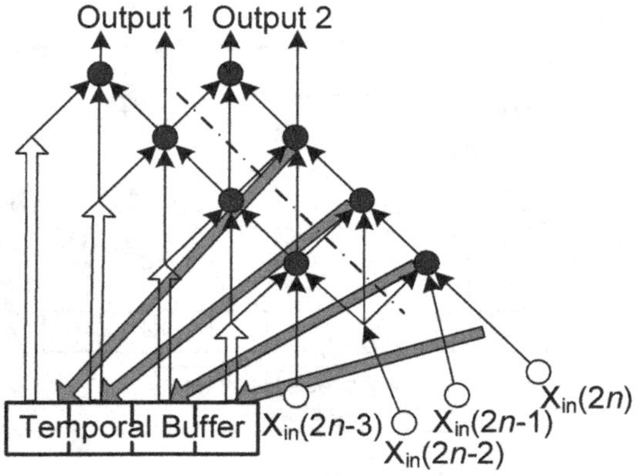

Fig. 4.30 Two-parallel processing implementation.

average memory bandwidth of temporal buffer thus can be halved compared with the architecture in Fig. 4.29. Continuing adding PEs in this way will result in similar multiple-parallel processing implementation, the average memory bandwidth of temporal buffer can be arbitrarily decreased.

The multiple-parallel processing implementation, however, results in increasing PE number that raises the cost of DWT core. Moreover, because one-read and one-write are still required within one cycle in multiple-parallel processing implementation, the temporal buffer still has to be a two-port RAM. The multiple-parallel processing thus trades the increase of area for the decrease of RAM access frequency.

4.5.2.2 *Two-lifting scheme*

To overcome the disadvantages of parallel processing implementation, the multiple-lifting scheme is proposed in [74]. The basic concept of multiple-lifting scheme is to maintain the clock rate as conventional line-based implementation discussed in Section 4.5.1 and average out the concentrated processing of multiple-parallel processing implementation into every cycle, thus only one set of PE is required and the maximum memory access within one cycle can be reduced.

Take Fig. 4.30 as an example, if the signals "Output 1"and "Output 2" show up in different cycles, only one set of PE is required. To maintain the low average memory bandwidth, registers are used to buffer the calculated data along the dashed line in Fig. 4.30. Moreover, the reading and writing of memory can be arranged in different clock cycles such that the maximum

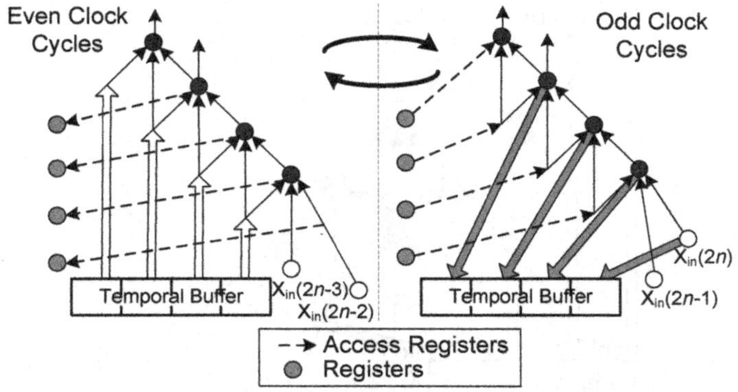

Fig. 4.31 The two-lifting scheme.

memory access within one clock cycle is one read/write, and the temporal buffer can be a single-port RAM.

The two-lifting scheme is shown in Fig. 4.31. In even cycles, data are read from temporal buffer, and the calculated data are buffered in registers. In odd cycles, data are read from registers, and the calculated data are written back into temporal buffer. The average memory bandwidth of temporal buffer is halved, and only one read or one write of temporal buffer is required per clock cycle. The two-lifting scheme thus combines three advantages: halved average memory bandwidth, only one set of PE, and single-port temporal buffer.

4.5.2.3 *N-lifting scheme*

The concept of the N-lifting scheme is quite similar to that of the two-lifting scheme. The N sets of PE in N-parallel processing implementation are folded into one PE, and this results in the N-lifting scheme. The scheduling of temporal buffer in four-lifting scheme is shown in Fig. 4.32 as an example of the multiple-lifting scheme. The average memory bandwidth of temporal buffer in four-lifting scheme thus can be further reduced to half of that in two-lifting scheme while still one full-utilized PE is needed.

In Table 4.7, the multiple-lifting schemes are compared with the conventional line-based scheme in Fig. 4.29 and multiple-parallel processing implementation in Fig. 4.30. The multiple-lifting schemes reduce the average memory bandwidth and change the temporal buffer from two-port RAM to single-port RAM while only one set of PE is needed.

Table 4.7 Comparisons of temporal buffer in different schemes with the same output throughput per second. B is the average memory bandwidth (number of memory access per second) of temporal buffer in conventional line-based implementation.

	Average Memory Bandwidth	Number of Processing Elements of Column DWT	Maximal Memory Access Within One Cycle	Type of Temporal Buffer
Convolutional Line-based	B	1	One Read and One Write	Two-port
Two-parallel Processing	B/2	2	One Read and One Write	Two-port
N-parallel Processing	B/N	N	One Read and One Write	Two-port
Two-Lifting Scheme	B/2	1	One Read/Write	Single-port
Four-Lifting Scheme	B/4	1	One Read/Write	Single-port
N-Lifting Scheme	B/N	1	One Read/Write	Single-port

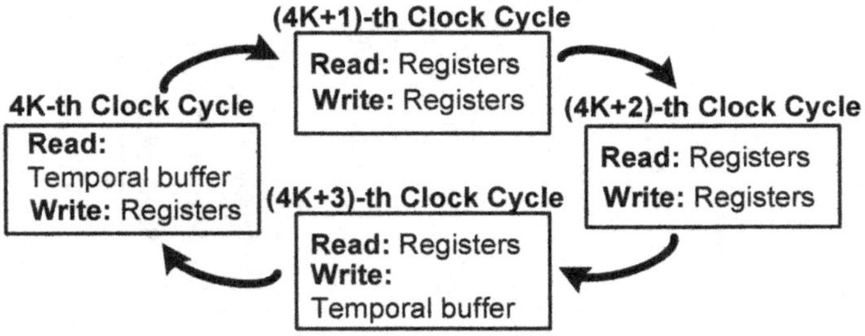

Fig. 4.32 The scheduling of memory access in the four-lifting scheme.

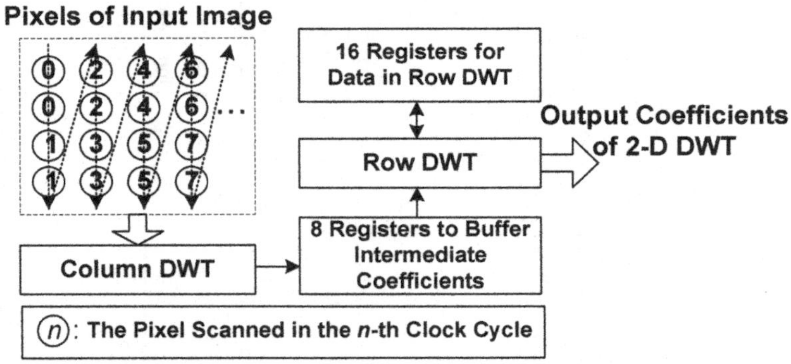

Fig. 4.33 The M-scan and 2-D implementation for two-lifting scheme with (9,7) filter.

4.5.3 *The M-scan for multiple-lifting scheme*

In Section 4.5.2, the multiple-lifting schemes reduce the power and area of temporal buffer. To eliminate the data buffer, the M-scan suited for multiple-lifting scheme is also introduced in this section.

4.5.3.1 *M-scan for two-lifting scheme*

Figure 4.33 shows the M-scan for two-lifting scheme. The main idea of this M-shape data scan is to use out the intermediate coefficients after column DWT as soon as possible and hence the storage requirement of intermediate coefficients after column DWT can be minimized. Because the scheduling of two-lifting scheme is periodic of two clock cycles as suggested in Fig. 4.31, the length in column direction of the M-scan has to be four pixels. The row DWT has to be performed right after the intermediate coefficients after column DWT are stored in registers for using out coefficients as soon as

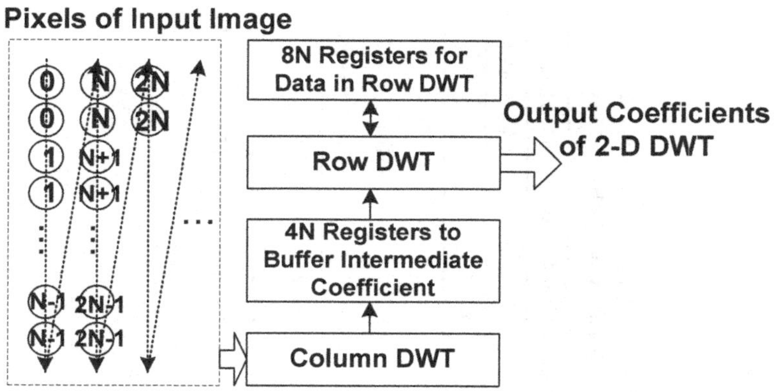

Fig. 4.34 The M-scan and 2-D implementation for N-lifting scheme with (9,7) filter.

possible. Because two pixels in row direction have to be fed in row DWT each cycle, eight ($2 \times 4 = 8$) intermediate coefficients after column DWT have to be buffered.

The register values of the row DWT core in each of the four rows in M-scan also have to be buffered. The functionality of this additional buffer in row direction is similar to that of temporal buffer in column direction. The dimension of this additional buffer is four times of the number of registers in row DWT core. If lifting-based (9,7) filter in Fig. 4.29 is adopted, the size of this buffer is sixteen words ($4 \times 4 = 16$). Registers are sufficient for this small buffer.

4.5.3.2 *M-scan for N-lifting scheme*

Figure 4.34 shows the M-data scan for N-lifting scheme to eliminate data buffer. As discussed in Section 4.5.2.3, the scheduling of N-lifting scheme is periodic of N clock cycles. The length in column direction of the proposed M-data scan for N-lifting scheme is thus 2N pixels.

Because two pixels in row direction have to be fed in row DWT each cycle, 4N ($2 \times 2N = 4N$) intermediate coefficients after column DWT have to be buffered. Register values of row DWT in each of the 2N rows also have to be buffered. The dimension of this additional register array is the product of 2N and the number of registers in 1-D DWT core. If lifting-based (9,7) filter is adopted, the size of this buffer is 8N ($2N \times 4 = 8N$) words as shown in Fig. 4.34.

Table 4.8 Comparisons between multiple-lifting scheme and conventional line-based scheme with eliminated data buffer under the same throughput per second. All three schemes have the same critical path and operate at clock frequency = 77MHz.

Implementation	Total Area (μm^2)	Area of RAM (μm^2)	Total Power (mW)	Power of RAM (mW)	Overhead	
					Area	Power
Convolutional Line-based	587737	288786	129	95.95	-	-
Two-lifting Scheme	422438	131435	79.44	37.6		
(Reduced Amount)	165298	157351	49.56	58.35	-7947	8.79
	(28%)	(54%)	(38%)	(61%)	(-1%)	(6.8%)
Four-lifting Scheme	452978	131435	64.52	21.02		
(Reduced Amount)	134758	157351	64.48	74.93	21593	10.45
	(23%)	(54%)	(50%)	(78%)	(3.7%)	(8.1%)

Overhead = Reduction of RAM - Total Reduction

4.5.4 *Experimental results*

This section presents the implementation results presented in [74]. Three schemes are implemented using (9,7) filter with the same throughput per second. Lifting-based is implemented by flipping structure [49] in all three schemes. The image width is 128 pixels. The first scheme is the conventional line-based lifting architecture in Fig. 4.29 with the non-overlapped stripe-based scan [76] of two pixels stripe width to eliminate the data buffer. The second and third schemes are the two-lifting scheme and four-lifting scheme introduced in this section with the corresponding M-scan, respectively. The comparisons of these three schemes are listed in Table 4.8 in which Artisan 0.18 μm cell library and Artisan 0.18 μm RAM compiler are used. The area information is reported by Synopsys Design Vision and the power information is reported by Synopsys PrimePower. All three schemes are synthesized in the same critical path of 13ns because all three schemes have the same critical path within 1-D DWT core.

Firstly, the total area is reduced by 28% in the two-lifting scheme, which mainly comes from the reduction in the area of RAM. This is due to the required temporal buffer is changed from two-port RAM to single-port RAM. The area of the four-lifting scheme is slightly larger than the two-lifting because there are more registers needed in four-lifting scheme as discussed in Section 4.5.3.2.

Secondly, the total power is reduced 38% and 50% with two-lifting scheme and four-lifting scheme, respectively. The power of RAM is reduced by 61% in two-lifting scheme because the average memory bandwidth is halved and temporal buffer becomes single-port. The power of RAM in four-lifting scheme is reduced by 78% because the average memory bandwidth is further decreased. The reduced power in RAM is always slightly higher than the reduced total power. Because some registers have to take over the task of buffering when temporal buffer is not accessed, some power is consumed.

Finally, the slight overhead is from the registers buffering the intermediate coefficients and data in row DWT. The overhead of area in two-lifting scheme in Table 4.8 is negative because of the variation of circuit synthesis. The power in these registers is reduced greatly by using the clock gating technique. As can be seen in the discussion above, the multiple-lifting scheme can reduce both total power and total area significantly. The temporal buffer size is proportional to image width, but the overhead and cores of 1-D DWT are independent of image width. Therefore, the reduction ratio will be further increased as longer image width is required.

4.5.5 *Summary*

The on-chip line buffer dominates the total area and power of line-based 2-D DWT. In this section, several schemes are discussed in terms of the total area and power of on-chip memory.

The multiple-lifting scheme is introduced to provide a memory-efficient scheme for line-based VLSI implementation. Under the same throughput per second, the two-lifting scheme and four-lifting scheme can halve and quarter the average memory bandwidth of temporal buffer, respectively. The temporal buffer can also be a single-port RAM instead of a two-port RAM. Moreover, the data buffer can still be eliminated with the proposed M-scan. From experiment results, the multiple-lifting scheme can reduce both the total area and total power significantly while maintaining the same throughput per second as anticipated. The M-scan is designed for line-based but degenerated into the category of non-overlapped stripe-based scan. However, the intention of detailed implementation is actually different.

Chapter 5

Practical Design Examples of 2-D DWT: JPEG 2000 Encoder Systems

In this chapter, we take the latest still image coding standard, JPEG 2000, as an example to illustrate the system integration issues of DWT module. Based on different system schedulings of JPEG 2000, various suitable architectures of DWT module can be developed by applying our analysis in previous chapters. The organization of this chapter is as follows. In Sec. 5.1, an overview of JPEG 2000 algorithm is given. What follows is the design issue of JPEG 2000 hardware architecture. In Sec. 5.3 and Sec. 5.4, two types of JPEG 2000 encoding systems and the corresponding DWT implementations are introduced. The first introduced encoding scheduling is the tile pipelined scheduling [77]. This tile-level pipeline implies the possibility of simple DWT implementation. The second introduced encoding scheduling is the tile pipelined scheduling [78, 103]. To eliminate the tile buffer required in tile pipeline scheduling, complex DWT control is required in the stripe pipeline scheduling.

5.1 Introduction to JPEG 2000 Algorithm

JPEG 2000 [79] [7] [80] is the latest still image coding standard. The goal of developing JPEG 2000 is to create a new image coding system for different types of image (bi-level, gray level, color, and multi-component), with different characteristics (natural images, scientific, medical, remote sensing, text, rendered graphics, *etc.*) allowing different imaging models (client/server, real-time transmission, image library archival, limited buffer and bandwidth resources, *etc.*) preferably within a unified system. Besides, JPEG 2000 can provide better coding efficiency or, equivalently, higher image quality than the existing standards. In this chapter, Part I, which is the core coding system, of the JPEG 2000 standard is presented. Unlike

JPEG [1], JPEG 2000 adopts the Discrete Wavelet Transform (DWT) as the transform unit and the Embedded Block Coding with Optimized Truncation (EBCOT) as the entropy coding engine. The EBCOT comprises of the Embedded Block Coding (EBC) and the Rate-Distortion Optimization (RDO). By use of the DWT and the EBCOT, the above goals can be achieved by a unified coding system without compromise of coding efficiency.

5.1.1 *Coding system overview*

The JPEG 2000 coding system is shown in Fig. 5.1. It has three major functional parts: the DWT, the uniform scalar quantization, and the EBCOT. In JPEG 2000, rate control is usually achieved by the RDO, and therefore the uniform scalar quantization is not used to control the bit rates. Instead, the quantization is usually used as the digitization of DWT coefficients when the floating points transform kernel, the 9-7 filter, is used. Thus, we will not discuss this part hereafter since it's not critical to the system.

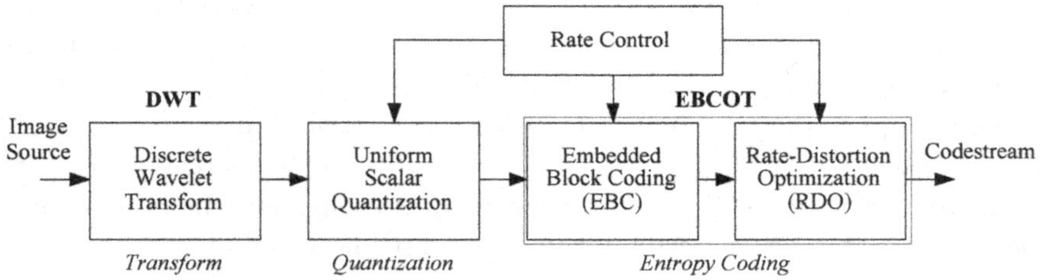

Fig. 5.1 JPEG 2000 encoder system. JPEG 2000 adopts the DWT as the transform unit and the EBCOT as the entropy coding engine.

In JPEG 2000, an image is decomposed into various abstract levels for coding, as shown in Fig. 5.2. An image is partitioned into tiles to be independently coded. By encoding each tile independently, the JPEG 2000 can provide random access to the whole image. Each tile is decomposed by the DWT into some subbands with certain decomposition levels. For example, seven subbands are generated by two-level decomposition. Resolution scalability can be supported by decoding bit-streams at various decomposition levels. One subband is further divided into code-blocks to be processed by the EBC. The DWT coefficients are represented as sign-magnitude for the

EBC. The detailed operations of the DWT and the EBC are described in the following sections.

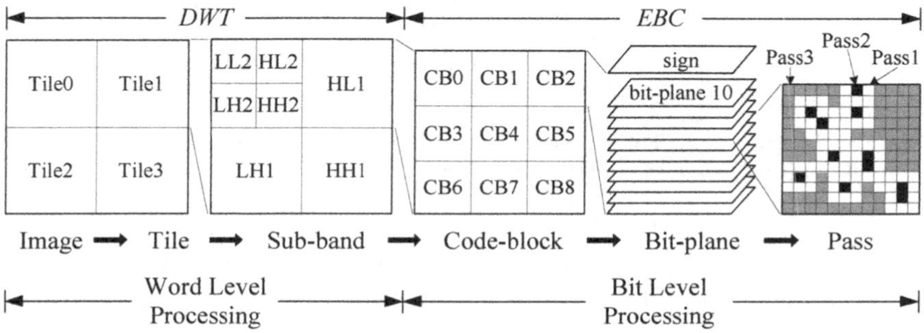

Fig. 5.2 Image decomposition in JPEG 2000. An image is decomposed into tiles, sub-bands, Code-Blocks (CB), bit-planes, and coding passes.

5.1.2 *Discrete wavelet transform*

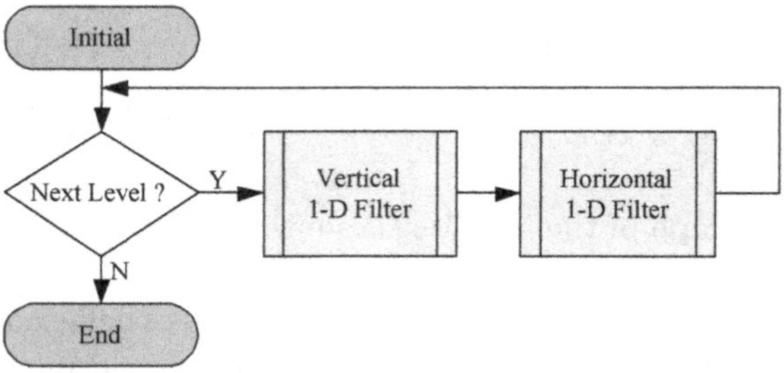

Fig. 5.3 Flowchart of the 2D DWT. The 2D DWT is accomplished by cascading two 1D DWT, vertical filter followed by horizontal filter.

The flowchart of the DWT is shown in Fig. 5.3. The two-dimensional (2D) DWT is accomplished by cascading two one-dimensional (1D) DWT. Please note that in JPEG 2000 encoder, the 2-D DWT must be accomplished in a column-row order as in Fig. 5.4. Multi-level decomposition is accomplished by recursively 2D decomposition on the LL band. After L decomposition levels, there will be $3L + 1$ subbands.

There are two types of 1-D DWT filter defined in JPEG 2000 standard.

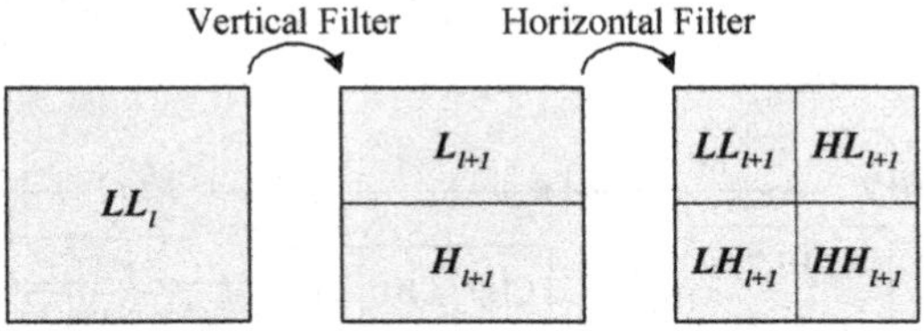

Fig. 5.4 Diagram of 2D DWT decomposition. For the l-th decomposition level, the LL band of the $(l-1)$-th level are decomposed into four subbands.

The first one is the integer 5-3 filter, and the second one is the 9-7 filter. In this section, both filters will be introduced.

5.1.2.1 *5-3 reversible filter*

The 5-3 reversible integer wavelet filter [81], also called the Le Gall 5-3 filter, described in this section is defined using lifting-based filtering. Let $x(\cdot)/y(\cdot)$ denote the input/output signal. The odd-indexed output is calculated by

$$y(2n+1) = x(2n+1) - \left\lfloor \frac{x(2n) + x(2n+2)}{2} \right\rfloor . \tag{5.1}$$

Then, the even-indexed output is calculated by

$$y(2n) = x(2n) + \left\lfloor \frac{y(2n-1) + y(2n+1) + 2}{4} \right\rfloor . \tag{5.2}$$

The signal flow graph of the 5-3 filter is shown in Fig. 5.5. The reason why the filter is called the 5-3 filter can be observed from the figure. The first number, 5, which comes from that every low-pass coefficient is obtained by computations of 5 input pixels. Similarly, the second number, 3, comes from that every high-pass coefficient is obtained by computations of 3 input pixels. Note that the low-pass and high-pass filters are performed in an interlaced order, in which even outputs are the low-pass coefficients and the odd outputs are the high-pass ones.

5.1.2.2 *9-7 irreversible filter*

The Daubechies 9-7 filter [82] is the other recommended filter in JPEG 2000. Its energy compaction capability is better than that of the Le Gall 5-3 filter. However, it is irreversible filter since its filter coefficients are floating points and the DWT coefficients are represented in finite precision. For the 9-7

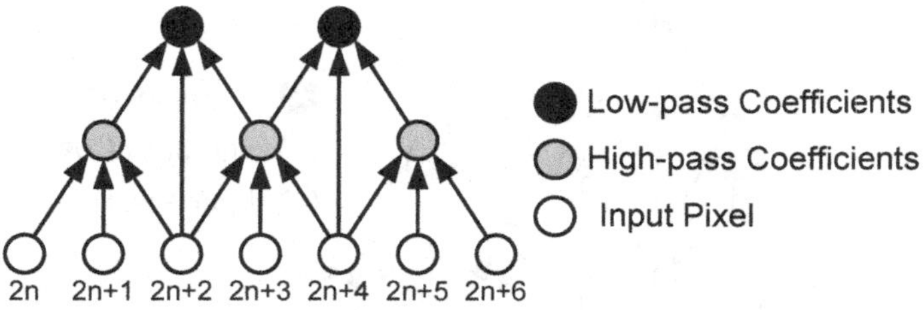

Fig. 5.5 Signal flow graph of the 5-3 filter. Even-indexed coefficients are low-pass coefficients and odd-indexed coefficients are high-pass coefficients.

Table 5.1 Filter Coefficients of the 9-7 Filter

Filter Coefficients	Value
α	-1.586134342059924
β	-0.052980118572961
γ	0.882911075530934
δ	0.443506852043971
K	1.230174104914001

filter, four lifting steps and two scaling steps are defined. At the first two lifting steps, $\hat{y}$ are defined by

$$\begin{cases} \hat{y}(2n+1) = x(2n+1) + \alpha[x(2n) + x(2n+2)] \\ \hat{y}(2n) = x(2n) + \beta[\hat{y}(2n-1) + \hat{y}(2n+1)] \end{cases} . \tag{5.3}$$

The last two lifting steps and the two scaling steps are combined as

$$\begin{cases} y(2n+1) = K\{\hat{y}(2n+1) + \gamma[\hat{y}(2n) + \hat{y}(2n+2)]\} \\ y(2n) = (\frac{1}{K})\{\hat{y}(2n) + \delta[y(2n-1) + y(2n+1)]\} \end{cases} . \tag{5.4}$$

The approximate value of filter coefficients is given in Table 5.1. For the exact expressions of the filter coefficients, please refer to the JPEG 2000 standard [7]. The signal flow graph of the 9-7 filter is shown in Fig. 5.6. Although having different number of filtering taps, the input and output of the 5-3 filter and the 9-7 filter are the same except for two additional latency of the 9-7 filter.

5.1.3 *Embedded block coding*

Embedded Block Coding with Optimized Truncation (EBCOT) [83] [84] is adopted as the entropy coding algorithm of JPEG 2000. EBCOT is a two-

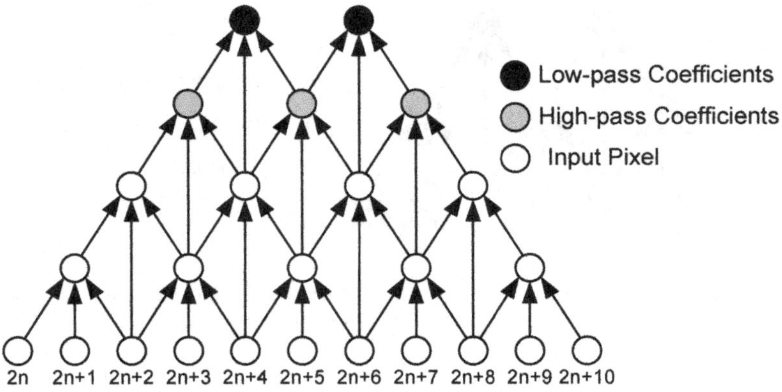

Fig. 5.6 Signal flow graph of the 9-7 filter. Even-indexed coefficients are low-pass coefficients and odd-indexed coefficients are high-pass coefficients.

tiered algorithm, as shown in Fig. 5.7. The tier-1 part is the EBC, which is composed of the Context Formation (CF) and the Arithmetic Encoder (AE). The bit stream formed by the EBC is called the embedded bit stream and is passed to the tier-2 for rate control. Given a target bit rate, tier-2 truncates the embedded bit streams to minimize the overall distortion.

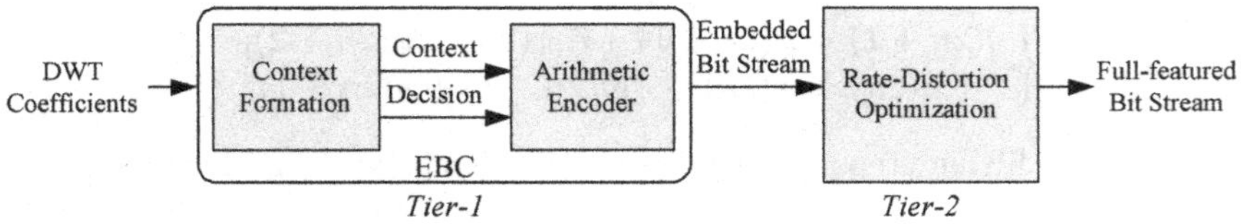

Fig. 5.7 Diagram of the EBCOT algorithm. It is a two-tiered algorithm, in which tier-1 is also called the embedded block coding.

The basic coding unit of the EBC is a code-block with size $N \times N \times W$, where N is the code-block width and W is the bit-width of a DWT coefficient. Figure 5.8 shows an example of $N = 64$ and $W = 11$. Unlike the DWT that processes a word per operation, the EBC is a bit-level processing algorithm. A code-block is coded in a bit-plane by bit-plane manner, from the Most Significant Bit (MSB) bit-plane to the Least Significant Bit (LSB) bit-plane. Each bit-plane is further divided into three coding passes, which will be elaborated in the next section. The division of a bit-plane to three coding passes has the advantages of high coding gain and fine granularity rate control, which will be evident in the following sections. A magnitude bit is called a sample coefficient to prevent from confusing with the coefficient that represents an entire word. Within a coding pass, sample coefficients are coded in a stripe-scan order as shown in Fig. 5.8.

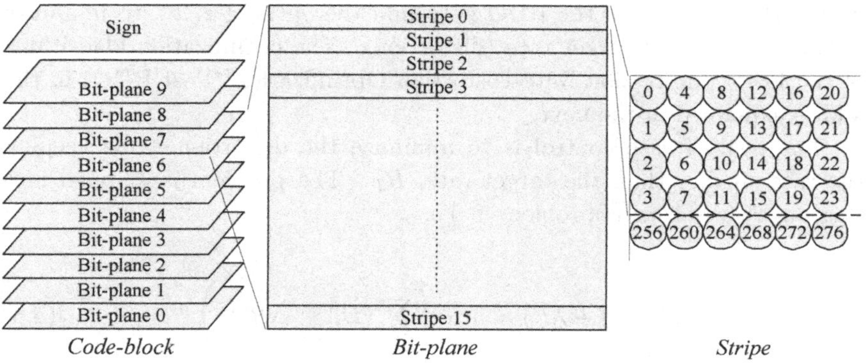

Fig. 5.8 Diagram of code-block, bit-plane, and stripes. A 64 × 64 bit-plane is divided into sixteen 4 × 64 stripes.

5.1.4 *Rate-distortion optimization*

In this section, the RDO algorithm in JPEG 2000 is reviewed. Each coding pass is a candidate of truncation point of a code-block. For convenience, we define a consecutive integer set to represent all candidates. The candidate corresponding to Pass m of the bit-plane k in the code-block i, B_i, is represented as

$$n_i(k, m) = 3k - m + 3. \tag{5.5}$$

In the following discussion, n_i is used to represent $n_i(k, m)$ for simplicity. Truncating B_i at n_i results in the rate $R_i^{n_i}$ and the distortion $D_i^{n_i}$. The total bit rate, R, and the total distortion, D, of the image are

$$R = \sum_i R_i^{n_i} \tag{5.6}$$

and

$$D = \sum_i D_i^{n_i}. \tag{5.7}$$

The set of selected truncation points for all B_i is denoted as z, i.e. $z = \{n_i\}$. The goal of the RDO is to find the optimal z, z^*, to minimize distortion (rate) at target rate (distortion). The optimization algorithms of the Post-compression Rate-Distortion Optimization (Post-RDO) in the VM is explained in the next.

The goal of rate control is to minimize the distortion while keeping the rate smaller than the target rate, R_T. The problem is mapped into Lagrange optimization problem [83] as

$$min(D + \lambda R) = min\left(\sum_i (D_i^{n_i} + \lambda R_i^{n_i})\right), \tag{5.8}$$

where λ is the Lagrange multiplier. To minimize $J = D+\lambda R$, the derivative of J,

$$\partial J = \partial D + \lambda \partial R = 0, \tag{5.9}$$

is set to zero. Thus, the optimal λ, λ^*, can be obtained as

$$\lambda^* = -\frac{\partial D}{\partial R}, \tag{5.10}$$

where $\frac{\partial D}{\partial R}$ is the slope of the R-D curve. Since the R-D curve is piece-wise linear, the slope corresponding to n_i in B_i, $S_i^{n_i}$, can be obtained by

$$S_i^{n_i} = \frac{\Delta D_i^{n_i}}{\Delta R_i^{n_i}} = \frac{D_i^{n_i} - D_i^{n_i+1}}{R_i^{n_i} - R_i^{n_i+1}}. \tag{5.11}$$

The physical meaning of $S_i^{n_i}$ is how fast the distortion is reduced with the increase of the rate when B_i is truncated at n_i. With decrease of the value of n_i, $S_i^{n_i}$ must be strictly decreasing. If some $S_i^{n_i}$ violates this property, the method about merging slopes [83] is used to guarantee the monotonic-decreasing property. In [83], it has been proved that λ^* and z^* are optimal if both

$$\begin{cases} -S_i^{n_i} \geq \lambda^*, \; n_i \geq n_i^* \\ -S_i^{n_i} < \lambda^*, \; n_i < n_i^* \end{cases} \tag{5.12}$$

and

$$\sum_i R_i^{n_i^*} \leq R_T \tag{5.13}$$

are satisfied, where n_i^* is the optimal truncation point for B_i, i.e. $z^* = \{n_i^*\}$. For convenience, the rate control problem is expressed by $\pounds(\lambda, D(R_T))$. There is an interesting property that only $\Delta D_i^{n_i}$ and $\Delta R_i^{n_i}$ are required to solve $\pounds(\lambda, D(R_T))$ instead of $D_i^{n_i}$ and $R_i^{n_i}$. That is to say the optimization can be achieved when available n_i is sufficiently close to n_i^* and the corresponding $S_i^{n_i}$ is also close to λ^*, even if the R-D information of the unavailable n_i is unknown.

5.1.5 *Coding efficiency of JPEG 2000*

In this section, we'll compare three coding standards, JPEG, H.264/AVC intra coder, and JPEG 2000, in various aspects, such as coding performance, computational complexity, and functionality. Although H.264/AVC is a video coding standard, its intra coder performs very well compared with the previous video standard. Thus, people may wish to use the H.264/AVC intra coder as a image coder. Thus, it's worth to evaluate the performance of the standard.

In order to make a fair comparison, all options lead to best coding performance are selected for all the standards. For the JPEG, the optimization option of the software in [85] is selected. For the H.264/AVC, the configuration file of main profile is used. Moreover, the "LevelIDC" is set as 51 to support large image size and the "RDOptimization" is turned on. For JPEG 2000, images are coded by 9-7 filter with 5 decomposition levels without tiling and the code-block size is 64×64. The RD curves of JPEG are obtained by varying quality index. For H.264/AVC, all the Macro-Blocks (MB) of an image are coded by the same Quantization Parameter (QP) to obtain a point on the RD curves. Since rate control is supported by the JPEG 2000, the RD curves are generated by directly assigning the target bit rate.

Figure 5.9 and Figure 5.10 show the RD curves of all the test images. Several phenomena can be observed. Firstly, the coding efficiency of JPEG is much lower than that of JPEG 2000 and H.264/AVC, and the difference ranges from 2 dB in low bit rate and 5 dB in high bit rate. Secondly, H.264/AVC always outperforms JPEG 2000 at image quality higher than 50 dB. This might because of the problem of rate control, which will be

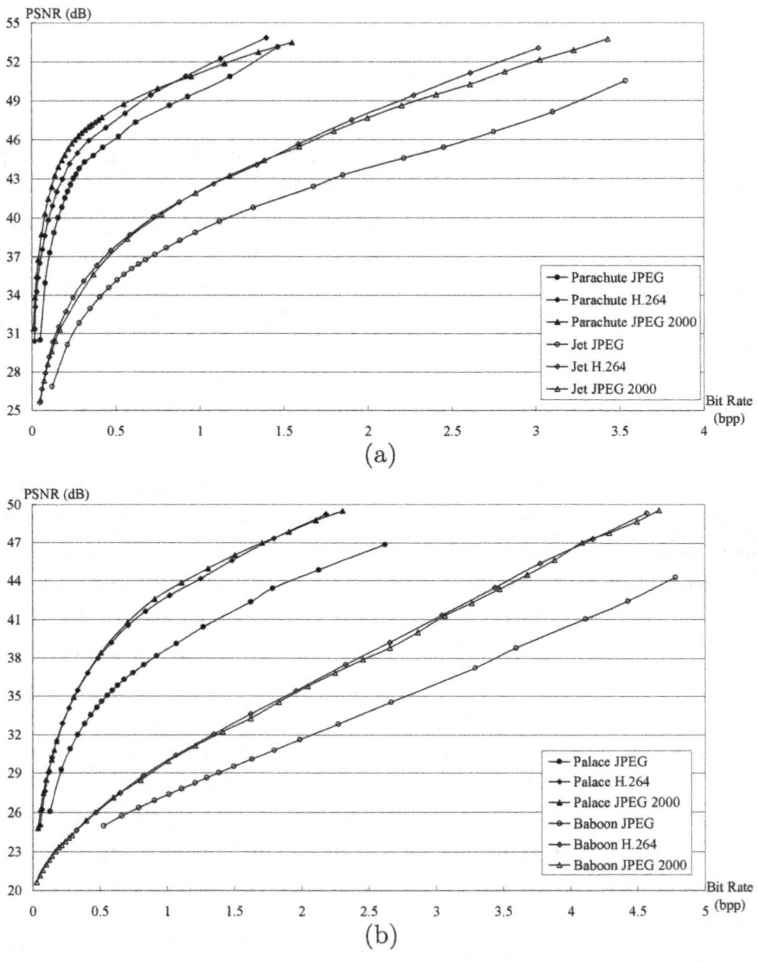

Fig. 5.9 Comparisons of JPEG, H.264/AVC, and JPEG 2000. (a) R-D curves of Parachute and Jet. (b) R-D curves of Palace and Baboon.

discussed later. Finally, the coding efficiency of JPEG 2000 is better than that of H.264/AVC for large images. The reason is that the DWT favors large image size.

It is very interesting that H.264/AVC always outperforms JPEG 2000 at high bit rate regardless of images or image sizes. This somewhat fits in with the results in previous rate control works [86] [87]. In the previous

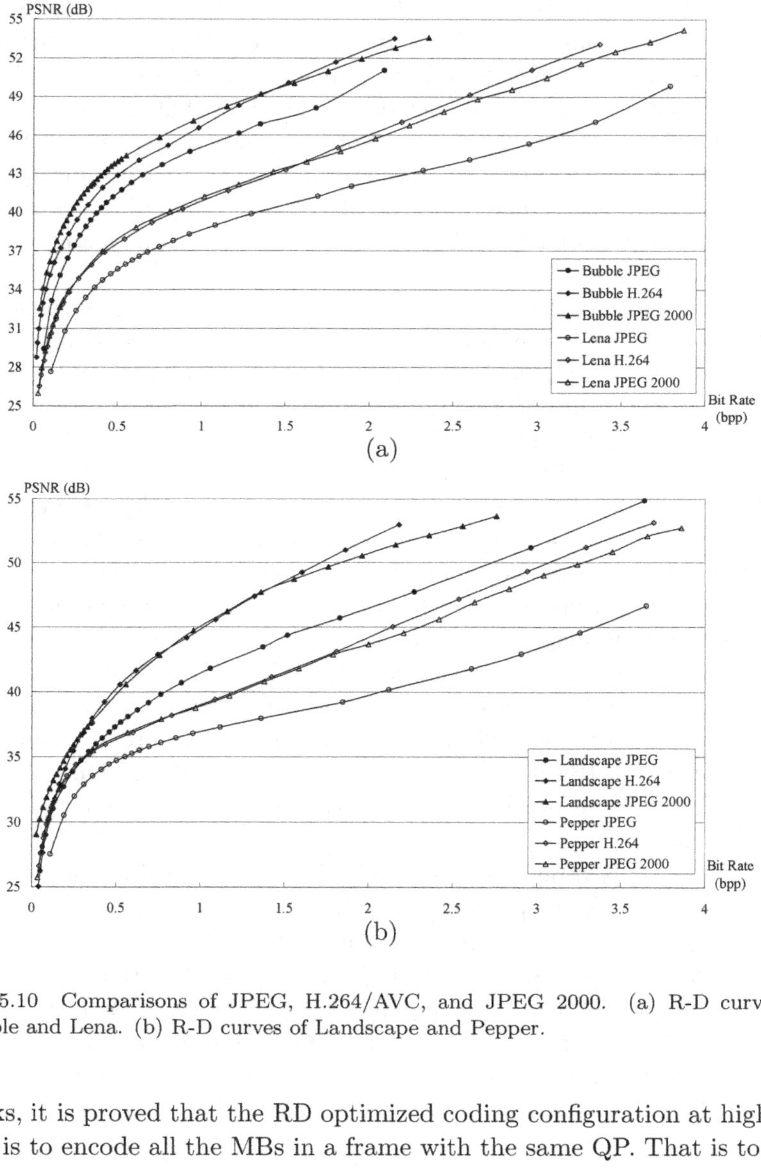

Fig. 5.10 Comparisons of JPEG, H.264/AVC, and JPEG 2000. (a) R-D curves of Bubble and Lena. (b) R-D curves of Landscape and Pepper.

works, it is proved that the RD optimized coding configuration at high bit rate is to encode all the MBs in a frame with the same QP. That is to say, if an image is coded by the same QP for all MBs, which results in certain bit rate, R, any other combinations of QPs for the MBs cannot result in better image quality with rate constraint, R. This result is quite interesting and can be observed for various coding algorithm and various images. In our case, the images are coded by H.264/AVC with single QP for all the MBs. Thus, this configuration is optimum at high bit rate, and therefore H.264/AVC outperforms JPEG 2000 at high bit rate. However, this advantage disappears when rate control is applied to H.264/AVC, which is already applied to JPEG 2000. In a word, the superiority of H.264/AVC over JPEG 2000 at high bit rate would disappear if rate control is applied. It's a pity that the reference software of H.264, JM9.0 [88], does not implement rate control for intra frames. Otherwise, we can experiment and prove this inference.

By the above observations and analyses, the coding efficiency of JPEG 2000 is almost the same as that of H.264/AVC and is much better than that of JPEG. For larger image size, JPEG 2000 is slightly better than H.264/AVC, since the DWT favors large image size. Moreover, the maximum frame size regulated in H.264/AVC [89] is 4096×2304, which is equivalent to 36864 MBs.

Besides the object comparisons by the RD curves, subjective comparisons are also important for image/video coding. Figure 5.11 shows the reconstructed images of Lena coded at ultra-low bit rate. It is obviously that the quality of image coded by JPEG is totally unacceptable, and is much poorer than images coded by the other two standards. It seems that almost all the blocks have only DC values. For H.264/AVC and JPEG 2000, it's hard to say which one is better than the other. However, the subjective views of the distortions produced by the two standards are quit different. The distortion of JPEG 2000 tends to be the blur effects. On the other hand, there are some abrupt intensity changes in the reconstructed image of H.264/AVC.

Another comparison is shown in Fig. 5.12, in which Baboon is coded at low bit rate. As in previous example, the image coded by JPEG is much poorer than images coded by the other two standards. The blocking artifacts can be easily seen. The subjective qualities of H.264/AVC and JPEG 2000 are also hard to compare with each other. For JPEG 2000, ringing effects appear in the hair region due to the ultra high frequency. For H.264/AVC, the pattern in the light region near the nose is disappeared for most part.

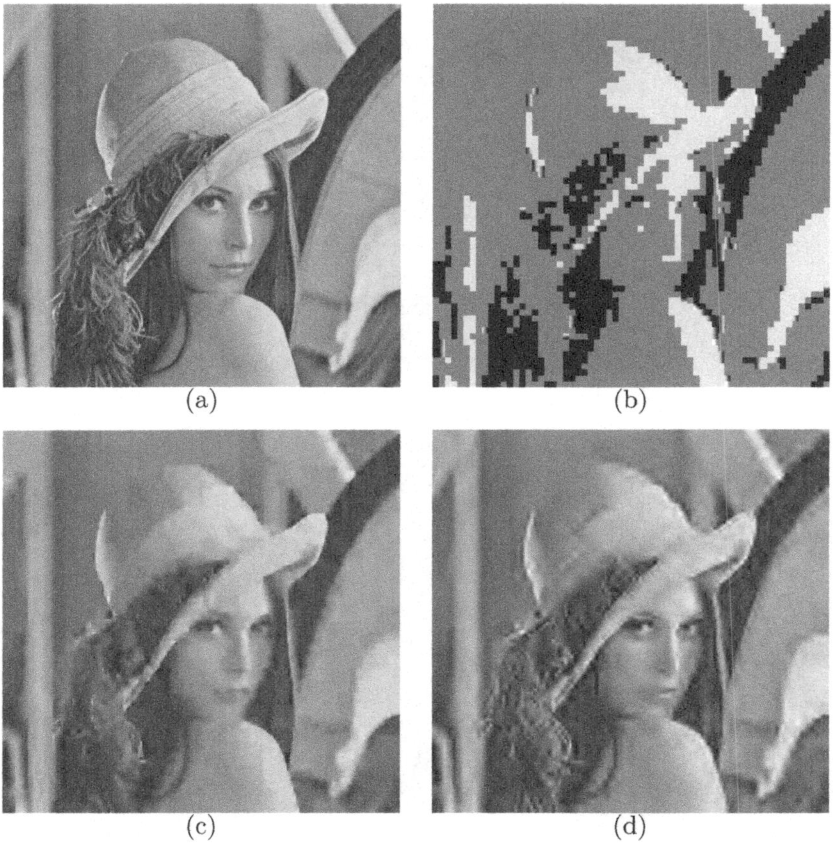

Fig. 5.11 Subject view comparisons for JPEG, H.264/AVC, and JPEG 2000 at ultra-low bit rate. (a) Original Lena. (b) Image coded by JPEG at 0.044 *bpp* and 17.8 *dB*. (c) Image coded by H.264/AVC at 0.038 *bpp* and 26.5 *dB*. (d) Image coded coded by JPEG 2000 at 0.038 *bpp* and 26.8 *dB*.

5.2 Design Issues of JPEG 2000 Encoding Systems

In this section, we'll briefly describe the design issues for the JPEG 2000 encoding system. In the follows, they are described in different sections for different algorithms since the design issues are quit different for different algorithms.

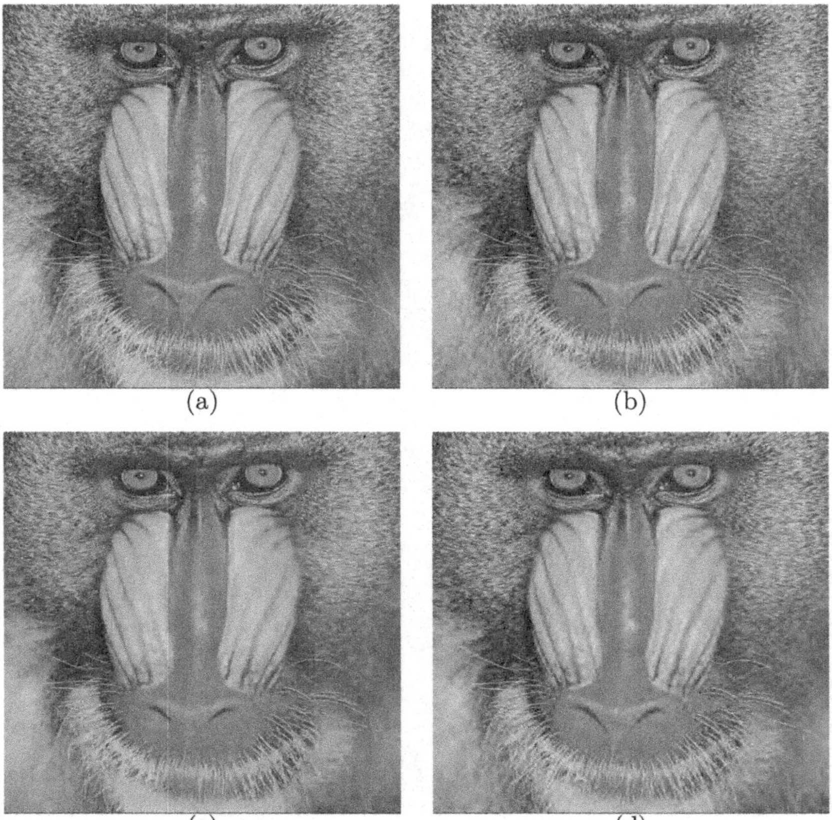

(a) (b) (c) (d)

Fig. 5.12 Subject view comparisons at low bit rate for JPEG, H.264/AVC, and JPEG 2000. (a) Original Baboon. (b) Image coded by JPEG at 0.361 *bpp* and 23.9 *dB*. (c) Image coded by H.264/AVC at 0.327 *bpp* and 24.6 *dB*. (d) Image coded coded by JPEG 2000 at 0.326 *bpp* and 24.6 *dB*.

5.2.1 *Discrete wavelet transform*

The major design challenge of the DWT is the memory issue. It can be further divided into off-chip memory bandwidth and on-chip buffer size, and the two issues are tradeoffs. In general, the memory bandwidth can be reduced by using some on-chip buffer. For 2-D DWT, the line-based architecture can minimize the memory bandwidth with some line buffers, which is not too large. On the other hand, LL band memory is required to reduce memory bandwidth for multi-level decomposition. However, the LL band memory size is very large, which may occupies more than 10% for typical JPEG 2000 encoder with small tile size. For future applications with large tile size, it is impractical to put the LL band memory on chip. But, putting the LL band memory outside the chip is also a big problem since memory bandwidth is very limited for large image applications. Therefore, this would be the major challenge of not only the DWT but also the whole JPEG 2000 encoder system.

Scan order is another issue for the DWT. This issue arises from that the scan order of the EBC is not the same as the scan order of the conventional DWT. If there is no special design, the data to be buffered would be as large as the tile size. Efficient scan order of DWT would alleviate this problem, even eliminate the use of tile buffer.

5.2.2 *Embedded block coding*

Unlike the DWT, the major challenge of the EBC is the computational complexity. Moreover, it requires extremely complicated control and sequential processing, which make it hard to increase the throughput. The EBC is a bit-level processing algorithm that a coefficient must be processed several times. Since the DWT is a word-level processing algorithm, the speed of the EBC is much lower than that of the DWT. Thus, the EBC is the speed bottleneck of the JPEG 2000 system. Moreover, it requires a code-block memory for data format conversion between the tile memory and the EBC. This memory is almost as large as the whole embedded block coding engine. As a result, increasing the throughput as well as reducing the memory requirement are the targets to design the EBC.

5.2.3 *Rate-distortion optimization*

In JPEG 2000, the RDO requires a large memory for storing the lossless code-stream and rate-distortion information. Moreover, it causes computational power waste since the EBC must losslessly encode all the code-blocks regardless of the compression ratio. The major problem lies on that the RDO is performed after the EBC, and it can only start after all the code-blocks have been encoded. Therefore, reducing the wasted computational power and the buffer requirement are the design issues of the RDO.

5.3 Tile Pipelined Scheme and the Corresponding DWT Architecture

5.3.1 *Preliminary*

There are three critical issues to design a high throughput JPEG 2000 encoder. Firstly, the DWT requires high memory bandwidth and enormous computational power. Secondly, the EBC requires extremely complicated control and sequential processing. Thirdly, the RDO requires a large memory for storing the lossless code-stream and rate-distortion information. Moreover, it causes computational power waste since the EBC must losslessly encode all the code-blocks regardless of the compression ratio. All of the above issues require high operating frequency, huge memory size, and high memory bandwidth for chip implementation of a high speed JPEG 2000 encoder.

Some JPEG 2000 designs have been reported in the literature [90, 91, 92, 94, 93]. However, they suffer from high operating frequency or large area. The designs in [91], [92], and [93] operate at frequency higher than 150 *MHz* to provide the throughput of about 50 MSamples/sec (*MS/s*). On the other hand, the design in [92] occupies 289 mm^2 to achieve about 50 *MS/s* throughput. In order to lower the operating frequency, Yamauchi [94] proposed an architecture, which achieves 21 *MS/s* at 27 *MHz* operating frequency. However, the area, which is 25 mm^2, is still too large.

All the above problems mainly come from the EBC. In the above designs, two techniques are adopted to increase the throughput of the EBC: increasing operating frequency and duplicating the EBC module. Increasing operating frequency is the simplest method to increase the throughput without increasing hardware cost. However, this technique directly leads to high power consumption. In order to avoid high power consumption, others adopt the technique of duplicating the EBC module to increase the throughput of their JPEG 2000 designs. However, this technique results in large silicon area, and therefore high hardware cost.

In this chapter, we introduce a high performance architecture for the JPEG 2000 encoder. For the EBC, the parallel architecture proposed by Fang [77] is used to increase the throughput without increasing operating frequency or silicon area. In order to reduce the I/O access power consumption, a line-based architecture is used to achieve two-dimensional (2-D) and two-level DWT operations. This architecture can reduce the memory access to only one read and one write per sample, which is the theoretical lower bound.

5.3.2 *System architecture*

The architecture of the tile-pipelined JPEG 2000 encoder is shown in Fig. 5.13. There are six functional blocks in this architecture: the main control module, the DWT module, the EBC module, the BSF module, the RDO module, and the SRAM Address Generator (AG) module. The SRAM AG module translates the addresses of the DWT, EBC, and BSF modules into real SRAM addresses. The main control module is a hardwired controller, which is composed of three Finite State Machines (FSM). The hardwired controller is much more cost-effective than general-purpose processors. The DWT, EBC, and BSF modules are pipelined at tile-level by use of the two off-chip SRAMs. The RDO module observes the output of the DWT module and truncates the input of the EBC module. In the subsequent sections, we will elaborate the architecture in detail.

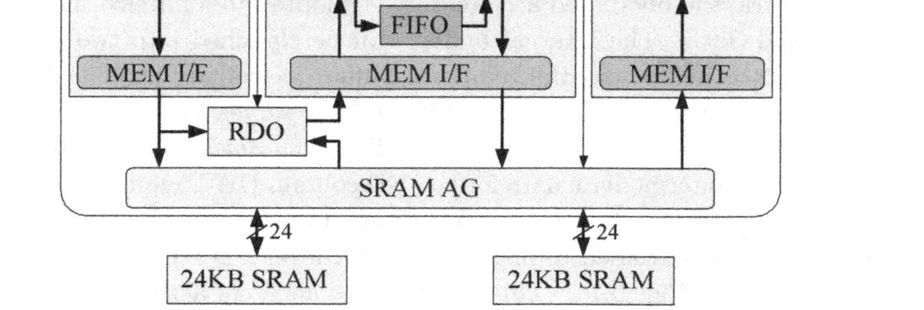

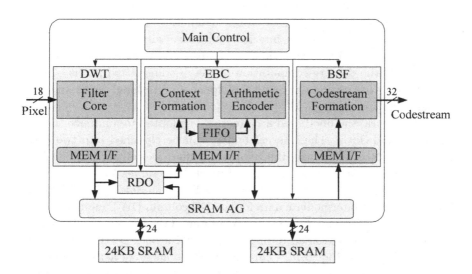

Fig. 5.13 System block diagram of the tile-pipelined JPEG 2000 encoder. The DWT, EBC, and BSF modules are pipelined at tile-level by use of the two off-chip SRAMs.

Table 5.2 Comparisons of Various 2-D DWT Architectures

Architecture	Bandwidth†		Internal Buffer
	Read	Write	(words)
Direct 2-D	2.5	2.5	0
Block-based [94]	$\frac{1.25B}{B-2K}$	1.25	LB
Line-based [95]	1	1	$1.5LN$

† Bandwidth is represented as access times per sample.
B: Block width N: Tile width K,L: Filter dependent constants

5.3.3 *Discrete wavelet transform*

Memory issues are most important for the DWT in JPEG 2000. Unlike the 8×8 Discrete Cosine Transform (DCT), the DWT operates on a much larger area. Therefore, the major goal has been reducing the memory requirements, which include off-chip memory bandwidth and on-chip memory size. Table 5.2 shows the comparisons of three 2-D DWT architectures: the direct 2-D, overlapped block-based, and line-based architectures. The B is the block size of the block-based architecture and the N is the tile width. The L and K depend on the filter type. Two levels of decompositions are assumed. The line-based architecture minimizes tile memory bandwidth with some inter buffers. On the other hand, the block-based and direct 2-D architectures reduce the internal buffer size with the increase of the tile memory bandwidth. Note that the increase of tile memory read is proportional to the data re-computation of the re-transmitted pixels. These computations are unnecessary, and therefore computational power and processing time are wasted.

In this work, the line-based architecture is adopted to minimize the tile memory bandwidth. The internal buffers can be classified into two categories: the data buffer and the temporal buffer, as defined in [95]. The data buffer, which requires 1.5 lines of pixel data, serves as the transpose memory between the 1-D row and column DWT modules. The temporal buffer stores the intermediate data for the 1-D column DWT module, which requires 2 lines of pixel data for the 5/3 filter. Two 1-level 2-D line-based DWT modules are cascaded to implement the 2-level 2-D DWT decomposition as shown in Fig. 5.14. This architecture achieves a throughput of two pixels per cycle since the 1-D DWT modules are implemented using the lifting scheme. To achieve the 128×128 tile size, 8512 bits of buffers are required. Three of the six buffers are implemented by two-port SRAM with 128×24 bits, 64×24 bits, and 64×28 bits, respectively. The other three are implemented by register files with 32×24 bits, 32×28 bits, and

16 × 28 bits, respectively.

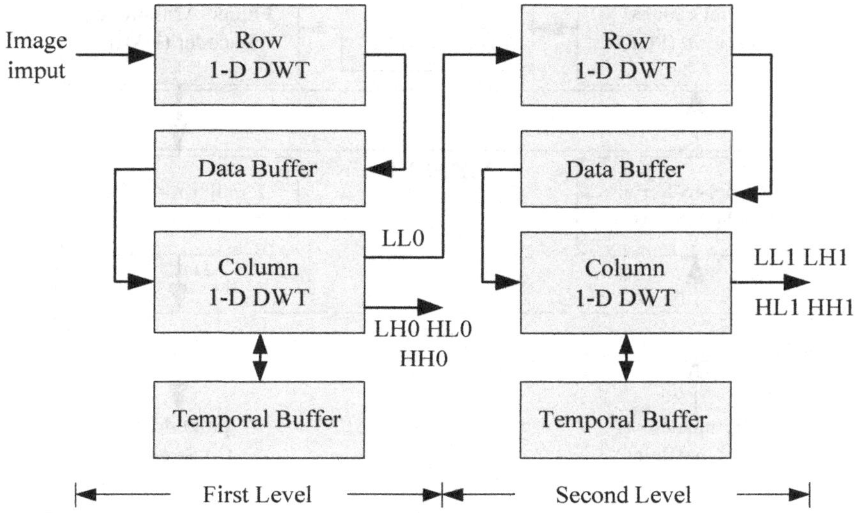

Fig. 5.14 Block diagram of the 2-level 2-D DWT architecture. The architecture can process two samples per cycle.

5.3.4 *Embedded block coding*

The most critical challenge to increase the throughput of a JPEG 2000 design is the EBC, which requires a lot of sequential operations and complicated controls. In this work, the parallel EBC architecture capable of processing all bit-planes of a DWT coefficient per cycle proposed by Fang is adopted [77]. The block diagram of the parallel EBC architecture is shown in Fig. 5.15. It contains two parts: the EBC engine and the memory interfaces (MEM I/F). The MEM I/F includes a Parallel-to-Serial Read (PSR) AG, a Parallel-to-Serial Write (PSW) AG, and an arbiter. The arbiter is used to make sure that only one AG is granted to access the SRAM and to prevent deadlocks from happening.

Fang proposed an EBC engine capable of processing a DWT coefficient in parallel, regardless of bit-width. Three new techniques are used to achieve the parallel processing. First, the Parallel Context Formation (PCF) approach is taken, instead of traditional sequential approaches, to

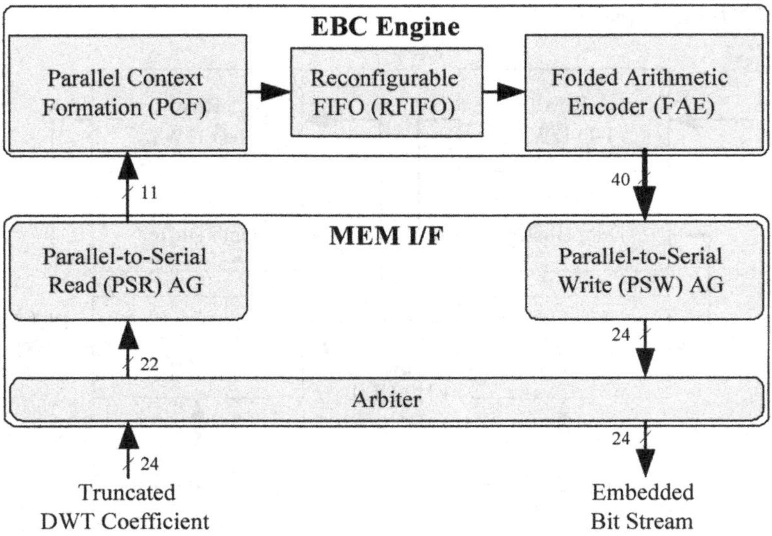

Fig. 5.15 Block diagram of the parallel EBC architecture. The architecture can process all bit-planes of a DWT coefficient per cycle.

increase the processing speed. Second, a Reconfigurable FIFO (RFIFO) architecture that reduces bubble cycles is obtained by exploiting the features of the EBC algorithm and the DWT algorithm. Third, a Folded Arithmetic Encoder (FAE) architecture is devised to reduce the area. Combing the three techniques, the parallel architecture is about six times faster than the best techniques described in the literature with similar hardware cost.

The block diagram of the parallel EBC engine is shown in Fig. 5.16. It can encode an 11-bit DWT coefficient per cycle. Therefore, 28 coding passes must be processed in parallel since each magnitude bit-plane, except the Most Significant Bit (MSB) bit-plane, contains 3 coding passes. These bit streams are encoded by the FAE, which can process 5 of them at a time. Thus, there will be at most 5 output bytes per cycle.

5.3.5 *Scheduling*

Figure 5.17 shows the system scheduling and the bandwidth usage of the off-chip SRAMs. Tile-level pipeline is chosen to achieve high throughput and high utilization. There are three pipeline stages: the DWT, the EBC, and the BSF modules. The RDO module neither forms a individual pipeline

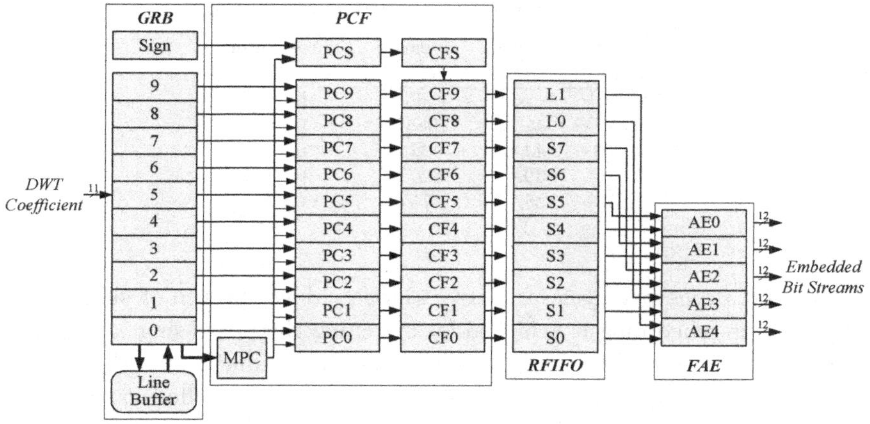

Fig. 5.16 Block diagram of the EBC engine. This architecture can process 11 bit-planes of a DWT coefficient per cycle. At most five of 28 embedded bit streams may be outputted in a cycle.

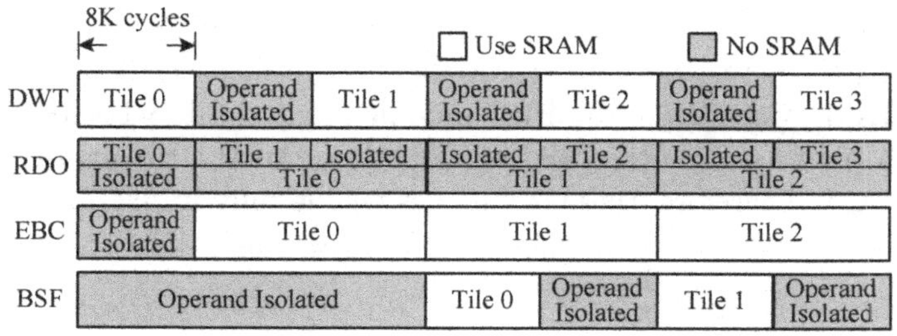

Fig. 5.17 System scheduling and bandwidth usage. The DWT, EBC, and BSF modules are pipelined at tile level by the two SRAMs. The block in gray and white colors represent that the corresponding operations need and need not access the SRAM.

stage nor uses any memory bandwidth. It observes the output coefficients of the DWT module to decide the truncation points, and on the other hand it truncates the input coefficients of the EBC module according to the truncation points. Thus, it operates at two pipeline stages for two tiles concurrently. In order to reduce power consumption, the DWT, the RDO, and the BSF modules are operand isolated at idle stages. Therefore, the switching power of the processing elements are saved.

By such efficient scheduling, the memory bandwidth of external SRAM

Table 5.3 Throughput vs. Bit Rate of Jet Image

Bit Rate (*bpp*)	PSNR (*dB*)	Cycles (*K*)	Throughput (Sample/Cycle)
11.91	∞	1165	0.66
8.37	48.37	1084	0.71
4.71	43.18	924	0.83
2.67	39.43	826	0.93
1.37	35.77	775	0.99

is two operations per cycle at most, which enables the use of single-port SRAM. The scheduling is achieved by matching the processing rate of the DWT, the EBC, and the BSF modules. The throughput of the EBC module depends on the truncation points and is about one coefficient per cycle. Adopting lifting scheme, the throughput of the DWT module is two coefficients per cycle. By using the ALL addressing scheme, the BSF module can finish its work in about 8 K cycles, which is approximately equal to the speed of the DWT module. Thus, the DWT and the BSF modules are designed to share the memory bandwidth of one SRAM. During a pipeline stage, the BSF module reads bit streams of the $(N-1)$-th tile from one SRAM and forms the codestream. After that, the DWT starts to transform the $(N+1)$-th tile and stores the transformed coefficients into the same SRAM. Meanwhile, the EBC module reads the DWT coefficients of the N-th tile from the other SRAM and stores the bit streams back to the same SRAM. Therefore, these techniques enable fully utilization of SRAM bandwidth and reduce the number of SRAM by one.

5.3.6 *Experimental results*

5.3.6.1 *Performance and chip feature*

Table 5.3 shows the throughput of the encoder at various bit rates. The test image is *Jet* of size 512×512 and 24 bits per pixel (*bpp*). In lossless mode, the throughput is about 0.66 $(=\frac{512\times512\times3}{1165\times1024})$ samples/cycle. The throughput can be greatly increased to 0.99 samples/cycle in lossy mode. The speedup in lossy mode comes from the pre-compression RDO algorithm that truncates the DWT coefficients before the EBC module. Thus, the data to be processed by the EBC module are reduced. In extreme cases, a code-block is entirely discarded by the RDO module, which greatly reduces the processing time.

The micrograph of the prototype chip is shown in Fig. 5.18. Table 5.4

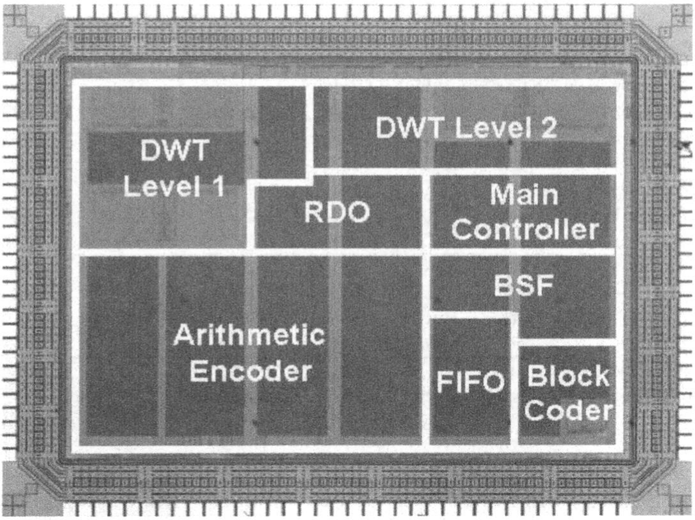

Fig. 5.18 Micrograph of the prototype chip. The core size is $2.73 \times 2.02\ mm^2$ by using TSMC 0.25 μm technology.

Table 5.4 Chip Specifications

Technology	TSMC 0.25 μm 1P5M CMOS	
Transistor Counts	914 K	
Core Size	$2.73 \times 2.02\ mm^2$	
Power Consumption	348 mW @ 81 MHz	
Operating Frequency	81 MHz	
Supply Voltage	Internal	2.8 V
	I/O	3.3 V
Throughput	Lossy	81 MS/s
	Lossless	54 MS/s
On-Chip SRAM	Two-Port	6400 b
	Single-Port	768 b
Logic Gates	Total	166479
	DWT	40665
	RDO	12291
	EBC	104137
	Others	9386

summarizes the chip specifications. This chip is fabricated with a $0.25\mu m$ CMOS 1P5M technology, in which 914 K transistors are integrated on $2.73 \times 2.02\ mm^2$. It consumes 348 mW at 81 MHz and 2.8 V supply voltage. Operating at 81 MHz, it can encode at least 54 MS/s in lossless

Table 5.5 Comparisons of Various JPEG 2000 Designs

Architecture	[90]	[91]	[92]	[94]	[93]	This Work
Category	Enc.	Codec	Codec	Enc.	Enc.	Enc.
Tech. (μm)	N/A	0.18	0.18	0.25	0.18	0.25
Area† (mm^2)	N/A	N/A	189_d	25_c	6.0_d	5.5_c
Rate‡ ($\frac{MS}{s}$)	-/10	60/36	50/-	21/-	60/-	81/54
Freq. (MHz)	100	150	180	27	150	81
Power (mW)	N/A	N/A	1944	N/A	280	348
Voltage (V)	N/A	1.5	1.8	2.5	1.8	2.8
Tile	256^2	2048^2	256^2	1024×512	128^2	128^2
Code-block	64^2	N/A	N/A	N/A	32^2	64^2
DWT	Both	Both	Both	9/7	Both	5/3
RDO	Aid	Aid	No	No	No	Yes

† d/c for die/core area
‡ processing rate in lossy/lossless mode

mode and 81 MS/s in lossy mode. It can support HDTV 720p (1280×720) 4:4:4 at 30 fps in real-time. Table 5.4 also shows the memory requirements and the logic gate counts (2-input NAND gate equivalent) of the encoder.

5.3.6.2 *Comparisons*

A Performance Index (PI), defined as processing rate per mm^2 and per MHz, is used to make a fair comparison to existing work. The PI of this work is 0.182 ($= \frac{81}{5.5\times81}$) S/mm^2, which means this work can process 0.182 samples per unit area per cycle. The area of the JPEG 2000 core in [94] [96] is estimated as 25 mm^2 and the PI will be 0.030 ($= \frac{20.7}{25\times27.4}$) S/mm^2. Hence, the developed chip is 6 times better than [94] [96] using this metric. Although the specification of the encoder in [96] is four times higher than that in [94], the improvement comes from doubling the area and the operating frequency. Thus, the efficiency of the architecture does not be improved. In fact, the architectures are exactly the same. Therefore, the PI can actually reflect the performance of an architecture, and won't be affected by such modifications. In order to make a complete comparison among various designs, important parameters for a JPEG 2000 encoder are summarized in Table 5.5.

5.3.7 *Summary*

Due to the parallel EBC, Fang's encoder chip can achieve equal processing rate between DWT and EBC. The line-based architecture is selected for

DWT implementation because of the off-chip access concern. Under the tile pipeline, the DWT can be performed tile-by-tile and level-by-level with a relatively simple control. The hardware area of DWT thus can be reduced.

5.4 Stripe Pipelined Scheme and the Corresponding DWT Architecture

Memory issues become the most critical problem to design a high performance JPEG 2000 architecture since the proposition of the parallel EBC architecture. In this chapter, a pipelined JPEG 2000 encoder architecture is introduced to reduce the tile memory size. The tile memory occupies more than 50% of area in conventional JPEG 2000 architectures. To solve this problem, Fang proposes a stripe pipeline scheme. For this scheme, a Level Switch Discrete Wavelet Transform (LS-DWT) and a Code-block Switch Embedded Block Coding (CS-EBC) are proposed. With small additional memory, the LS-DWT and the CS-EBC can process multiple levels and code-blocks in parallel by an interleaved scheme. As a result of above techniques, the overall memory requirements of this architecture can be reduced to only 8.5% compared with conventional architectures.

Many architecture for JPEG 2000 has been proposed [90, 93, 97, 91, 94, 96, 77]. All the above architectures focus on how to overcome the computation complexity, especially the Embedded Block Coding (EBC). The solutions can be classified into two categories. The first one is to use multiple EBC engines [90, 93, 97, 91], which process multiple code-blocks in parallel. The second one is to increase the processing rate of the EBC engine [94, 96, 77] by processing multiple bit-planes in parallel. The major disadvantage of using multiple EBC engines is that this method needs to use multiple code-block memory, which size is commonly 6 KB $(64 \times 64 \times 12)$ for a code-block. The parallel EBC architecture can greatly increase the processing rate of the EBC while maintain similar hardware cost with architectures that use single EBC engine. Since the parallel EBC architecture can process one DWT coefficient per cycle with even less cost than conventional EBC architecture, the problems of insufficient computational power of the EBC are solved in my opinion. On the other hand, memory issues of the DWT are also key factors of a JPEG 2000 design. Block-based scan for DWT [94, 98] is proposed to eliminate the use of tile memory, which size is commonly 96 KB $(256 \times 256 \times 12)$, at the cost of the increase of memory bandwidth. Although the tile memory is eliminated, the scan order of the block-based scan is not optimized such that the memory requirements are still too high. Therefore, the hardware cost of JPEG 2000 is still too high to let JPEG 2000 take place of JPEG regardless of the large coding gain by use of JPEG 2000.

In this chapter, we will introduce a stripe pipeline scheme for the DWT and the EBC to solve the above problems. The stripe pipeline scheme takes the throughputs and the dataflows of the DWT and the EBC into joint consideration. The main idea is to match the throughputs and the dataflows of the two modules so that the DWT coefficients generated are processed by the EBC as soon as possible. Thus, the size of local buffers between the two modules is minimized. To achieve the stripe pipeline scheme, a Level Switch DWT (LS-DWT) and a Code-block Switch EBC (CS-EBC) are proposed by Fang. The CS-EBC can process 13 code-blocks in parallel, and LS-DWT can accomplish multi-level two-dimensional DWT concurrently. As a result of the stripe pipeline scheme, the memory requirements are reduce to only 8.5% comparing with conventional architectures.

5.4.1 *Preliminary*

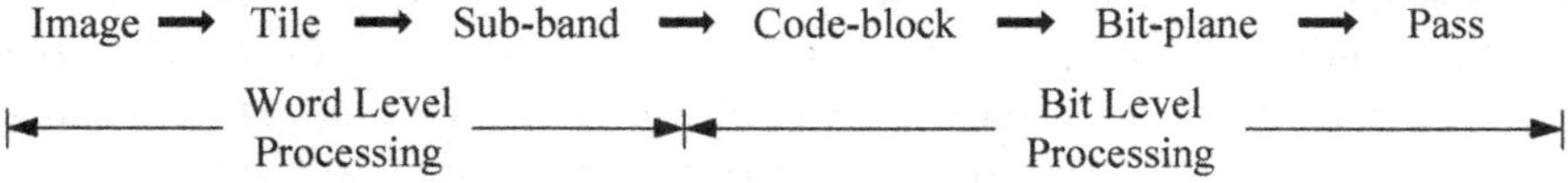

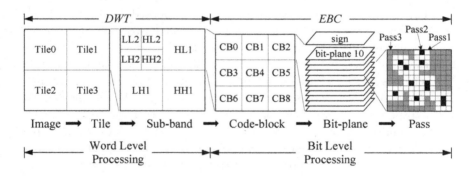

Fig. 5.19 Decomposition of an image into various abstract levels. These abstract levels include tile, subband, code-block, bit-plane, and coding pass.

In this section, we'll briefly describe the JPEG 2000 coding system, especially the dataflow. Figure 5.2 is re-drawn here; Fig. 5.19, which shows how an image is decomposed into abstract levels, which include tile, subband, code-block, bit-plane, and coding pass. The original image is partitioned into several rectangular tiles, which are independently coded. The DWT decomposes a tile into L levels. Except for the L-th level that has four subbands, each level has three subbands, which are the HL, LH, and HH bands. In general, the DWT coefficients co-located at each subband are generated consequently. Figure 5.20 shows an example of a 8×8 tile. Each circle represents a DWT coefficient, and the number within the circle indicates the order it is generated. The order of the DWT coefficients generated within each subband depends on the scan order of the DWT engine. However, the co-located DWT coefficients are always generated consequently.

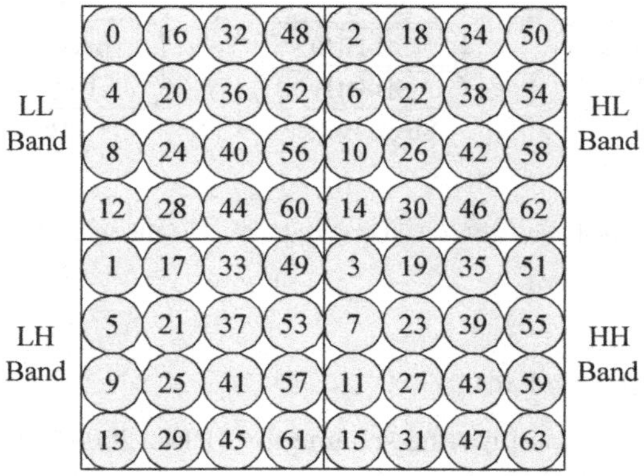

Fig. 5.20 Output order of DWT coefficients. The co-located DWT coefficients in all subbands are generated consequently.

For the EBC, each subband is further partitioned into code-blocks. The DWT coefficients in the code-block are sign-magnitude represented. The code-block is processed in a bit-plane by bit-plane manner, from the Most Significant Bit (MSB) bit-plane to the Least Significant Bit (LSB) bit-plane. Every bit-plane has three coding passes called Pass 1, Pass 2, and Pass 3. A special coding order called stripe scan is used within any coding pass. A stripe is a $N \times 4$ rectangle, where N is the width of the code-block. The coefficients are scanned stripe by stripe from top to bottom in a coding pass, and column by column from left to right in a stripe.

5.4.2 *System architecture*

In this section, the stripe-pipelined JPEG 2000 architecture is presented. The block diagram of the architecture is shown in Fig. 5.21. Seven Stripe Buffers (SB) are used for the stripe pipeline, each buffer has 256×11 bits.

The Level Switch DWT (LS-DWT) generates 256 DWT coefficients for each subband at every pipeline stage. The resulting coefficients are stored in the SBs, and then processed by the Code-block Switch EBC (CS-EBC).

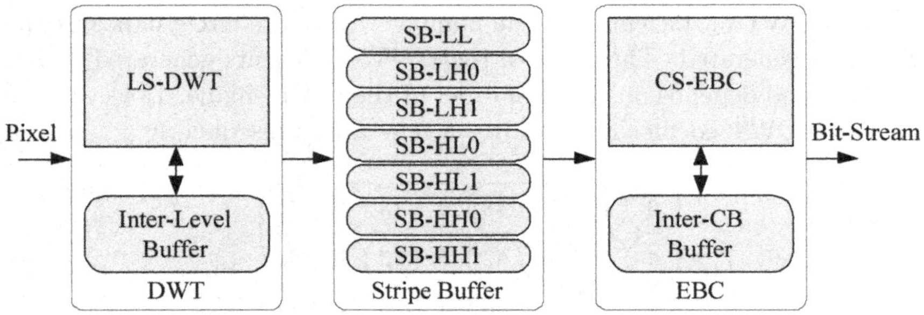

Fig. 5.21 Stripe-pipelined JPEG 2000 architecture. No tile memory is required in this architecture.

5.4.2.1 *Stripe pipeline scheme*

In this section, a stripe pipeline scheme for JPEG 2000 is introduced. The key concept is to design a scheduling that can minimize the memory requirement while maintain reasonable complexity and overhead. As described in Section 5.4.1, the memory issues are arisen from the mismatch between output dataflow of the DWT and the input scan order of the EBC. The mismatch can be solved by using a buffer between the two modules. In conventional architecture [97], the whole tile and three code-block are buffered. Wu et al. [98] proposed a Quad Code-Block (QCB) scheduling scheme that reduces the memory requirements to $\frac{1}{4}$ tile and six code-blocks. However, the memory requirements are still too high. This stripe pipeline scheme can fully eliminate the use of tile memory and code-block memory. It only requires stripe memory, which size is $\frac{1}{16}$ of a code-block memory for a 64×64 code-block.

The detail of the stripe pipeline scheme is shown in Fig. 5.22. Each rectangle represents a computation state of the LS-DWT or the CS-EBC. The state of LS-DWT is indicated by, for example, $T_kL_i : R_{s-t}\text{-}L$, which means that the LS-DWT is processing left half of the s-th row to the t-th row in the i-th level of the k-th tile. On the other hand, the state of CS-EBC is indicated by, for example, $T_kCB_{s-t} : S_i$, which means that the CS-EBC is processing the i-th stripe of the s-th code-block to the t-th code-block of the k-th tile. The order of execution is from top to bottom. All the computation states require 768 cycles except when the CS-EBC is at T_kCB_{0-3} state, which needs 1024 cycles. In fact, the cycles required in each state is exactly the number of DWT coefficients the CS-EBC must process.

For the stripe pipeline schedule, seven stripe buffers are required as shown in Fig. 5.21. Each stripe buffer is 256×11 bits, where 11 is the bit-width of a DWT coefficient. While the LS-DWT is writing coefficients into SB-LH0, SB-HL0, and SB-HH0, the CS-EBC is reading coefficients from SB-LH1, SB-HL1, and SB-HH1, or vice versa. When the LS-DWT is processing L_2 or the CS-EBC is processing CB_{0-3}, SB-LL must be accessed by the corresponding module. Therefore, the stripe-pipelined scheduling only requires about 2.4 Kilo-Bytes (KB) or 1.75 Kilo-Words (KW), equivalently.

5.4.2.2 *Level switch DWT*

In this section, a Level Switch DWT (LS-DWT) is introduced. It can greatly reduce the memory requirements of the DWT in JPEG 2000. Figure 5.23 shows the architecture of the LS-DWT. It has four major parts, including the two 1-D DWT cores, the line-buffer, and the LL-band buffer. The LL-band buffer serves as tile buffer of other conventional architectures. In order to achieve the level switch with efficient memory usage, the line-based implementation [99] combined with non-overlapped stripe-based scan [100] is adopted. In the following, the dataflow and memory requirement of the adopted line-based scheme for 2-D decomposition is presented, and the memory requirement for level switch is analyzed. In the following analyses, the 2-D DWT is accomplished in column-row order to be compatible with JPEG 2000.

Figure 5.24 shows a generic line-based 2-D DWT architecture in column-row order. The line buffer contains data buffer and temporal buffer. The size of data buffer depends on the scheduling of 1-D column and row DWT. At the extreme case that row DWT starts after complete column filtering, the size of data buffer is the same as the tile size. To reduce the size of data buffer, row DWT must start as soon as possible to reduce the life time of intermediate coefficients. Figure 5.25 shows the data flow of the adopted non-overlapped stripe-based scan in the line-based DWT. Each circle represents either a pixel or an intermediate coefficient between 1-D column and row DWT. The number in the circle indicates which cycle

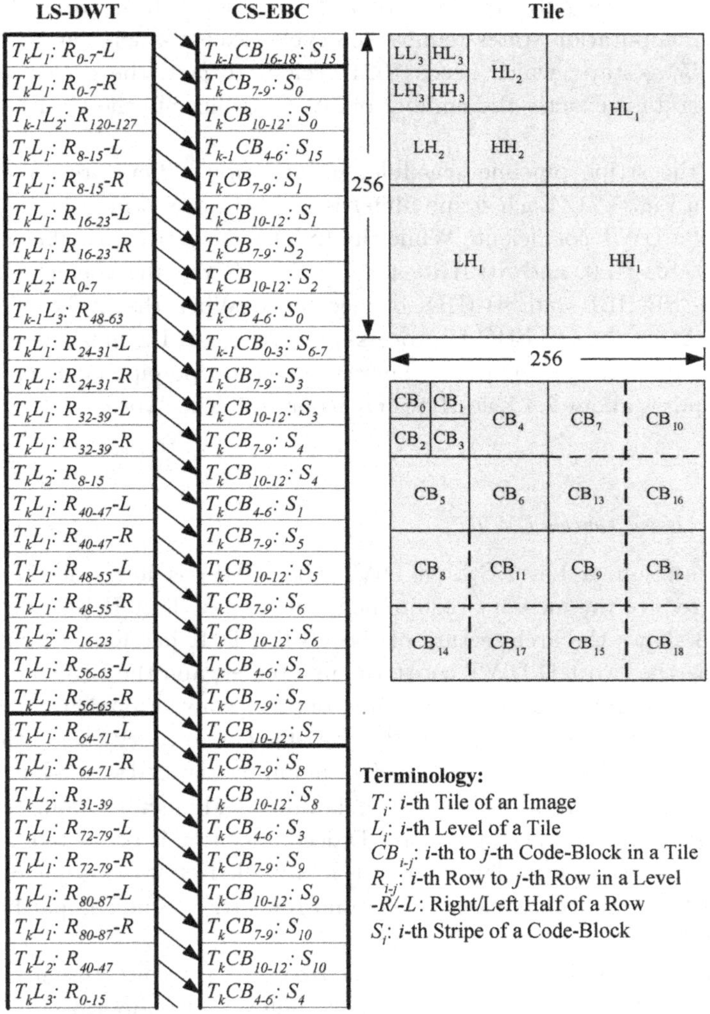

Fig. 5.22 Stripe pipeline scheme. The LS-DWT and CS-EBC are pipelined at stripe level, and therefore the buffer size is reduced to the same as the stripe size.

it is scanned. The intermediate coefficients are generated right after the co-located original pixels are scanned. For example, the two coefficients denoted by 3 and 4 in the first column are generated when pixels denoted by 0 are scanned. Thus, eight coefficients are required to be buffered since

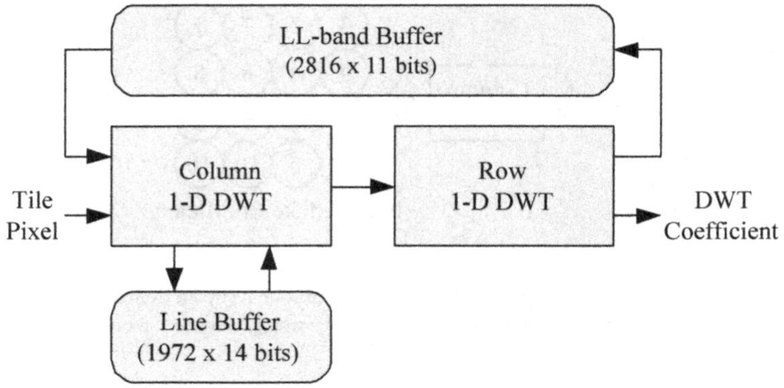

Fig. 5.23 Block diagram of the LS-DWT. It can accomplish multi-level decomposition by two 1-D DWT core.

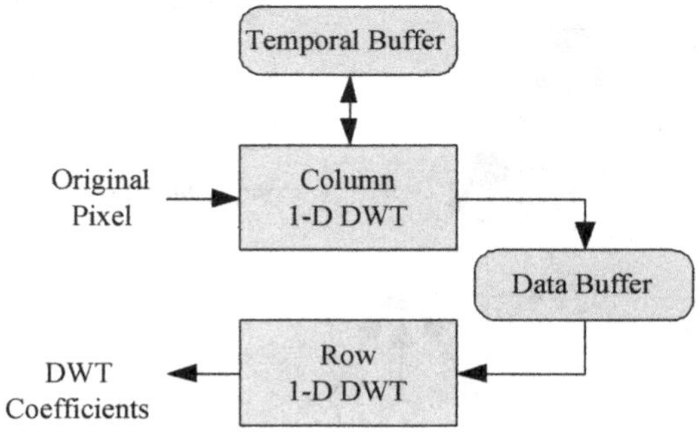

Fig. 5.24 Generic line-based 2-D DWT architecture. The line buffer contains data buffer and temporal buffer.

they are no longer needed after row DWT computations. Therefore, the data buffer is eliminated with the non-overlapped stripe-based scan, and only a few extra registers are needed.

Because the non-overlapped stripe-based scan requires that the column DWT switches between columns, the intrinsic registers inside column DWT should also be buffered. This is the temporal buffer depicted in Fig. 5.24. Figure 5.26 shows the lifting-based architecture for 1-D DWT [101, 102] in 9-7 filter. There are four intrinsic registers in this case, and therefore the size of the temporal buffer equals to four lines of the tile. Assume that the

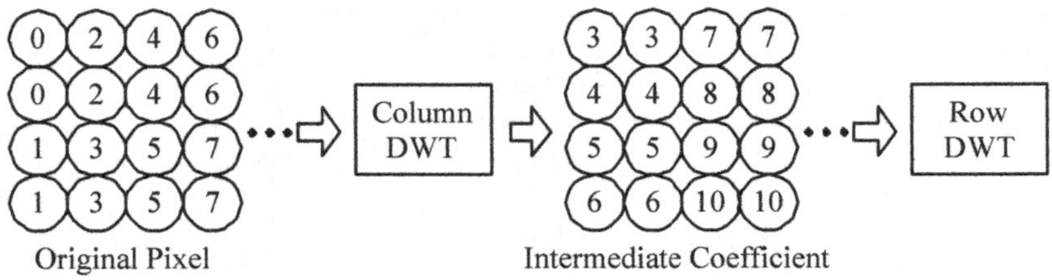

Fig. 5.25 Non-overlapped block-based scan. The number in cycle denote which cycle the coefficient is scanned. The intermediate coefficients are generated when the co-located pixels are scanned.

tile width is 256 pixels, the temporal buffer is 1024 ($= 4 \times 256$) words.

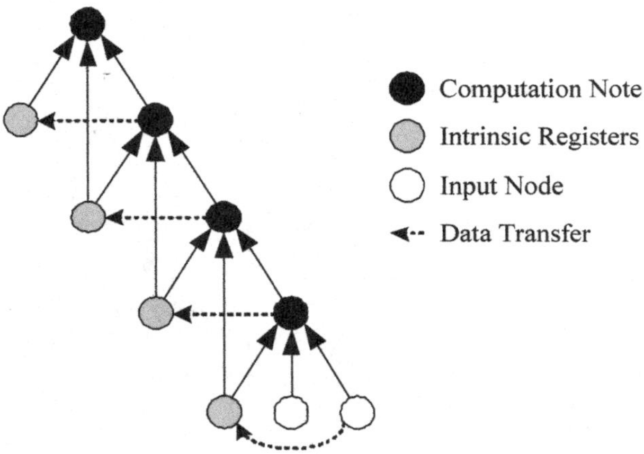

Fig. 5.26 Lifting-based implementation of 9-7 filter for line-based column DWT. It requires 4 intrinsic registers.

5.4.2.3 *Memory requirement for LS-DWT*

In order to reduce the memory bandwidth and computational complexity, the intermediate data stored in line-buffer must be buffered when the LS-DWT switches to next level. Thus, the DWT can continue its operation seamlessly after it switches back to previous level. Thus, for level-switch DWT with L decomposition levels, the line-buffer requirement is $4 \times W \times (1 + \frac{1}{2} + \cdots + \frac{1}{2^L})$ words, where W is the tile width and 9-7 filter is assumed.

For example, for 3-level DWT, the line buffer size is 1792 ($=4 \times 256 \times (1 + \frac{1}{2} + \frac{1}{2^2})$) words. Therefore, it requires 3136 bytes for the line buffer since the coefficient is 14 bits in the architecture.

Since LL_l is the input of $(l + 1)$-th level DWT, the coefficients in LL-band have to be buffered in preparation for the next decomposition level. In conventional architectures, all the coefficients in LL-band are buffered since they start the decomposition of next level after the finishing of previous level. In this level-switched architecture, the LS-DWT can switch to next level within the decomposition of previous level. Thus, the memory requirement is reduced. The size of memory is equal to the life time of coefficients in each level, i.e. the period between the generation and consumption of the coefficients. As shown in Section 5.4.2.1, the LS-DWT switches to next level whenever 1024 coefficients are generated. Thus, memory for 1024 coefficients is required. However, this is not enough since there is latency arisen from the 1-D DWT filter. For 9-7 filter, the latency is four coefficients, i.e. the first coefficient is generated after the fifth pixel is read as shown in Fig. 5.26. The life time of the coefficients is actually $1024 + 4 \times W_{LL}$, where W_{LL} is the width of the corresponding LL-band. In the LS-DWT architecture, the bit-width of the coefficients is 11 bits and the number of decomposition levels is three with 256×256 tile. Thus, the memory requirement for all LL-bands is 30976 ($= 11 \times ((1024 + 4 \times 128) + (1024 + 4 \times 64))$) bits. Therefore, the total memory requirement for the three-level LS-DWT is about 7 KB.

5.4.2.4 *Code-block switch EBC*

The block diagram of the Code-block Switch EBC (CS-EBC) is shown in Fig. 5.27. It comprises of four functional modules, the Gobang Register Bank (GRB), the Parallel Context Formation (PCF), the Sorting First-In-First-Out (SFIFO), and the Code-block Switch Arithmetic Encoder (CSAE). The CS-EBC is based on the parallel EBC architecture, and evolved to increase the throughput and to support the code-block switch function. As the LS-DWT, a coding state buffer will be needed to store the temporary data during the stripe-pipeline scheduling.

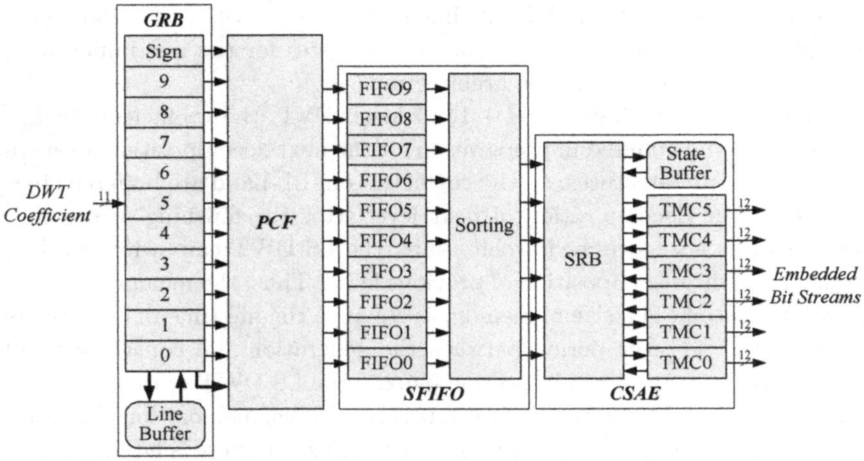

Fig. 5.27 Block diagram of the CS-EBC. It is based on the parallel EBC architecture.

Table 5.6 Memory Requirement Comparison.

Architecture	Memory Requirement (KB)				
	Tile	CB	DWT	EBC	Total
Amphion [93]	128	48	-	-	176
Andra's [97]	128	24	-	-	152
Wu's [98]	32	48	-	-	80
Stripe-Pipeline	2.4	0	5.1	7.5	15

5.4.3 *Experimental results*

5.4.3.1 *Memory reduction*

To show the performance on memory reduction of the stripe pipeline scheme, we compare the memory requirements for DWT coefficients between the DWT and the EBC in various architectures. The memory requirements depend on the specification of the architecture. Without loss of generality, we assume that the tile size is 256×256, and the code-block size is 64×64. The memory requirements of various architectures are shown in Table 5.6. In this table, memory requirements within the DWT and the EBC are not shown since the scheduling will only affect the tile memory requirements. In Table 5.6, the Tile column is the memory size for storing DWT coefficients, and the CB column is the code-block memory for the EBC. The DWT column and the EBC column are the additional memory

Table 5.7 Comparison with the Parallel Architecture in Section 5.3

Architecture	Area	Mem. (gates)	Freq. (KB)	Rate (MHz)	DWT ($\frac{MS}{s}$)	Level	Tile Filter
Parallel	166479	48.9	81	54	2	5-3	128 × 128
Pipeline	243792	16.7	124	124	3	5-3/9-7	256 × 256

requirements for the DWT and the EBC to support the stripe pipeline schedule. By the table, the memory requirements are reduced to only 8.5% comparing with Amphion's architecture [93] and 18.8% comparing with Wu's architecture [98].

There is another important advantage of the stripe pipeline scheme that the memory requirements are proportional to the square-root of the tile size. On the other hand, memory requirements of conventional architectures are proportional to the tile size. Thus, for tile size of 512 × 512, the memory requirements of the stripe-pipeline architecture is only 4.2%.

5.4.3.2 *Comparison*

In this section, the pipeline architecture is compared with the parallel architecture introduced in Section 5.3. Since detailed hardware costs of other JPEG 2000 encoders are not available, comparisons with other architectures are not shown. However, a complete comparison of the parallel architecture with others is shown in Table 5.5. Thus, it is easy to compare the pipeline architecture with others through the parallel architecture. Table 5.7 shows the comparisons of hardware cost, performance, and encoding parameters. Although the area of the pipeline architecture is 1.5 times larger than that of the parallel architecture, its memory requirement is only 30%. According to our RAM architecture, the overall silicon area of the two architectures will be similar. The rate stands for the processing rate in lossless mode. The throughput, i.e. samples per cycle, of the pipeline architecture is 1 while that of the parallel architecture is about 0.66. This advantages comes from the processing rate of the AE has been increased.

Besides the hardware cost and processing rate, coding performance is also an important issue for a encoder. The decomposition level and tile size of the pipeline architecture has been enhanced. Moreover, it can also support 9-7 filter. Thus, the coding performance of the pipeline architecture is about 2 dB higher than that of the parallel architecture. Intuitively, this advantage has nothing to do with the architecture. However, it is the superiority of the pipeline architecture that can support a large tile size with small overhead. If the tile size of the parallel architecture also increases to 256×256, its memory requirement will increase to 195 KB, which will triple the silicon area. By making the coding performance of the two architectures the same, the cost of the pipeline architecture becomes only 30% of that of the parallel architecture while the throughput of the pipeline architecture is 1.6 times higher than that of the parallel architecture. Therefore, the pipeline architecture is about 4.8 times better than the parallel architecture by this matrix at this spec.

5.4.4 *Summary*

In this section, the memory efficient JPEG 2000 architecture with stripe pipeline scheme is introduced. The stripe pipeline scheme takes the dataflow of the DWT and the EBC into joint consideration. By matching the dataflow of both modules, the tile memory is replaced by the stripe memory with additional memory requirements in the DWT and the EBC. The overall memory requirements are reduced to only 8.5% of the conventional architecture.

For the stripe pipeline scheme, the DWT module has to be able to shift between levels. The overhead of this level-switch DWT (LS-DWT) is the LL-band buffer and the larger size of line buffer. There is also similar overhead in the EBC module. Overall, the stripe-pipeline JPEG 2000 system only needs much less memory and die size.

5.5 Summary

In this chapter, two types of scheduling in JPEG 2000 encoding systems are introduced. According to the adopted JPEG 200 encoding system scheduling, there are suitable implementations of DWT module. In the tile pipelined scheduling [77], the tile buffer is required to buffer the data between pipeline stages. The DWT module thus can process one tile at a time. Line-based DWT is selected to avoid the repeated loading of image pixels. Multi-level decomposition is achieved by iteratively processing LL band coefficients. In the pipelined scheduling [78, 103], the tile buffer is eliminated by use of pipeline stage with smaller size. To eliminate the tile buffer required in tile pipeline scheduling, the DWT module has to process coefficients at different decomposition level in a interlace manner. This level-switch DWT (LS-DWT) has a more complex control and a on chip LL-band buffer. But in the system point of view, these overheads are small compared with the elimination of the tile buffer.

Chapter 6

Introduction to MCTF

In this chapter, the introduction to motion-compensated temporal filtering (MCTF) is given, including its development, basic operations, and the related open-loop video coding schemes. The original MCTF is based on the convolution algorithm, and it can be further improved by using lifting scheme to be lifting-based MCTF. We will introduce these two kinds of MCTF in Section 6.1 and 6.2, respectively. In Section 6.3, the detailed operations of the most common used MCTF schemes, 5/3 MCTF and 1/3 MCTF, are presented. Next, two categories of open-loop video coding schemes developed based on MCTF are explored in Section 6.4 and 6.5. Finally, the video coding standard of MCTF, Scalable Video Coding (SVC), is discussed in Section 6.6.

6.1 Convolution-Based MCTF

If we view a video sequence as a set of 3D video, the DWT filter not only can be applied in the spatial domain but also can be performed in the temporal domain. Therefore, the temporal filtering is developed. However, the direct implementation of the temporal filter has a low coding efficiency. This is because the positions of one object in different frames are different. In order to improve the performance of the temporal filtering, a temporal filtering along the motion trajectory is proposed by Taubman and Zakhor [104], and Ohm [13, 105]. The former applies a frame-based motion model, which is similar to global motion estimation and compensation [11, 106] in close-loop video codings. The latter adopts a block-based motion model, which is similar to block-based motion estimation and compensation [9, 107] in close-loop video codings. The frame-based motion model describes the motion trajectories of all pixels in one frame by only one unique motion model. Contrarily, in the block-based motion model, each block in one frame can have its motion trajectory. Hence the temporal filtering with block-based motion model has a better performance than that with a frame-based motion model.

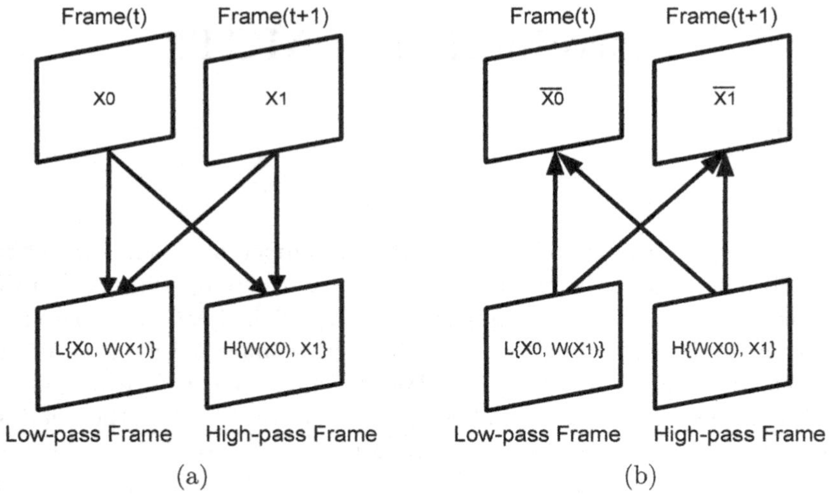

Fig. 6.1 Convolution-based MCTF. Two-tap Haar filter are adopted for example. (a) Forware MCTF decomposition. (b) Inverse MCTF recontruction.

The convolution-based MCTF is the earliest proposed MCTF, where the temporal filtering is implemented by the convolution-based method with a block-based motion model. Figure 6.1(a) shows an example which is a convolution-based Haar filter, and the operations of convolution-based Haar filter are as follows. First, because of the Haar filter, two frames are consisted of one pair, such as $X0$ and $X1$ frames. Based on the block-based motion model, each frame in one pair is divided into many small blocks, and for each block, it is matched in the other frame to find its motion trajectory. As for the much more detail of the block-based motion model, we will illustrate them in Chapter 7. After finding the motion trajectories, the filter is applied along the motion trajectories, and the equations of convolution-base Haar filter are

$$L\{X0, W(X1)\} = \frac{1}{2}(X0[m,n] + \widetilde{X1}[m + d_{0->1,m}, n + d_{0->1,n}]), \quad (6.1)$$

$$H\{X1, W(X0)\} = X1[m,n] - \widetilde{X0}[m + d_{1->0,m}, n + d_{1->0,n}], \quad (6.2)$$

where $L\{X0, W(X1)\}$ and $H\{X1, W(X0)\}$ are low-pass (L) and high-pass (H) frames, $(d_{0->1,m}, d_{0->1,n})$ and $(d_{1->0,m}, d_{1->0,n})$ are the displacements of the pixel (m, n) from $X0$ frame to $X1$ frame and from $X1$ frame to $X0$ frame, and $\widetilde{X1}$ and $\widetilde{X0}$ are interpolated frames of $X1$ and $X1$ frames, respectively. The interpolation is required because the motion can be fractional pixels. The inverse convolution-based Haar filter is

$$X0[m,n] = (L[m,n] - \frac{1}{2}\widetilde{H}[m + d_{0->1,m}, n + d_{0->1,n}]), \quad (6.3)$$

$$X1[m,n] = (\frac{1}{2}H[m,n] + \widetilde{L}[m + d_{1->0,m}, n + d_{1->0,n}]). \quad (6.4)$$

Figure 6.1(b) shows the flow of the inverse Haar filter.

Note that although we can reconstruct the $X0$ and $X1$ frames according to (6.3) and (6.4), the reconstructed frames are not exactly equal to the original frames. We illustrate this point more clearly by (6.1) and (6.2). When we want to reconstruct $X0$ and $X1$ frames, only L and H frames are available at the decoder. Hence there are four variables, $X0$, $X1$, $\widetilde{X0}$, and $\widetilde{X1}$ in (6.1) and (6.2). Although $\widetilde{X0}$ and $\widetilde{X1}$ can be derived from $X0$ and $X1$, it is hard to formulate $\widetilde{X0}$ and $\widetilde{X1}$ by $X0$ and $X1$ when the fractional-pixel interpolation is involved. Hence $X0$ and $X1$ frames cannot be exactly solved from L and H frames in (6.1) and (6.2). That is to say, the perfect reconstruction is not guaranteed due to the interpolation of the fractional-pixel motion, and the data loss exists after filtering and inverse filtering, even if there is no quantization. This induces a low coding performance of convolution-based MCTF.

6.2 Lifting-Based MCTF

Lifting-based DWT filter is also applied in MCTF [14, 108]. The operations of lifting-based MCTF are shown in Fig. 6.2(a). Similar to lifting-based 2D DWT, lifting-based MCTF consists of a series of prediction and update stages. The prediction stage is processed and followed by the update stage. The filtering equations are

$$P\{W(X0), X1\} = X1[m,n] - \widetilde{X0}[m + d_{1->0,m}, n + d_{1->0,n}], \quad (6.5)$$

$$U\{X0, W(H0)\} = X0[m,n] + \frac{1}{2}\widetilde{P}[m + d_{0->1,m}, n + d_{0->1,n}], \quad (6.6)$$

where $P\{W(X0), X1\}$ and $U\{X0, W(H0)\}$ are high-pass (H) and low-pass (L) frames respectively, $(d_{0->1,m}, d_{0->1,n})$ and $(d_{1->0,m}, d_{1->0,n})$ are the

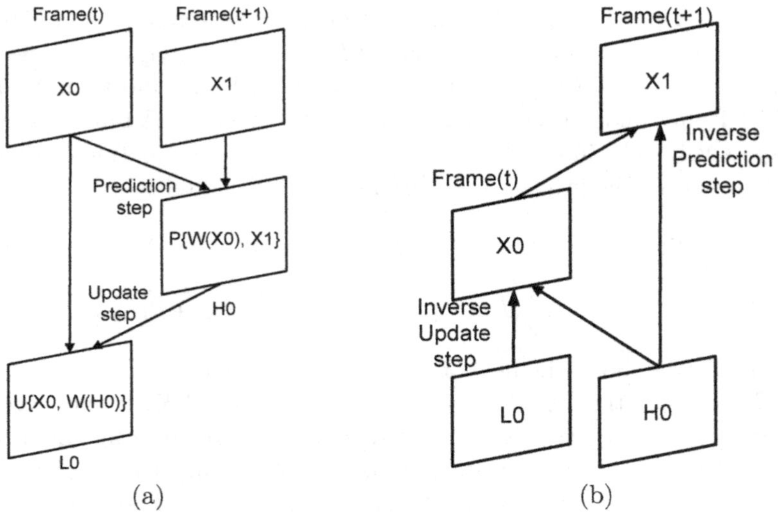

Fig. 6.2 Lifting-based MCTF. Two-tap Haar filter are adopted for example. (a) Forward MCTF decomposition. (b) Inverse MCTF reconstruction.

displacements of the pixel (m, n) from $X0$ frame to $X1$ frame and from $X1$ frame to $X0$ frame separately, and $\widetilde{*}$ is the interpolated frame of $(*)$ frame because the motion can be fractional pixels.

The inverse filtering equations can be directly derived from (6.5) and (6.6), and they can be written as

$$X0[m,n] = U[m,n] - \frac{1}{2}\widetilde{P}[m + d_{0->1,m}, n + d_{0->1,n}], \tag{6.7}$$

$$X1[m,n] = P[m,n] + \widetilde{X0}[m + d_{1->0,m}, n + d_{1->0,n}]. \tag{6.8}$$

The flow of inverse lifting-based MCTF is shown in Fig. 6.2(b). When reconstructing frames, because P and U are available at the decoder, then we can easily derive $\widetilde{P}$. Therefore, $X0$ frame can be perfectly reconstructed according to (6.6) or (6.7). When $X0$ frame is available, $\widetilde{X0}$ also can be derived and $X1$ frame can be reconstructed in (6.5) or (6.8). Hence in the lifting-based algorithm, perfect reconstruction can be guaranteed after the operations of filtering and inverse filtering, and the coding performance of MCTF is improved significantly.

Note that in lifting-based MCTF or convolution-based MCTF, two sets of motion information are required for L and H frames. However, in the update stage of lifting-based MCTF, the data in H frames are the prediction error and those in $X0$ frames are the object content. Therefore, it is hard to perform motion estimation and find the motion trajectory between H and $X0$ frames. Moreover, the bitrate overhead of motion information is also large. For the above reasons, the motion information of the update stage is usually derived from that of the prediction stage, so not only the motion estimation can be skipped but also the bitrate of motion information for the update stage can be saved.

6.3 5/3 MCTF and 1/3 MCTF

After the introduction to the development of MCTF, we further introduce the detailed operations of MCTF. The coding performance of MCTF depends on which wavelet filter is adopted. From recent experimental results [16, 21], MCTF is usually implemented by use of 5/3, 1/3, or Haar filter with the lifting scheme. 5/3 MCTF can achieve a better coding performance than 1/3 MCTF but requires a longer encoding delay [109]. For simplicity, MCTF represents the lifting-based MCTF using 5/3 or 1/3 filter in the following.

5/3 MCTF can be simply illustrated by Fig. 6.3, in which only two lifting stages are involved. The prediction stage uses even frames to predict odd frames, and the residual frames are high-pass frames (H frames). The update stage uses the H frames to update even frames, and the derived frames are low-pass frames (L frames). The detailed operations of the prediction stage, update stage, and multi-level MCTF will be introduced in the following subsections. 1/3 MCTF is just to skip the update stage of 5/3 MCTF and treat the even frames as the L frames. The open-loop MCTF means the frames used to predict or update are the original or filtered frames, instead of reconstructed or coded frames in the close-loop motion compensated prediction (MCP) scheme.

6.3.1 *Prediction stage*

The prediction stage uses even frames to predict odd frames, and the residual frames are the high-pass frames (H frames). As shown in Fig. 6.3, H frames are similar to B-frames, which are predicted by neighboring frames in the traditional MCP scheme. In the prediction stage, the block-based motion model is usually adopted for motion estimation. For every block in the odd frames, ME should be performed to find the best motion vectors,

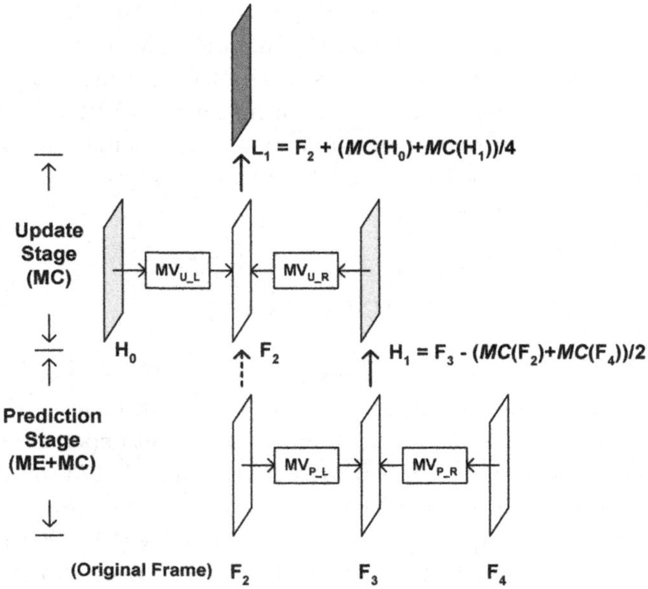

Fig. 6.3 The 5/3 MCTF scheme, where MV_{P_L} and MV_{P_R} represent the motion vectors from the left and right neighbor frames for the prediction stage, respectively, and so represent MV_{U_L} and MV_{U_R} for the update stage. The light gray frames (H) are the high-pass frames, and the heavy gray frames (L) are the low-pass frames.

MV_{P_L} and MV_{P_R}. Because of bi-prediction, these two motion vectors can be found by individual optimization or joint optimization. The individual optimization is that MV_{P_L} and MV_{P_R} can be found separately by the following criteria

$$\min\{COST_1(F_3, MC(F_2), MV_{P\_L})\},$$
$$\min\{COST_1(F_3, MC(F_4), MV_{P\_R})\},$$

where $COST_1(*)$ is the cost function to select the best motion vectors in the individual optimization. And based on the sought MV_{P_L} and MV_{P_R}, the filtering equations of the prediction stage are performed. The joint optimization is to refine the search results of the individual optimization in a bi-iterative way like SVC WD1.0 [110]. That is, MV_{P_L} and MV_{P_R} can be refined, based on the following equation,

$$\min\{COST_2(F_3, MC(F_2), MV_{P\_L}, MC(F_4), MV_{P\_R})\},$$

where $COST_2(*)$ is the cost function to select the best motion vectors in the joint optimization.

In the prediction stage, motion estimation and compensation are the major operations. Motion estimation is also a hot topic in the last two decades. We will introduce more about ME in Chapter 7.

6.3.2 *Update stage*

Although motion vectors are also required in the update stage, the motion vectors of the update stage are derived from those of the prediction stage (MV_{P_L} and MV_{P_R}). This is because of the data heterology between H frames and the original frames. The concept of motion estimation is hard to be performed in the update stage. Hence the computations of the update stage are to derive motion vectors and perform motion compensation. Many algorithms [111, 112, 113, 114, 20, 18, 19] are proposed to derive the motion vectors of the update stage. In the following, we only illustrate the algorithm of deriving the motion vectors in SVC WD1.0. As for the others, interested readers can study the above references.

Figure 6.4 shows the relationships of motion vectors in the prediction and update stages. We want to derive the motion vectors, MV_{U_R}, which are from F_2 frame to F_3 frame, but we only have the motion vectors, MV_{P_L}, which are from F_3 frame to F_2 frame, after the motion estimation of the prediction stage. For each motion vector in the prediction stage, it has a corresponding reference block in F_2 frame. For each current block in F_2 frame, it overlaps several reference blocks. Among these overlapped reference blocks, one reference block with the largest overlapped area is selected. And the motion vector of this current block in the update stage is set as the inverse of the corresponding motion vector. Based on the derived motion vector, the filtering equations are performed to update the current block. Note that it is possible that a current block has no overlapped reference blocks. If this condition occurs, the update stage of this current block is skipped. Moreover, because of no motion estimation, the computation complexity of the update stage is much less than that of the prediction stage.

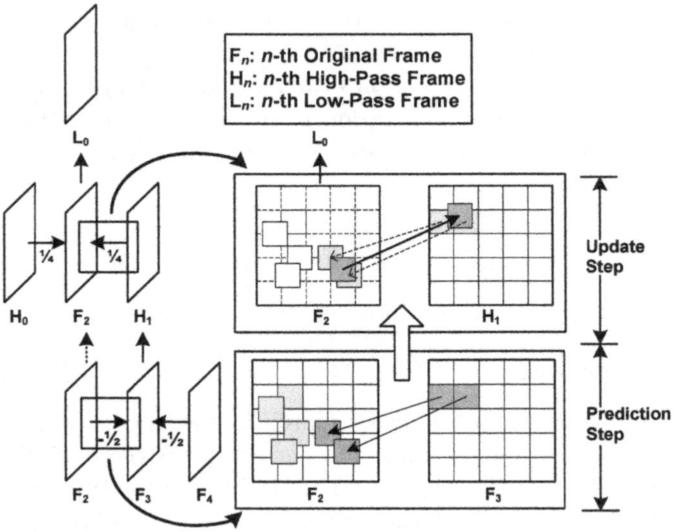

Fig. 6.4 The concept of deriving motion vectors in SVC WD1.0.

6.3.3 *Multi-level MCTF*

Figure 6.3 only shows the one-level MCTF scheme. The multi-level MCTF can be derived by recursively performing one-level MCTF on the L-frames, as shown in Fig. 6.5, which is an example for two-level MCTF. From Fig. 6.5, the temporal scalability of MCTF is apparently observed. If the original frame rate is 30 frames per second (fps), we can provide 15 fps after one-level MCTF. That is, only the L frames are required to be decoded and displayed for the half frame rate. If J-level MCTF is performed, $(J+1)$-level temporal scalability can be provided. This kind of temporal scalability does not require extra computations, so we call it an embedded temporal scalability in MCTF.

6.4 Different MCTF Schemes with DWT for Video Coding

Based on lifting-based MCTF, several new open-loop video coding schemes [115, 116, 117, 118, 119, 120, 121] are developed. We classified them into two categories, inter-wavelet video coding schemes and the pyramid scheme. The former consists of MCTF and 2D DWT, and the latter is composed of MCTF and discrete cosine transform (DCT). In inter-wavelet video coding

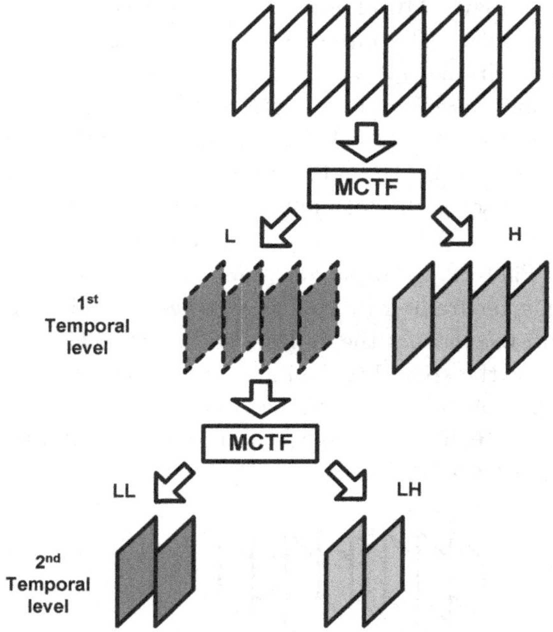

Fig. 6.5 Two-level MCTF that applies one-level MCTF on L-frames recursively.

schemes, the processing order of MCTF and 2D DWT can be interchanged, and then various scalabilities can be provided by arranging the processing orders of MCTF and 2D DWT. Moreover, based on the processing orders of MCTF and 2D DWT, the coding schemes can be classified into three types, including multi-level MCTF (t+2D), in-band MCTF (2D+t), and hybrid MCTF (2D+t+2D), in which "2D" is the abbreviation of 2D DWT and "t" is the abbreviation of temporal filtering, MCTF. In the following subsections, we will introduce their characteristics and illustrate their scalabilities.

As for the pyramid scheme, lifting-based MCTF is used to instead of MCP scheme in the close-loop video codings to become an open-loop video coding scheme, which will be introduced in the next section.

6.4.1 *Multi-level MCTF scheme*

In the multi-level MCTF schemes, the basic coding flow is that MCTF is executed first and followed by the process of 2D DWT. Figure 6.6 is an example of multi-level MCTF with two-level decomposition in temporal and spatial domains. The input video sequence is decomposed into two groups, L and H frames, by the first decomposition level of MCTF. The generated L frames are processed again by the second decomposition level of MCTF to get the LL and LH frames. After MCTF, two-level 2D DWT is executed in these LL, LH, and H frames, as shown in Fig. 6.6.

The temporal scalability of multi-level MCTF is embedded in MCTF, and similarly, the spatial scalability of multi-level MCTF is also embedded in 2D DWT. That is, by displaying these LL frames and dropping other frames, the quarter frame rate can be provided. Or if we get the LL and LH frames and reconstruct the L frames, then the half frame rate can be provided. As for the spatial scalability, we can show the LLL subband or reconstruct LL subband of each frames to provide a one-sixteen or quarter frame resolution. Hence the temporal and spatial scalabilities can be easily realized in multi-level MCTF.

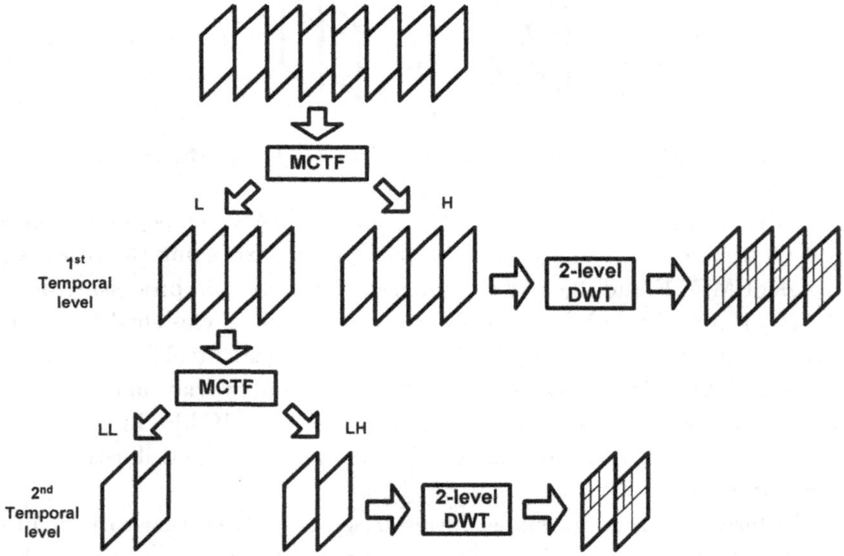

Fig. 6.6 Multi-level MCTF scheme.

We use a figure to describe the decoding path and illustrate the scalability of different coding schemes, in which one axis is frame size and the other is frame rate. Figure 6.7 is an example. Because the encoding order

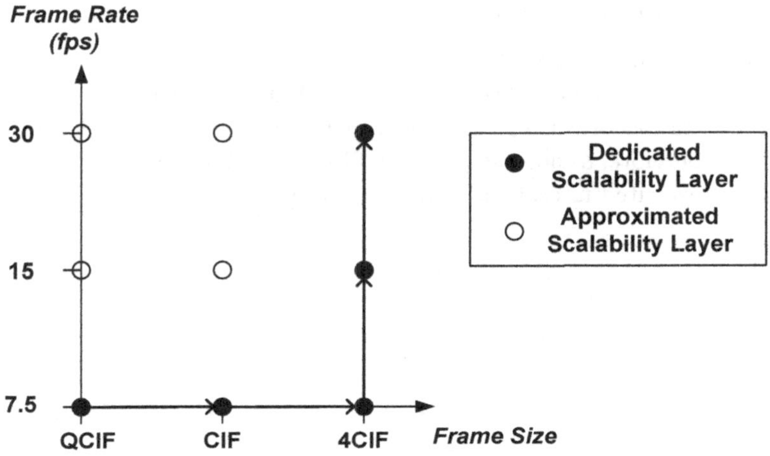

Fig. 6.7 The decoding path and scalability of multi-level MCTF scheme.

of multi-level MCTF is MCTF first, the decoding order is inverse and it is similar to Fig. 6.7. In fact, all points in Fig. 6.7 are the scalability layers of multi-level MCTF. Based on the decoding path, we classify these scalability layers into two categories, dedicated or approximated scalability layers. If the scalability layer is one point of the decoding path, this scalability layer is a dedicated scalability layer. Contrarily, if the scalability layer is not one point of the decoding path, this scalability layer is one approximated scalability layer. The performances of the dedicated scalability layers is better than those of the approximated scalability layers. This is because the dedicated scalability layers can be exactly decoded, but the approximated scalability layers can not. They have to be generated by the approximation from neighboring dedicated scalability layers, so their visual qualities are worse. For example, for the scalability layer (CIF, 15 fps), we do not have the exact motion vectors for CIF frames, but we can downsample the motion vectors of 4CIF frames to approximate the required motion vectors in CIF. Then, the scalability point (CIF, 15 fps) can be provided. Finally, Figure 6.7 shows that multi-level MCTF has a good temporal scalability but a bad spatial scalability.

6.4.2 *In-band MCTF scheme*

Compared to multi-level MCTF, we can interchange the processing order of MCTF and 2D DWT. We can process 2D DWT first and next perform the computation of MCTF, as shown in Fig. 6.8, which is called in-band MCTF. Therefore, a video sequence is filtered by 2D DWT first, and then MCTF is executed in each subband, respectively.

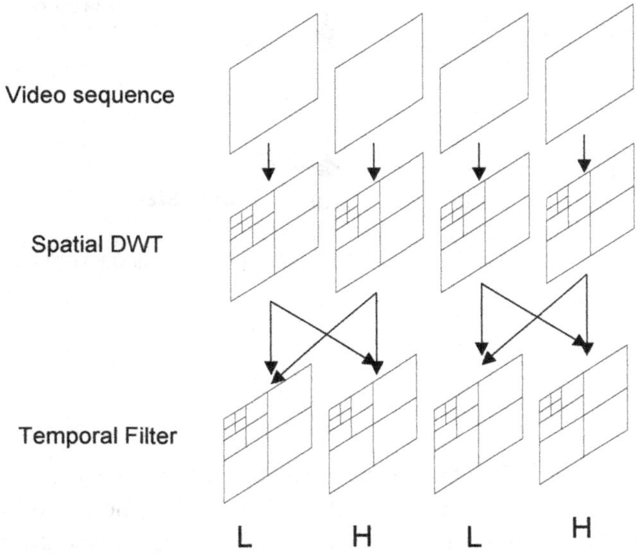

Fig. 6.8 In-Band MCTF scheme.

Two important issues are required to be explored in in-band MCTF scheme. The first one is how to do motion estimation in DWT domain. This is because DWT is a shift-variant transformation. Therefore, the filtered results of one object depends on its positions, and then it is hard to use motion estimation and compensation to align the objects. In multi-level MCTF, this problem does not exist, because motion estimation is performed in the spatial domain. Hence multi-level MCTF usually has a better coding performance than in-band MCTF does. In order to overcome the shift-variant problem of DWT transformation, the complete-to-overcomplete DWT (CODWT) [122, 123] with a shift-invariant property is proposed for motion estimation. Although the performance of in-band MCTF can be improved, the computation complexity and memory bandwidth are increased largely and the performance is still worse than that of multi-level MCTF.

The second problem is how to do motion estimation in H subband. The data in H subbands are the components of high frequency and similar to the prediction residual, so they are less correlated with each other. Hence it is hard to find the motion trajectories between two H subbands. Many methods [120, 115] are proposed to solve this problem. For example, we can use the motion vector of L subband or not perform MCTF in H subband. The former may induce more energy in H subbands if the motion vector is not suitable, and the latter can not reduce the temporal redundancy between two H subbands.

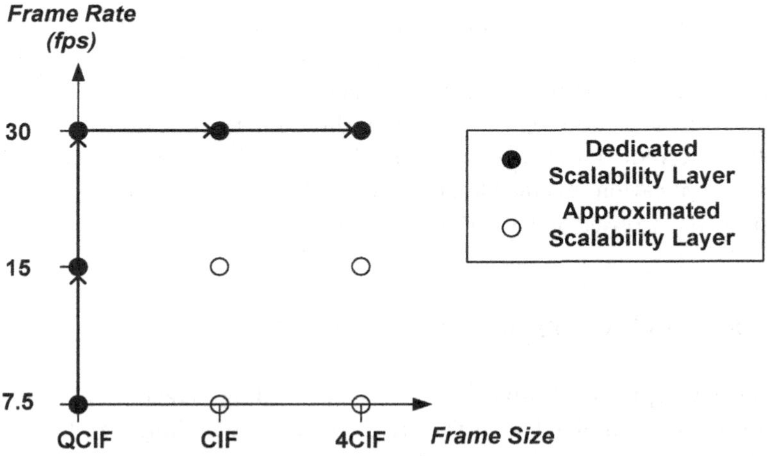

Fig. 6.9 The decoding path and scalability of In-Band MCTF scheme.

Figure 6.9 shows the decoding path and scalability of in-band MCTF scheme. Compared to Fig. 6.7, the dedicated scalability layers of in-band MCTF are opposite to those of multi-level MCTF. Hence in-band MCTF scheme has a good spatial scalability but a bad performance about temporal scalability.

6.4.3 *Hybrid MCTF scheme*

If we use "2D" and "t" to represent the operations of one-level 2D DWT and MCTF, respectively, then the processing orders of multi-level MCTF and in-band MCTF can be written as "t+t..+t+2D+2D+...+2D" and

"2D+2D+...+2D+t+t..+t", in which the number of "2D" or "t" depends on the decomposition levels of 2D DWT or MCTF, respectively. However, there are other hybrid MCTF schemes, besides multi-level MCTF and in-band MCTF. In the hybrid MCTF schemes, the decomposition levels of MCTF and 2D DWT can be arbitrarily partitioned and reorganized to be different processing orders.

We take two-level MCTF with two-level 2D DWT as an example to illustrate the hybrid schemes. Two-level MCTF with two-level 2D DWT totally has six possible kinds of processing orders. Two of them are multi-level MCTF and in-band MCTF, and the others are shown in Fig. 6.10. In Fig. 6.10(a), the processing order is "2D+t+t+2D". That is, in the beginning, we process one-level 2D DWT, and next two-level MCTF are adopted. Lastly, the remainder decomposition level of 2D DWT is performed. Figure 6.10(b), (c), and (d) show the related processing order of "t+2D+2D+t", "t+2D+t+2D" and "2D+t+2D+t", respectively. Different processing orders can provide different decoding paths, and then various scalabilities can be achieved. Therefore, based on the required scalability layers of the specific application, a suitable decoding path can be designed by arranging the processing order of MCTF and 2D DWT.

6.5 Pyramid MCTF with DCT for Video Coding

In the development of MCTF-based video coding schemes, lifting-based MCTF is also combined with the traditional video coding standards, such as H.264, to become a new scalable video coding scheme, pyramid MCTF, as shown in Fig. 6.11. In pyramid MCTF, temporal scalability is provided by MCTF. As for spatial scalability, it adopts the concept of layer coding in MPEG-2 [10]. Based on the requirement of spatial scalability, several downsampled video sequences of different frame sizes and frame rates are generated from the original sequence first. Therefore, the spatial scalability is decided after the downsample filter is performed. Note that the temporal scalability of each downsampled sequence is constrained if the corresponding frame rate is simultaneously downsampled.

After generating these dowsampled sequences, each sequence is coded by MCTF and DCT from the smallest frame size to the original size. However, because the spatial scalability is provided by the layer coding, the redundancy between different spatial layers is also induced. This problem doesn't exist in inter-wavelet video coding schemes, because 2D DWT

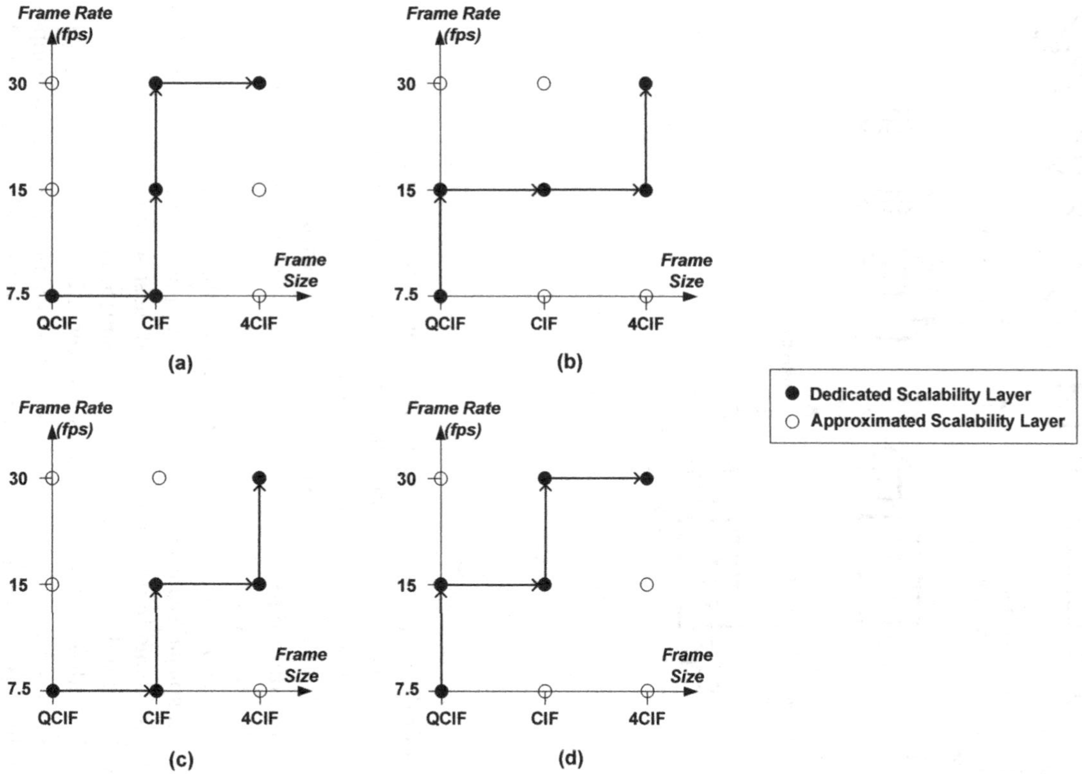

Fig. 6.10 The decoding path and scalability of Hybrid MCTF schemes: (a) "2D+t+t+2D"; (b) "t+2D+2D+t"; (c) "t+2D+t+2D"; (d) "2D+t+2D+t".

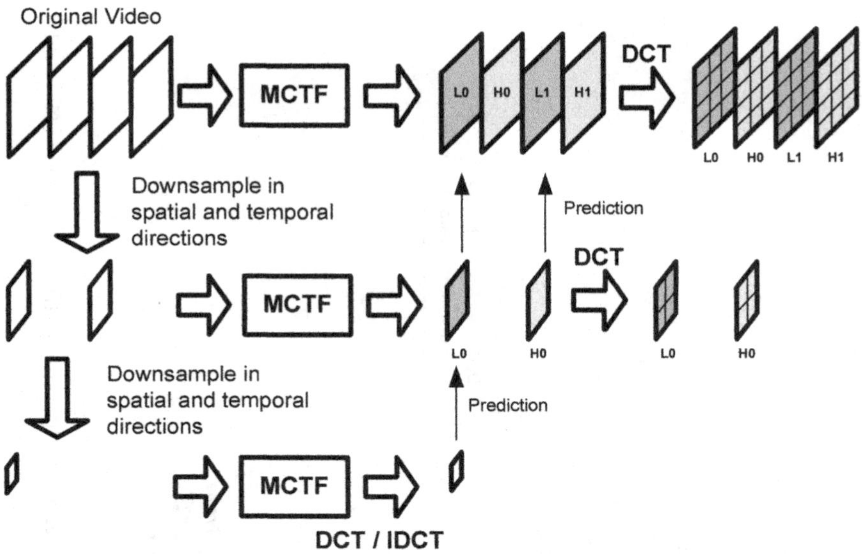

Fig. 6.11 Pyramid MCTF scheme.

has the embedded spatial scalability. In order to remove the redundancy between spatial layers, a new prediction tool, inter-layer prediction, is developed. The concept of inter-layer prediction is that when coding one sequence with the larger frame size, one sequence with the smaller frame size can be upsampled to be one kind of prediction modes. Hence the coding efficiency of pyramid MCTF can be improved.

Figure 6.12 shows the decoding path and scalability of pyramid MCTF. Because each spatial scalability is a dedicated sequence in pyramid MCTF, not a DWT subband in inter-wavelet video coding schemes, pyramid MCTF can provide a good spatial scalability and subjective view, compared to inter-wavelet video coding schemes. Moreover, MCTF is directly applied in each spatial layer, so pyramid MCTF also can provide a good temporal scalability. However, the disadvantage of pyramid MCTF is that the scalability is constrained after the downsample filter is applied. And much more redundant information has to be removed, because extra sequences with smaller frame sizes exist.

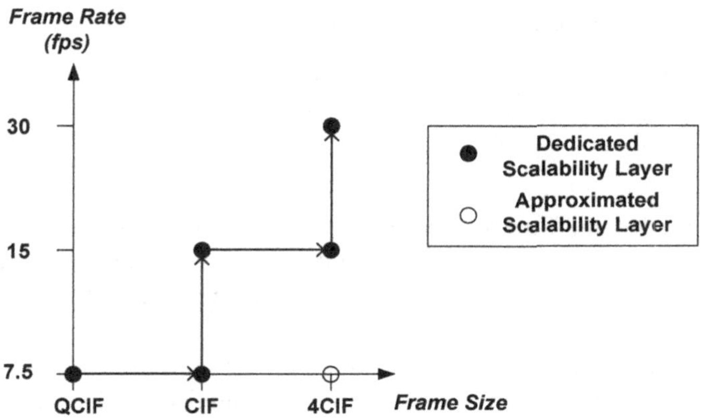

Fig. 6.12 The decoding path and scalability of pyramid MCTF scheme.

6.6 Scalable Video Coding

Many video coding standards, such as MPEG series [9, 10, 11] and H.26x series [107, 124, 12], have been made one after another from 1990 to now. The revolution between two video coding standards is a significant improvement in the compression ratio. For example, H.264 can provide double compression ratio, compared with H.263. However, besides the compression ratio, some specific functionality becomes more and more important, as the internet and multimedia devices are more and more popular. For instance, in order to communicate by wireless network, error resilience and concealment are demanded to overcome the transmission noise and error. Because the communication bandwidth is variant and there are many different display devices, such as PC, PDAs, and mobile phones, the scalable capability of a video bitstream becomes necessary. Hence scalable video coding (SVC) standard [17, 18, 19] is being made by MPEG in order to provide a scalable bitstream and better error resilience. Table 6.1 shows the schedule of SVC standard in MPEG meeting, and the whole SVC standard will be finalized at January, 2007.

MPEG also has identified many future applications and related requirements of SVC. The requirements of scalability in SVC include temporal scalability, spatial scalability, coarse/fine SNR scalability, and complexity scalability. Temporal scalability means that single bitstream can support different frame rates. Spatial scalability is to support various frame sizes

Table 6.1 The timeslot of scalable video coding.

Milestone	CfP	WD	CD	FCD	FDIS
Time (Year/Month)	03/10	05/07	06/04	06/07	07/01

in single bitstream. Coarse/Fine SNR scalability means that the single bitstream can be adapted to be various bitrate or visual quality. Complexity scalability is that the more computation power at the decoder is, the better quality can be decoded.

As for the applications of SVC, there are three major proposals, home entertainment, broadband video distribution, and digital video surveillance. In home entertainment, by use of SVC, we only store one single bitstream, and it can be adapted and decoded for different display devices, such as HDTV, DTV, PDA and mobile phones. The storage size can be significantly saved. In broadband video distribution, there are various communication bandwidths and display devices. When broadcasting a video program, we have to broadcast many bitstreams for different specifications in traditional video codings. If a scalable bitstream is available, only one bitstream is required to be transmitted. By a simple adaption, the scalable bitstream can be adapted to fit the communication bandwidth or the application requirements.

In the future, more and more camera sensors exist in a digital video surveillance system, so many video sequences are required to be stored. But in a surveillance system, the importance of video sequences is decreased, as the time increases. Therefore, we can use a smaller frame size or a low frame rate to store those older video sequences. For example, if a sequence is recorded in this morning, we may hope that it can provide the highest spatial and temporal resolutions such as D1 Format and 30 frame per second (fps). But for a sequence which is recorded in the last week, it may only require medium spatial and temporal resolutions like CIF Format and 15 fps. For a sequence in the last month, maybe its specification is only QQCIF Format and 0.1 fps. We called this characteristic an erosion storage, which means the storage size of a video sequence could be eroded as the time increases. In traditional video coding standards, the erosion storage is provided by transcoding, which requires a huge computation complexity and makes it impossible. But in SVC, we can utilize the characteristics of scalable bitstream to provide the erosion storage. That is, we can directly discard the part of high spatial and temporal resolution in a bitstream to change the specification of a sequence, and no additional computations are required.

In SVC CfP [17], many kinds of coding schemes with lifting-based MCTF are proposed including multi-level MCTF, in-band MCTF, and pyramid MCTF. After comparing the performances of three coding schemes, pyramid MCTF [20] is adopted in the working document [19] and reference software [125, 110]. In SVC WD1.0, the coding scheme is composed of pyramid MCTF and coding tools of H.264. The coding flow of Scalable Video Model (SVM), which is the reference software of SVC, is shown in Fig. 6.13. Four basic components of SVM 3.0 are *MCTF*, *DCT/Q*, *Sub-bitplane CABAC*, and *Inter-layer Prediction*. *MCTF* is the temporal prediction, *DCT/Q* is the spatial transform and quantization, and *Sub-bitplane CABAC* is the entropy coding. *Inter-layer Prediction* is used to remove the redundancy between two spatial layers. The processing order is that *MCTF* is applied first and followed by *DCT/Q* and *Sub-bitplane CABAC*. If *Inter-layer Prediction* is allowed, the prediction modes of *Inter-layer Prediction* are added into *MCTF* and *DCT/Q*.

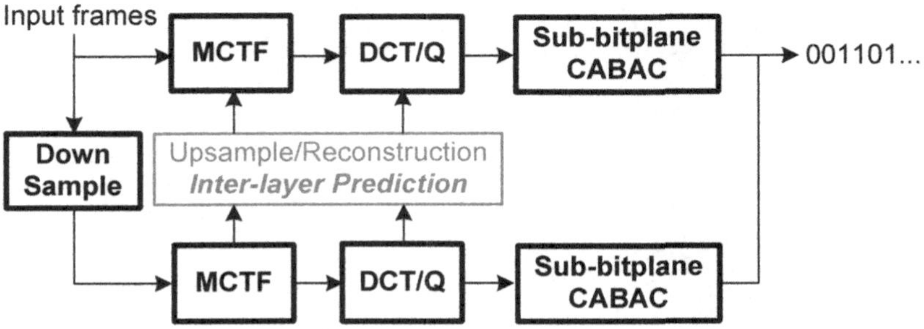

Fig. 6.13 The coding flow of SVM 3.0.

In SVC, there are three kinds of prediction schemes, which are extended from *MCTF*. They are 5/3 MCTF, 1/3 MCTF, and Hierarchical B-frames (HB) . In each scheme, not only bi-prediction but also uni-prediction are allowed. The operations of 5/3 MCTF and 1/3 MCTF are introduced in Section 6.3. The operations of HB are similar to 1/3 MCTF, and the difference between both is the coding order. Multi-level MCTF is performed in a bottom-to-top order, which is from higher to lower frame rates, as shown in Fig. 6.5. HB is to perform multi-level MCTF in a top-to-bottom way, which is from lower to higher frame rates. That is, the processing order of multi-level MCTF in Fig. 6.5 is from decomposition level 1 to decomposition level 2. Then the processing order of HB is from decomposition level 2 to decomposition level 1. Note that in SVC, the top-to-bottom decomposition is possible, only when all update steps are ignored. Therefore, the coding performance of HB is close to that of 1/3 MCTF. By changing the processing order of multi-level MCTF, HB can provide the advantage of being compatible with the generic B-frames of H.264/AVC.

As for the SNR scalability, the coarse SNR scalability is provided by *DCT/Q* which is to perform different quantization values to get different quality layers. The fine SNR scalability is achieved by *Sub-bitplane CABAC* which combines the concept of context-based adaptive binary arithmetic coding (CABAC) in H.264, and bit-plane coding of embedded block coding with optimized truncation (EBCOT) in JPEG2000. Therefore, SVC can realize three kinds of scalability, and now many new coding tools are still proposed in every MPEG meeting for the improvement of compression ratio and increasing the scalability.

Chapter 7

Introduction to Motion Estimation

Motion estimation (ME) and motion compensation (MC) is an important technique to remove the temporal redundancy in a video sequence. By use of ME and MC, the compression ratio of traditional motion-compensated prediction (MCP) can be significantly improved. In MCTF, motion estimation and compensation are used to align the object with different positions in different frames for the temporal filtering. The accuracy of object alignments seriously impacts the performance of MCTF. Therefore, we will introduce ME first before the analysis of MCTF.

Many ME algorithms and hardware architectures are proposed in the last two decades. In the following, we will introduce ME from algorithms to hardware architectures. The ME algorithms are classified into three types, full search, fast full search, and fast search algorithms. In each category, only one or two typical algorithms are introduced because of the limited space in this book. Next, we classify ME hardware architectures into several categories and discuss the tradeoffs between the required memory bandwidth and on-chip memory size of different data re-use schemes. There are many research reports about ME, so the interested reader can refer to them.

7.1 The Concept of Motion Estimation and Compensation

Motion estimation plays an important role in a video coding system, and it is adopted in many video coding standard, such as MPEG-X series [9, 10, 11] and H.26X series [107, 124, 12]. Because the time distance between two successive frames of a sequence is very short like 1/30 or 1/15 second, the content of the neighboring frames are similar. Therefore, there are many redundancies between two continuous frames. In ME and MC, we use the previous frame as the reference frame to predict the current frame, as shown in Fig. 7.1. For a block in the current frame, $Cur.MB$, we find one reference block which is the most similar to $Cur.MB$ from the searching region in the reference frame. And only the differences between two blocks and the displacement used to describe the position of the reference block need to be coded. Therefore, the amount of coded data is much less than the original, and a high compression ratio can be achieved. The operation of ME is to find the most similar reference block, and that of MC is to reconstruct the reference block based on the displacement. In MCTF, ME and MC are used to align the positions of a object in different frames, so the performance of ME/MC seriously impacts the coding performance of MCTF.

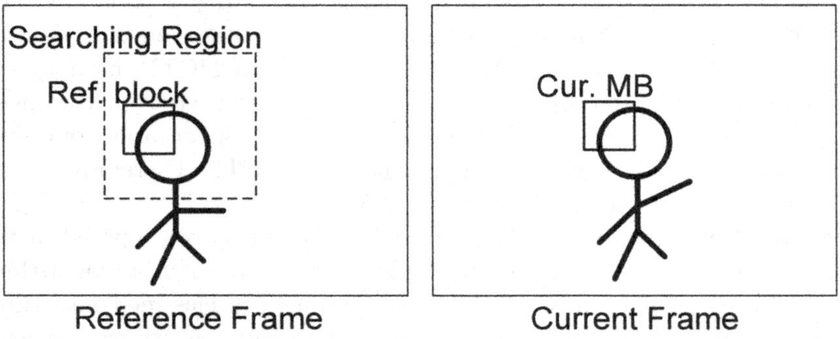

Fig. 7.1 The concept of ME.

7.2 Block Matching Algorithm

Among various ME algorithms, block matching algorithms (BMAs) are usually selected and adopted in all video coding standards because of its simplicity and good quality. In BMAs, the current frame is divided into many small macroblocks (MBs), and each MB in the current frame (current MB) is matched in the searching range of the reference frame by calculating the distortion. Figure 7.2 shows the spatial relationship between the current MB and searching region. Among many proposed distortion models, the sum of absolute differences (SAD) is the most common used, and it can be written as

$$SAD(k,p) = \sum_{j=1}^{B_V} \sum_{i=1}^{B_H} Distortion(i,j,k,p), \tag{7.1}$$

$$Distortion(i,j,k,p) = |cur(i,j) - ref(i+k, p+j)|, \tag{7.2}$$

$$-P_H \le k < P_H, \quad -P_V \le p < P_V, \tag{7.3}$$

where B_H and B_V are the block sizes of current MB, the searching range is $[-P_H, P_H)$ and $[-P_V, P_V)$ in the horizontal and vertical directions, respectively, (k,p) is one position in the searching range (search candidate), its corresponding block is called reference block, $cur(i,j)$ is the pixel value in the current MB (current pixel), $ref(i+k, j+p)$ is the pixel value in the reference block (reference pixel), $Distortion(i,j,k,p)$ is the difference between the current pixel $cur(i,j)$ and the reference pixel $ref(i+k, j+p)$, and $SAD(k,p)$ is the summation of all distortions in the current MB for the search candidate (k,p). The row SAD is the summation of B_H distortions in a row, and the column SAD is the summation of B_V distortions in a column. Finally, the search candidate which has the smallest SAD is selected as the best reference MBs, and the associated (k,p) is the motion vector of this current MB.

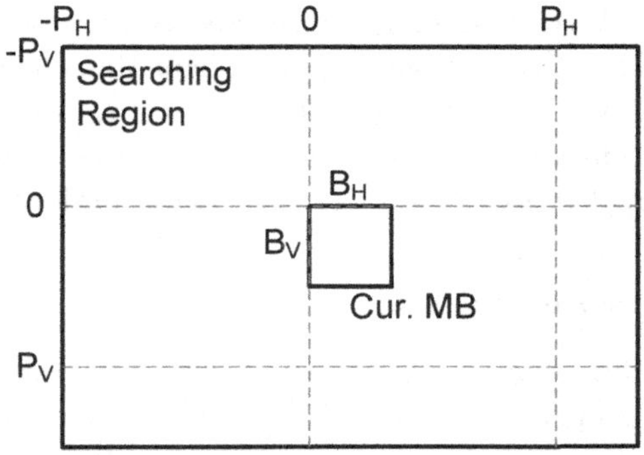

Fig. 7.2 The relationship between current macroblock and searching range.

For a video sequence, the procedure of ME in a video coding system can be decomposed into seven loops, as shown in Fig. 7.3. The first loop (*Frame-level loop*) is the number of frames in a video sequence, and the second and third loops (*MB-level loop*) are the number of current MBs in

```
for Number-of-Frame   ( Frame-level loop )

    for Number-of-MBV   ( MB-level loop in the vertical direction)
    for Number-of-MBH   ( MB-level loop in the horizontal direction)

        for Number-of-SRV   ( SR-level loop in the vertical direction)
        for Number-of-SRH   ( SR-level loop in the horizontal direction)

            for Number-of-CBV   ( CurBlock-level loop in the vertical direction)
            for Number-of-CBH   ( CurBlock-level loop in the horizontal direction)
                ... ...

                ...

            end of Number-of-CBH
            end of Number-of-CBV

        end of Number-of-SRH
        end of Number-of-SRV

    end of Number-of-MBH
    end of Number-of-MBV

end of Number-of-Frame
```

Fig. 7.3 The procedure of ME for a video sequence in a video coding system.

one frame. The fourth and fifth loops (*SR-level loop*) are the number of search candidates in the searching region, and the last two loops (*CurBlock-level loop*) are the number of pixels in one current MB for the computation of distortions. Many block matching algorithms are proposed to speed up the computation of ME, and different types of algorithms focused on different loops. In the following subsections, ME algorithms are classified into full search algorithm, fast full search algorithms, and fast search algorithms, based on the provided quality and focused operation-level loops.

7.2.1 *Full search algorithm*

In the full search block matching algorithm (FSBMA), all search candidates in the searching range are examined, and the search candidate with the smallest distortion in the searching range is selected as the final motion vector. Because all search candidates are examined in FSBMA, FSBMA can guarantee that its distortion is the smallest in the searching range. However, its price is the ultra huge computation complexity. For example, if we want to real-time compute motion estimation for CIF Format, 30 frame per second (fps) video with the searching range of size $[-16, 16)$, the computation complexity is 9.3 Giga-operation per second (GOPS). If the frame size becomes D1 Format and the searching range is enlarged to

$[-32, 32)$, the required computation complexity is increased to 127 GOPS. Therefore, many fast full search or fast algorithms are proposed to reduce the required computation complexity.

7.2.2 *Fast full search algorithm*

Many fast full search algorithms are proposed to speed up the computation of FSBMA without any quality drop. Most of them focus on the computation in the *CurBlock-level loop*. This is because all search candidates are still required to be examined to keep the full search quality, and then only the computation in the *CurBlock-level loop* can be changed. These algorithms try to avoid the unnecessary computation in the *CurBlock-level loop* in order to save the computation. In this subsection, partial distortion elimination (PDE) [126] and successive elimination algorithm (SEA) [127] are taken as examples.

7.2.2.1 *Partial distortion elimination*

The concept of PDE is simple and effective. The computation of FSBMA is the accumulation of distortions between the current pixels and reference pixels for each search candidate. If the partial SAD of this search candidate is larger than the current minimum SAD, it cannot be the optimal one. Hence the accumulation of the partial SAD can be terminated, and this search candidate can be skipped. By the early termination, the operations of ME can be speeded up.

Note that the performance of PDE depends on the current minimum SAD. If the current minimum SAD is closer to the final minimum and is found earlier, the reduction ratio is higher. In order to improve the reduction ratio, PDE is usually combined with the motion vector predictor which will be illustrated in Section 7.2.3.3. The scan order of search candidates also can be changed from raster scan to spiral scan, as shown in Fig. 7.4. This is because the search candidate with the minimum SAD is probably located on the original point $(0, 0)$ or motion vector predictor in the searching range.

Many other algorithms are also developed to enhance the performance of PDE. For example, in [128], an adaptive scanning order of pixels in the current MB is proposed for the accumulation of partial SAD to further speed up the computation of PDE. In [129], the partial distortions and the current minimum distortion are normalized to increase the probability of

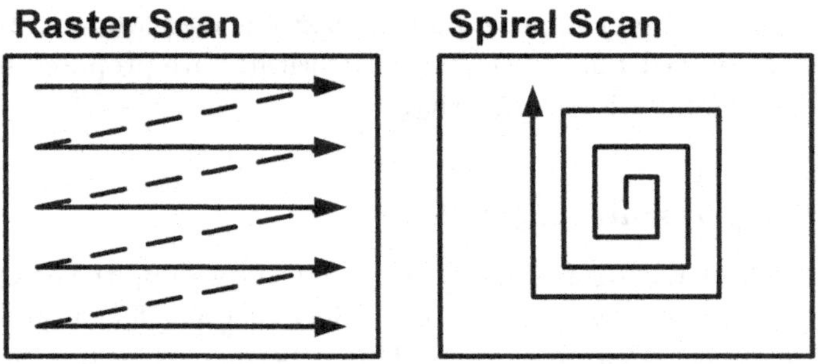

Fig. 7.4 Different scan orders.

early rejection of non-possible candidate MVs.

7.2.2.2 *Successive elimination algorithm*

In SEA , the inequality of the absolute difference between the sum of current pixels in the current block and the sum of reference pixels for a search candidate is used to skip the unnecessary computation. We can write the inequality as

$$\begin{aligned} SAD(k,p) &= \sum_{j=1}^{B_V}\sum_{i=1}^{B_H} |cur(i,j) - ref(i+k, j+p)| \\ &\geq \left| \sum_{j=1}^{B_V}\sum_{i=1}^{B_H} cur(i,j) - \sum_{j=1}^{B_V}\sum_{i=1}^{B_H} ref(i+k, j+p) \right| . \end{aligned} \tag{7.4}$$

If the absolute difference of the search candidate is larger than the current minimum SAD, then its SAD is also larger than the current minimum SAD. Hence this search candidate is impossible to be the optimal one, and the computation of this search candidate can be skipped. On the contrary, if this absolute difference is smaller than the current minimum SAD, the SAD for this search candidate has to be computed.

The sum of current pixels in the current MB is only computed once and can be re-used for all search candidates. The sum of reference pixels for different search candidates can be easily calculated by reusing the partial result. Because the computation complexity of this detecting procedure is small, the computation complexity of FSBMA can be reduced by skipping the SAD computations of those impossible search candidates with little computation overhead. Similar to PDE, a good initial search candidate can provide a better reduction ratio in SEA, so several methods, like motion vector predictor, spiral scanning order and so on, are also adopted to improve the performance of SEA. In [130, 131, 132], multilevel successive elimination algorithm (MSEA) are proposed to further improve the performance of SEA by changing the checking procedure.

7.2.3 *Fast search algorithm*

The fast full search algorithms can speed up the computation time of FS-BMA, but it is still hard to achieve the real-time computation with these algorithms, especially for a large frame size or searching range. Therefore, fast search algorithms are developed, which require much less computation with a little quality drop. Fast search algorithms can be roughly classified into four categories, including *Simplification of Matching Criterion*, *Reduction on Search Candidates*, *Predictive Search*, and *Hierarchical Search*, based on their characteristics. These four categories are not conflicted with each other, so they can be combined with each other to provide a better performance than the original does. In the following, we will introduce these categories and take some typical algorithms or methods as examples for illustration.

7.2.3.1 *Simplification of matching criterion*

Simplification of Matching Criterion is reducing the computation complexity of *CurBlock-level loop* to save the required computation complexity of ME. We take two examples to explain the concept of *Simplification of Matching Criterion.* The first one is Subsampling [133, 134], in which not all current pixels in the current MB are used to calculate the sum of distortions for each search candidate. That is, only a part of current pixels in the current MB are required to be computed. For example, if we subsample the current block by two, only one pixel in every two current pixels is used to calculate the distortion and SAD, and then the computation complexity is reduced to half. Figure 7.5(a), (b), and (c) show three cases, no subsampling, subsampling by two, and subsampling by four, respectively. The larger the subsample ratio is, the more computation can be saved, but the more quality is lost. In general, subsampling by two almost has the same performance as the original, but subsampling by four has some degree of quality loss.

There is another kind of *Simplification of Matching Criterion*, pixel

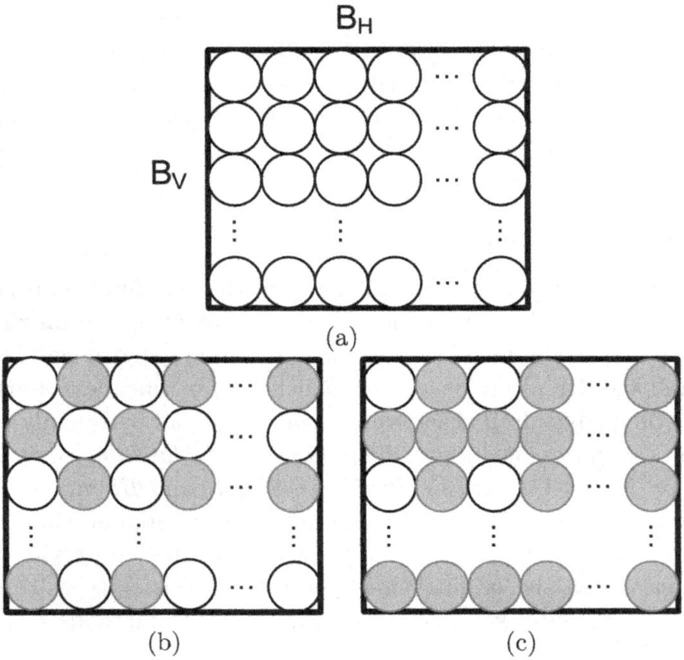

Fig. 7.5 The subsampling of current MB; (a) The original current MB. (b) The current MB with subsampling by two; (c) The current MB with subsampling by four, where only the white pixels are required to compute.

truncation [135]. In general, each current or reference pixel has eight bits, so the word length of absolute difference between current and reference pixels is also eight bits. Pixel truncation is truncating the number of bits in each pixel to achieve the computation reduction. For example, if the number of bits in each pixel is truncated from eight bits to five bits, then the required computation is only 5/8 of the original. Note that pixel truncation not only can reduce the computation complexity but also can save the hardware cost and the consumption power of ME hardware accelerator. This is because we can use a subtractor with less bits instead of that with eight bits. In most of video sequences, only six or five bits are required for one pixel.

7.2.3.2 *Reduction on search candidates*

The second category is *Reduction on Search Candidates.* In this category, they focus on the computation reduction of *SR-level loop*, and there is an important and common assumption for these algorithms. These algorithms assume that the distortion monotonically decreases as the search candidate approaches to the optimal one. That is, even if we does not match all the search candidates, the optimal search candidate can be achieved by following the search candidate with the smaller distortion. This category is the major part of fast search algorithms, and there are many proposed algorithms, such as center-biased diamond search [136, 137], advanced diamond zonal search [138, 139], three step search [140], two dimensional logarithmic search [141], one dimensional full search [142], new three step search [143], four step search [144], block-based gradient descent search [145], predictive line search [146, 147], and so on. Because of the limited space in this book, we only introduce two typical algorithms, diamond search and three step search, as examples.

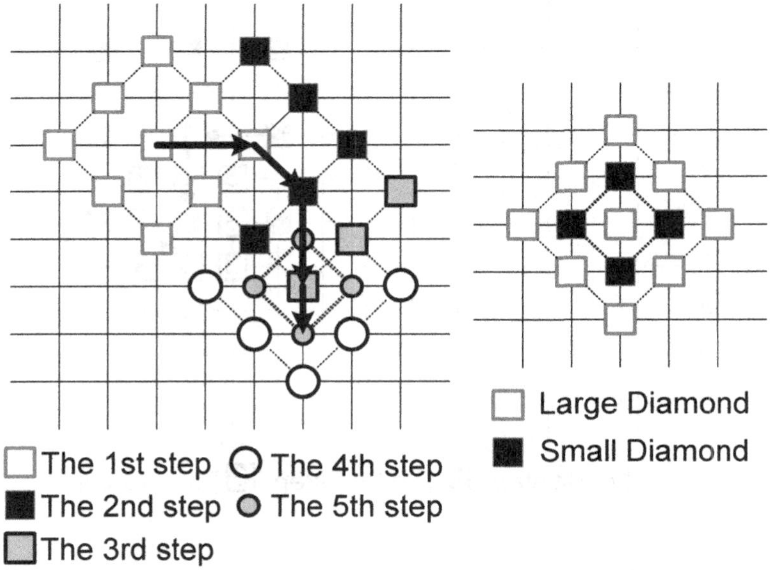

Fig. 7.6 The searching procedure of diamond search.

Figure 7.6 shows the searching procedure of diamond search. Diamond search has two search steps, large diamond and small diamond, as shown in the right-hand part of Fig. 7.6. In the searching procedure, the large diamond is applied first. Diamond search moves the large diamond, until the center search candidate has the smallest distortion among the nine candidates of the large diamond. Next, the small diamond is used to refine the searching result of the large diamond. The left-hand part of Fig. 7.6 is an example of diamond search. The arrow is the direction which the large diamond moves toward, and after the searching result of the large diamond converges in the fourth step, the small diamond is adopted to refine the searching result in the fifth step.

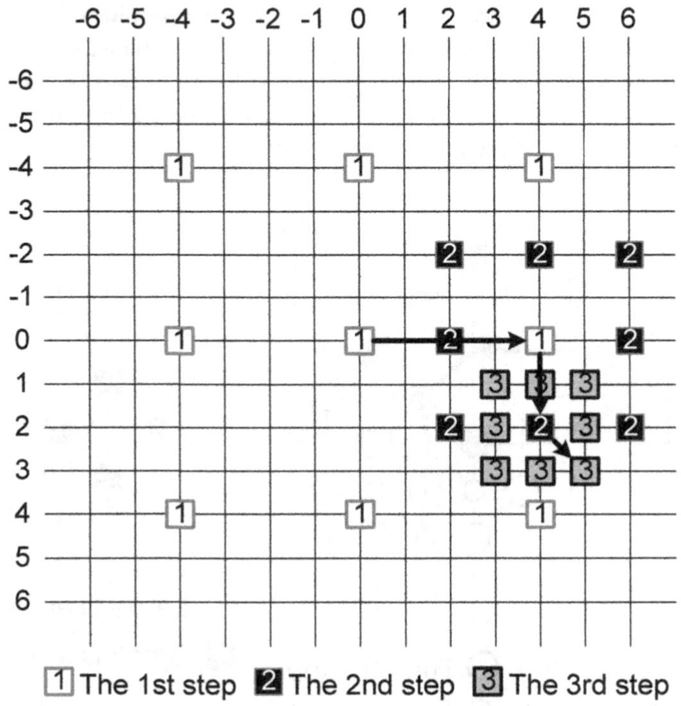

Fig. 7.7 The searching procedure of three step search.

Three step search is another typical fast search algorithm and is shown in Fig. 7.7. If the searching range is $[-P, P]$ in the both directions ($P_H = P_V = P$), the number of steps (NoS) in three step search is $log_2(P+1)$. And the interval between two search candidates in the n-th step is $2^{(NoS-n)}$. In each step, three step search calculates the distortion of nine search candidates and moves the center to the position with the smallest distortion for the next step, until all search steps are computed. For example, we assume that the searching range is $[-7, 7]$, so the number of steps is three and the intervals between two search candidates in three steps are 4, 2, and 1, respectively. The processing flow is as shown in Fig. 7.7.

Compared to diamond search, three step search has a fixed computation complexity for each current MB. The computation complexity of diamond search is variant and depends on the contents of the current MB and searching range. Therefore, the computation reduction of three step search is fixed, but for diamond search, its performance is variant.

7.2.3.3 *Predictive search*

In various fast search algorithms, there is a common assumption, which is that the distortion monotonically decreases as the search candidate approaches to the optimal one. However, this assumption may be failed, and then these fast search algorithms are usually trapped into the local minimum. Therefore, in order to avoid this condition, *Predictive Search* is developed and combined with other fast search algorithms. The concept of *Predictive Search* is that the motion vectors of neighboring MBs are correlated and similar, so we can use them to predict the motion vector of the current MB. Besides the spatial information, the temporal information also can be applied to be prediction because of the motion continuity in the temporal direction. Therefore, the motion information of neighboring blocks in the spatial or temporal space is used to be the initial search candidate of fast search algorithms instead of the original point. In brief, we can view *Predictive Search* as a method which utilizes the information of *MB-level loop* and *Frame-level loop* to predict the motion vector of the current MB and then save the computation of *SR-level loop*.

Motion vector predictors can be derived from many different methods and sources. For example, in [139], the initial search candidate can be the motion vectors of the blocks on the top, left, and top-right, their median, zero motion vector, the motion vector of the collocated block in the previous frame, and the accelerated motion vector of the collocated block in the previous two frames. By this way, the searching range can be reduced and constrained, so not only the computation complexity but also the bitrate of motion vector can be saved.

7.2.3.4 *Hierarchical search*

The last one is *Hierarchical Search*, which is a multi-resolution structure. The multi-resolution structure consists of several frame resolutions, including the original frame resolution and several downsampled frame resolutions. In *Hierarchical Search*, an initial estimation at the coarse level is processed first, and then a refinement at the next fine level is executed. Usually, two-level or three-level *Hierarchical Search* is adopted [148, 149, 150], and the downsample ratio of the current MB and searching range between two levels is usually set as two in the horizontal and vertical directions, as shown in Fig. 7.8. At the coarse level, because of subsampling in the current MB and searching region, the required computation complexity becomes small and acceptable. Therefore, full search is usually adopted to find the optimal motion vector in the subsampled searching region at the coarse level. As for the computation at the fine level, by using the searching result at the coarse level as the initial search candidate, only a local refinement is required. Hence the searching range at the fine level is reduced, and then the computation complexity is saved.

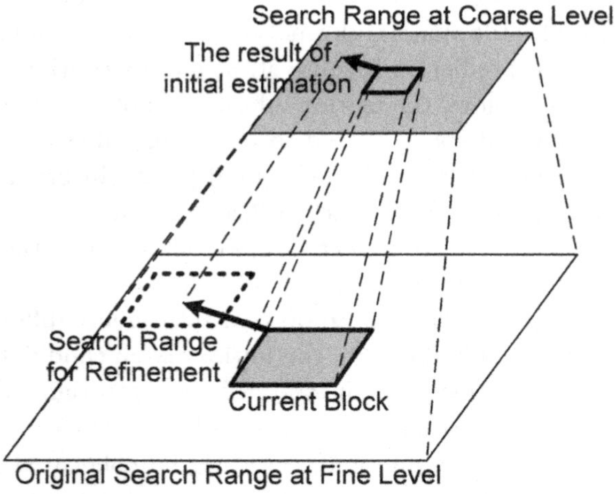

Fig. 7.8 The searching procedure of hierarchical search.

Compared to the seven loops of ME, *Hierarchical Search* creates a virtual loop for the multi-resolution structure between *MB-level loop* and *SR-level loop*. In general, *Hierarchical Search* is adopted in the applications with a high frame resolution or a huge searching range.

7.2.4 *Summary*

In a word, ME algorithms can be simply classified into three categories. The first one is FSBMA, which provides the best quality but requires large computation complexity. The second one is the fast full search algorithm which uses a simple check to detect whether a search candidate is possible to be the optimal one. And only the SADs of possible search candidates can be further calculated. By this method, the computation of those impossible search candidates can be saved, and no quality is lost. The third category is the fast search algorithm, in which the computation complexity can be saved largely with a little quality degradation. Based on the characteristics of fast search algorithms, they can be further categorized into four parts, *Simplification of Matching Criterion*, *Reduction of Search Candidates*, *Predictive Search*, and *Hierarchical Search*. *Simplification of Matching Criterion* and *Reduction of Search Candidates* focus on the computation reduction of *CurBlock-level loop* and *SR-level loop*, respectively. *Predictive Search* is to use the motion information of *MB-level loop* or *Frame-level loop* to speed up the computation. *Hierarchical Search* is to create a virtual loop for the multi-resolution structure between *MB-level loop* and *SR-level loop*, which can save the required computation complexity. Finally, these algorithms can be combined with each other to provide a better performance.

In the last years, the development of ME algorithms is changed from fixed block size ME to variable block size ME which means the current MB can be divided into several small current blocks with individual motion vectors. Variable block size ME can provide more coding gain but the required computation complexity is also increased. Besides variable block size ME, the bitrate overhead of motion vector is also considered when selecting one search candidate as motion vector [151]. That is, the cost function to select motion vector consists of two factors, the distortion of the reference block and the bitrate of its motion vector. By adding the bitrate overhead of the motion vector, the coding performance of video coding systems can be improved at least 1 dB.

7.3 Architecture of Motion Estimation

There are other methods to achieve the real-time computation of ME, and the hardware acceleration is the most commonly used due to the required computation complexity and memory bandwidth of ME. Hence many ME hardware accelerators are proposed in the last years. A general ME architecture can be roughly divided into two parts, *Processing Element Array* and *On-Chip Memory*, as shown in Fig. 7.9. *Processing Element Array* is the major operation core and responsible for the calculation of SAD in (7.1) and (7.2). The required data are loaded through *Data Bus*. Some of them are stored in *On-Chip Memory* for data re-use, so the required memory bandwidth can be reduced. For each MB, *Processing Element Array* gets the required data from *Data Bus* and *On-Chip Memory* and computes the corresponding SADs. At the same time, the data in the *On-Chip Memory* are updated for the data re-use of the next MB or search candidate.

Based on the different ME algorithms and adopted searching range data re-use schemes, *Processing Element Array*, the size of *On-Chip Memory* and the required memory bandwidth are very different. In the following, based on different ME algorithms and the characteristics of *Processing Element Array*, we classify ME architectures into three types, inter-level, intra-level, and tree-based architectures. For simplicity, we assume that the searching range is $[-2, 2)$ and the current block size is 2×2 to illustrate the operations of each ME architecture. Figure 7.10 shows the related data symbols of the current block and searching range. After the introduction of *Processing Element Array*, the tradeoffs between *On-Chip Memory* size and the required memory bandwidth in different searching region data re-use schemes are discussed.

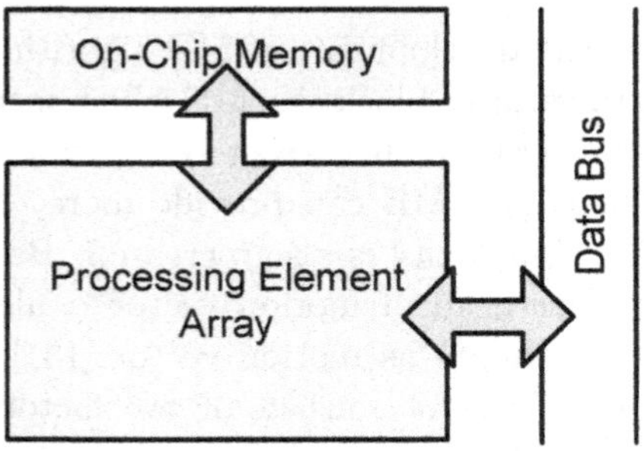

Fig. 7.9 The block diagram of a motion estimation architecture.

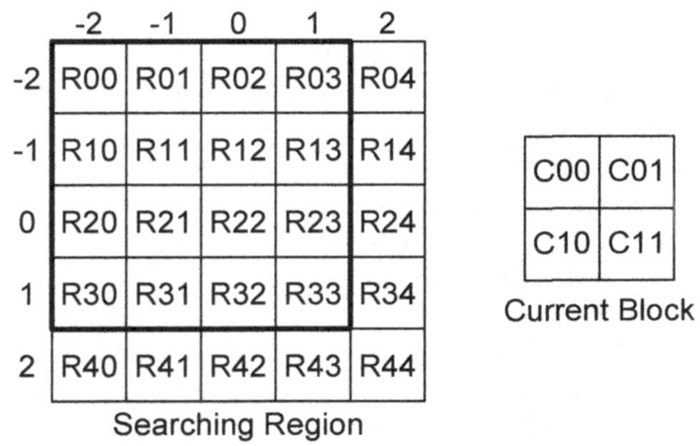

Fig. 7.10 The searching region and current block.

7.3.1 *Architecture for full search algorithm*

Among various ME algorithms, full search algorithms can provide the best quality but with a huge computation complexity overhead. Although full search requires a large computation complexity, full search is easy to be accelerated by a hardware architecture, because of its simple operations and regular data flow, compared to fast full search or fast search algorithms. Therefore, many different architectures are proposed for full search algorithm. Among of them, inter-level and intra-level architectures are the most common used. In the following, we will introduce these two kinds of ME architectures, respectively.

7.3.1.1 *Inter-level architecture*

Yang *et al.* implement the first VLSI architecture of ME [152] for full search algorithm in the world. They propose a family of inter-level ME architectures. In the inter-level architecture, the computations of *SR-level loop*, different search candidates, are computed in parallel but the computations of *CurBlock-level loop*, all current pixels, are processed sequentially. Figure 7.11(a) shows a processing element (PE) in inter-level architectures. The PE in inter-level architectures is responsible for the computation of one search candidate. One PE computes the differences of all current pixels in the current block and accumulate the SAD pixel by pixel, as shown in

(7.1).

Figure 7.11(b) shows the architecture of Yang *et al.'s* for full search algorithm. This architecture is an one-dimensional inter-level architecture which can compute all search candidates in a row at the same time. In Fig. 7.11(b), there are four processing elements for four search candidates in a row, because the searching region in the horizontal direction is $[-2, 2)$. The data flow of this architecture is as follows. Current pixels, *Cur.Pixel*, are input in the raster scan and propagated by the shift registers, *D*. By selection signals, *Sel0*, *Sel1*, and so on, the corresponding reference pixels, *Ref.Pixel0*, *Ref.Pixel1* and so on, are selected and input into PEs. The partial SAD is stored in each PE, until the SAD accumulation of one search candidate is finished. *Comparator* is responsible for selecting the minimum SADs among all generated SADs.

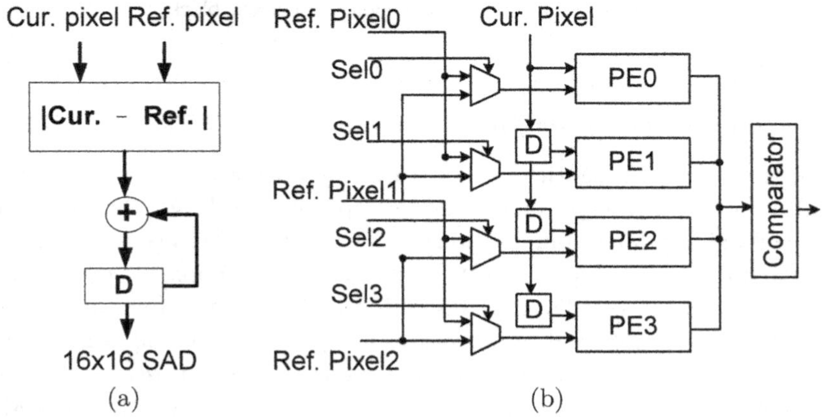

Fig. 7.11 (a) The processing element of inter-level motion estimation architectures. (b) The architecture of Yang *et al.'s*.

The detailed data flow of current input, reference inputs, and PE operations is shown in Fig 7.12. In each cycle, each PE calculates the distortion between one current pixel and one reference pixel and accumulates this distortion to the partial SAD of its search candidate. After 2×2 cycles, the first PE, *PE0*, generates the SAD of the top-left search candidate. And in the following cycles, the SADs of search candidates from left to right in a row are generated sequentially. The PEs which have generated the SADs can process the search candidates in the next row, until all search candidates are processed.

Cycle	Cur.Pixel	Ref.Pixel0	Ref.Pixel1	Ref.Pixel2	PE0	PE1	PE2	PE3
0	C00	R00	-	-	|C00-R00|	-	-	-
1	C01	R01	-	-	|C01-R01|	|C00-R01|	-	-
2	C10	R10	R02	-	|C10-R10|	|C01-R02|	|C00-R02|	-
3	C11	R11	R03	-	|C11-R11|	|C10-R11|	|C01-R03|	|C00-R03|
4	C00	R10	R12	R04	|C00-R10|	|C11-R12|	|C10-R12|	|C01-R04|
5	C01	R11	R13	-	|C01-R11|	|C00-R11|	|C11-R13|	|C10-R13|
6	C10	R20	R12	R14	|C10-R20|	|C01-R12|	|C00-R12|	|C11-R14|
7	C11	R21	R13	-	|C11-R21|	|C10-R21|	|C01-R13|	|C00-R13|
8	C00	R30	R22	R24	|C00-R30|	|C11-R22|	|C10-R22|	|C01-R14|
......		......					......	

Fig. 7.12 The scheduling of Yang et al.'s.

7.3.1.2 *Intra-level architecture*

Besides the inter-level architecture, the intra-level architecture is another kind of architectures for full search algorithm. In the intra-level architecture, the computations of *CurBlock-level loop*, all current pixels, are computed in parallel but the computations of *SR-level loop*, search candidates, are processed one by one.

In [153], Komarek and Pirsch contribute a detailed systolic mapping procedure from the dependency graph to various full search algorithm architectures. Among their proposed architectures, AB2 is a two-dimensional intra-level architecture. The PE in the intra-level architectures is responsible for the distortion between one specific current pixel and the corresponding reference pixel for all search candidates, as shown in (7.2) and Fig. 7.13(a). Figure 7.13(b) shows the architecture of AB2, which consists of four intra-level PEs corresponding to 2×2 current pixels in the current block.

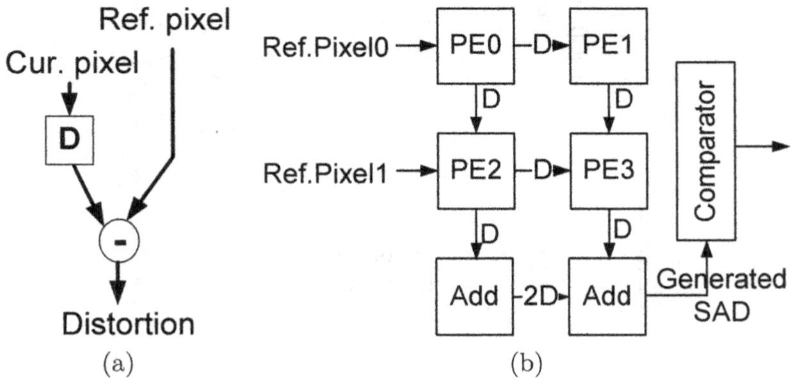

Fig. 7.13 (a) The processing element of intra-level motion estimation architectures. (b) The architecture of Komarek and Pirsch's.

The data flow is as follows. Current pixels are stored in corresponding PEs, and reference pixels are propagated PE by PE in the horizontal direction. The partial column SADs are propagated and accumulated in the vertical direction first. After the vertical propagation, the column SADs are propagated and accumulated in the horizontal direction. The detailed flow of reference inputs and PE operations is shown in Fig. 7.14. In each PE, the distortion of a current pixel in current MB is computed and added

<table>
<tr><th>Cycle</th><th>Ref.Pixel0</th><th>Ref.Pixel1</th><th>PE0</th><th>PE1</th><th>PE2</th><th>PE3</th><th>Generated SAD</th></tr>
<tr><td>0</td><td>R00</td><td>-</td><td>|C00-R00|</td><td>-</td><td>-</td><td>-</td><td>-</td></tr>
<tr><td>1</td><td>R01</td><td>R10</td><td>|C00-R01|</td><td>|C01-R00|</td><td>|C10-R10|</td><td>-</td><td>-</td></tr>
<tr><td>2</td><td>R02</td><td>R11</td><td>|C00-R02|</td><td>|C01-R01|</td><td>|C10-R11|</td><td>|C11-R10|</td><td>-</td></tr>
<tr><td>3</td><td>R03</td><td>R12</td><td>|C00-R03|</td><td>|C01-R02|</td><td>|C10-R12|</td><td>|C11-R11|</td><td>-</td></tr>
<tr><td>4</td><td>R04</td><td>R13</td><td>|C00-R04|</td><td>|C01-R03|</td><td>|C10-R13|</td><td>|C11-R12|</td><td>(-2, -2)</td></tr>
<tr><td>5</td><td>R10</td><td>R14</td><td>|C00-R10|</td><td>|C01-R04|</td><td>|C10-R14|</td><td>|C11-R13|</td><td>(-2, -1)</td></tr>
<tr><td>6</td><td>R11</td><td>R20</td><td>|C00-R11|</td><td>|C01-R10|</td><td>|C10-R20|</td><td>|C11-R14|</td><td>(-2, 0)</td></tr>
<tr><td>7</td><td>R12</td><td>R21</td><td>|C00-R12|</td><td>|C01-R11|</td><td>|C10-R21|</td><td>|C11-R20|</td><td>(-2, 1)</td></tr>
<tr><td>8</td><td>R13</td><td>R22</td><td>|C00-R13|</td><td>|C01-R12|</td><td>|C10-R22|</td><td>|C11-R21|</td><td>(-1, -2)</td></tr>
<tr><td>......</td><td>......</td><td></td><td></td><td></td><td>......</td><td></td><td></td></tr>
</table>

Fig. 7.14 The scheduling of Komarek and Pirsch's.

with the partial column SAD which is propagated in PEs from top to bottom in the vertical direction. In the horizontal propagation, two column SADs are accumulated one by one by two adders and four registers. After initial cycles, the SADs are generated one by one and *Comparator* selects the minimum of them.

7.3.1.3 *Summary*

Inter-level and intra-level architectures are two types of architectures for full search algorithm. The former computes the search candidates in parallel in the *SR-level loop* and sequentially estimates the distortions of all current pixels in the *CurBlock-level loop*. On the contrary, the latter computes the search candidates in sequential in the *SR-level loop* and estimates the distortions of all current pixels in the *CurBlock-level loop* in parallel. In general, inter-level architectures have a short critical path with a large set of registers, and intra-level architectures have a long critical path but fewer registers. Moreover, inter-level architectures require fewer data inputs by use of broadcasting or propagating reference pixels and current pixels, and intra-level architectures require much more data input than inter-level architectures do.

Besides the above-mentioned architectures, many architectures are proposed based on these two basic architectures. For example, Reference [154] is the extension of [152], and besides one-dimensional inter-level architectures, two two-dimensional inter-level semi-systolic architectures are proposed in [155, 156]. Reference [157] is the extension of [153]. Reference [158] and [159] are another two intra-level architectures with large registers for fewer data inputs and memory bandwidth. Many proposed architectures are not discussed due to the limited space in this book, and interested readers can read them by themselves.

7.3.2 ***Architecture for fast full search and fast search algorithms***

After the introduction of the architectures for full search algorithm, we introduce the architectures for fast search and fast full search algorithms. Although the computation complexity of fast search and fast full search algorithms is much smaller than that of the full search algorithm, the design challenges of VLSI architectures for fast search and fast full search algorithms are much more difficult than those of the full search algorithm.

This is because the data flow of fast search and fast full search algorithms is irregular and the processing order of search candidates is dynamic, which depends on the last searching result. For example, in three step search or diamond search, we can not know the center position of the next searching step, until the minimum of this searching step is found. Therefore, latency and pipelining bubble cycles become critical issues. A short latency, supporting random access in search candidates, and no pipelining bubble cycles after skipping some search candidates are required for ME architectures of fast search and fast full search algorithms.

7.3.2.1 *Tree-based architecture*

Tree-based architectures [160] have the above-mentioned advantages, a short latency, supporting random access in search candidates, and no pipelining bubbles cycles. Figure 7.15 shows the tree-based architectures with different degrees of parallelism. Tree-based architectures are similar to intra-level architectures. The difference between tree-based and intra-level architectures is the focused operation loop. Intra-level architectures process the computations in the *CurBlock-level loop* in parallel. Tree-based architectures not only can process the computations in the *CurBlock-level loop* in parallel but also can process the search candidates in the *SR-level loop* at the same time. That is to say, the processing order in the *CurBlock-level loop* and *SR-level loop* can be reordered for different degrees of parallelism in tree-based architectures.

For example, if the degree of parallelism in the tree-based architecture is two dimensions of the current MB, the tree-based architecture is equal to the intra-level architecture. If the degree of parallelism is only one dimension of current block, then it only processes the distortions of current pixels in a row at the same time. In the following, we take two examples to illustrate the data flow and characteristics of tree-based architectures.

The first case is that the degree of parallelism is two dimensions of current MB, as shown in Fig. 7.15(a). It is equal to the intra-level architecture. Each PE in tree-based architectures is corresponding to one current pixel and is responsible for the calculation of the difference between one current pixel and one corresponding reference pixel for all search candidates. The data flow is shown in Fig. 7.16. In this architecture, it can generate the SAD of one search candidate in one cycle. The latency of this architecture is dependent on the memory access of reference pixels, which can be shortened with the interleaved memory arrangement in [160]. Moreover,

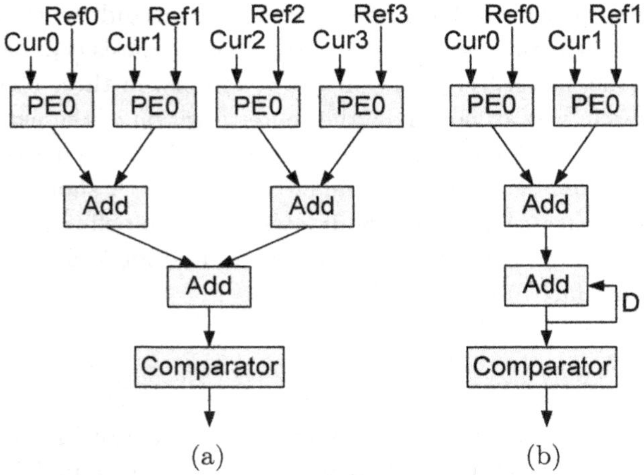

Fig. 7.15 (a) The architecture of tree. (b) The architecture of 1/2 tree.

no pipelining bubble cycles and no data dependency between the current and next search candidates exist in this architecture. Hence it is suitable for the hardware implementation of fast searching algorithms which require the property of random access in the searching region.

If the degree of parallelism in the tree-based architecture is only one dimension of current block, as shown in Fig. 7.15(b), the tree-based architecture is a hybrid architecture of inter-level and intra-level architectures. For example, Figure 7.15(b) is derived by folding Figure 7.15(a) by 2 (B_V). Then, it can calculate one row SAD of the search candidates in one cycle, and after generating and accumulating all row SADs, the total SAD of one search candidate can be derived. In this architecture, partial distortion elimination (PDE) can be easily integrated. The comparison between the partial SAD and the current minimum SAD of PDE is changed from the distortion of one pixel to one row SAD. Although this change degrades the performance of PDE, it is still an efficient method and the lost of performance is very small. Moreover, because of no pipelining bubble cycles and no data dependency in tree-based architectures, the early termination of one search candidate does not degrade the performance of this architecture.

The tree-based architecture has a good flexibility to support various reordering or rescheduling in the *CurBlock-level loop* and *SR-level loop*, so it is usually adopted in many architectures of fast search algorithms. We introduce two tree-based architectures for diamond search and three step

Cycle	Ref0	Ref1	Ref2	Ref3	PE0	PE1	PE2	PE3	Generated SAD
0	R00	R01	R10	R11	|C00-R00|	|C01-R01|	|C10-R10|	|C11-R11|	(-2, -2)
1	R01	R02	R11	R12	|C00-R01|	|C01-R02|	|C10-R11|	|C11-R12|	(-2, -1)
2	R02	R03	R12	R13	|C00-R02|	|C01-R03|	|C10-R12|	|C11-R13|	(-2, 0)
3	R03	R04	R13	R14	|C00-R03|	|C01-R04|	|C10-R13|	|C11-R14|	(-2, 1)
4	R10	R11	R20	R21	|C00-R10|	|C01-R11|	|C10-R20|	|C11-R21|	(-1, -2)
5	R11	R12	R21	R22	|C00-R11|	|C01-R12|	|C10-R21|	|C11-R22|	(-1, -1)
6	R12	R13	R22	R23	|C00-R12|	|C01-R13|	|C10-R22|	|C11-R23|	(-1, 0)
7	R13	R14	R23	R24	|C00-R13|	|C01-R14|	|C10-R23|	|C11-R24|	(-1, 1)
8	R20	R21	R30	R31	|C00-R20|	|C01-R21|	|C10-R30|	|C11-R31|	(0, -2)
......		......					......		

Fig. 7.16 The scheduling of tree-based architecture.

search respectively.

7.3.2.2 *Architecture for diamond search*

In [161], the authors utilize the tree-based architecture to propose an architecture which can support diamond search and fast full search algorithms. In diamond search, there are many duplicated search candidates between two successive steps, as shown in Fig. 7.6. After each moving the large diamond pattern, only five or three search candidates need to be calculated and the others are calculated at the last large diamond pattern. Hence an ROM-based solution which uses a ROM to check if the search candidate is required to be computed is proposed in [161] to avoid the duplicated search candidates. By the ROM-based solution, 24.4% search candidates in the diamond search algorithm can be saved, and the area overhead is little.

This architecture also can support fast full searching algorithms, such as PDE and SEA. The computation of SEA for one search candidate is executed by the processor first, and then if the SEA is smaller than the current minimum SAD, the real SAD of search candidate is calculated in this architecture. Otherwise, the SAD of this candidate is skipped. The degree of parallelism in this architecture is only half row ($B_H/2$), so PDE is easily integrated with less overhead, and the unit of comparison between the partial SAD and the current minimum SAD is changed to a half row SAD.

7.3.2.3 *Architecture for three step search*

In [160], the authors not only introduce the characteristics of the tree-based architectures but also propose a fully pipelined tree-based architecture for three step search. The fully pipelined architecture requires $log_2(B_H \times B_V) + 2$ cycles to process one search candidate. Therefore, for three step search algorithm, if the fully pipelined architecture has a two dimensional degree of parallelism and the searching range is $[-7, 7]$, the total required cycles are $3 \times (9 + log_2(B_H \times B_V) + 2)$, where "3" is the number of steps, "9" is the total search candidates in each step, and the others are the cycles for computing one searching candidate. However, the memory access becomes an important design challenge, because $B_H \times B_V$ reference pixels are required at the same time. The authors develop the interleaved memory arrangement to satisfy the memory access requirement.

7.3.2.4 *Summary*

Besides tree-based architectures, there are many other proposed architectures for fast full and fast search algorithms. For instance, in [162], Dutta and Wolf modify the data flow of the 1-D linear array in [152] to support FSBMA, three step search, and conjugate direction search in the same architecture. In [163], Lin, Anesko, and Petryna propose a joint algorithm-architecture design of a programmable motion estimator chip. In [164], Cheng and Hang use a universal systolic arrays structure to realize many BMAs. Interested readers can refer to them by themselves.

In a word, we classify the ME architectures into inter-level, intra-level and tree-based architectures based on their computation characteristics. Inter-level architectures can compute the search candidates in the *SR-level loop* in parallel, intra-level architectures can process all current pixels in the *CurBlock-level loop* in parallel, and tree-based architectures can reorder the processing order between the *SR-level loop* and *CurBlock-level loop.* In general, for the full search algorithm, because of its regular computation and data flow, inter-level and intra-level architectures are usually adopted. For fast full search and fast search algorithms, tree-based architectures are usually adopted because of no pipelining bubble cycles, no data dependency, and supporting random access in searching region. In fact, these three kinds of architectures can be applied into any types of ME algorithms, including full search, fast full search, and fast search algorithms with some suitable modifications.

7.3.3 *Block-level data re-use scheme*

In the previous subsections, we introduced the processing elements (PE) in the ME architectures. Besides PE designs, the tradeoff between on-chip memory size and the required memory bandwidth is another important issue in the hardware design of ME. The required memory bandwidth of ME for reference pixels is very huge, so how to re-use the reference data becomes a critical issue of hardware design for ME. Moreover, for full search and fast full search, because all search candidates are examined, the whole searching region data are required to be loaded. But for fast search algorithms, the required reference data are only a part of the searching region. Hence there are two methods to load the reference data in the hardware architectures of fast search algorithms. One is only to load the required data, and the other is to load the whole searching range data. The former has less memory bandwidth but its memory bandwidth may be irregular and unpredictable, so the efficiency of data re-use is low. Although the latter requires a large memory bandwidth, the required memory bandwidth can be significantly saved after adopting block-level data re-use schemes and the memory access is regular. Hence the memory bandwidth of the latter is usually equal to or less than that of the former, after applying the block-level data re-use scheme. In the following subsection, we will discuss the block-level data re-use schemes for loading the whole searching range data.

7.3.3.1 *Redundancy access factor*

Before introducing the block-level data re-use schemes, the concept of redundancy access factor [29] [30], Ra_{ME}, should be introduced first. We use the redundancy access factor (Ra_{ME}) to represent the required memory access of reference frames in ME with different block-level data re-use schemes. The redundancy access factor (Ra_{ME}), is defined as

$$Ra_{ME} = \frac{Total\ memory\ bandwidth\ for\ reference\ frame}{Minimum\ memory\ bandwidth\ (pixel\ count\ in\ total)}, \quad (7.5)$$

which means that the required memory bandwidth is Ra_{ME} times of the minimum memory bandwidth. Because the whole searching range data are required to be loaded for full search, the minimum memory bandwidth is equal to the number of pixels in one block for one current block. Hence in another view points, Ra_{ME} can be interpreted as that if we want to process one current pixel, Ra_{ME} reference pixels are required.

In general, if we want to have a small redundancy access factor, the required on-chip memory size becomes large. Hence a tradeoff exists between the required memory bandwidth and on-chip memory size. Several block-level data re-use schemes are surveyed or proposed in [29, 30, 165]. Different block-level data re-use schemes provide different tradeoffs between the required memory access and on-chip memory size. We will introduce these block-level data re-use schemes, from Level A to Level D and Level C+ schemes, respectively. Moreover, in order to simplify the analyzed equations, we set SR_H=$2P_H$, SR_V=$2P_V$, and B_H=B_V= N, in which the searching range is $[-P_H, P_H)$ and $[-P_V, P_V)$ in the horizontal and vertical directions and the block size is $B_H \times B_V$.

7.3.3.2 *Level A scheme*

Level A scheme is the weakest block-level data re-use scheme, and its concept is shown in Fig. 7.17(a). Level A scheme is the data re-use of *SR-level loop* in the horizontal direction and re-uses the overlapped region between two reference blocks of successive search candidates in the horizontal direction. As shown in Fig. 7.17(a), two reference blocks have a large common region, $N \times (N-1)$, and then only N pixels are different. Therefore, only N reference pixels are required to be updated for the next search candidate in the horizontal direction. For a current MB, the required memory access ($Ra_{ME,\ Level\ A}$) is

$$\begin{aligned} Ra_{ME,\ Level\ A} &\approx \frac{N \times (SR_H + N - 1) \times (SR_V)}{N \times N} \\ &\approx (SR_V) \times (1 + \frac{SR_H}{N}). \end{aligned} \tag{7.6}$$

In Level A scheme, because only $N \times (N-1)$ reference pixels are re-used, the on-chip memory size is only $N \times (N-1)$ reference pixels. Level A scheme can totally re-use the overlapped region between two reference blocks of successive search candidates in the horizontal direction.

7.3.3.3 *Level B scheme*

Level B scheme further improves the data re-use of Level A scheme. Compared to Level A scheme, Level B scheme presents the data re-use of *SR-level loop* in the horizontal and vertical directions, so Level B scheme not only can totally re-use the overlapped region in the horizontal direction but also can re-use the overlapped region in the vertical direction. Figure 7.17(b) shows the concept of Level B scheme. Therefore, for one current MB, the searching range is only required to be input once, and then the $Ra_{ME,\ Level\ B}$ is

$$\begin{aligned} Ra_{ME,\ Level\ B} &\approx \frac{(SR_H + N - 1) \times (SR_V + N - 1)}{N \times N} \\ &\approx (1 + \frac{SR_V}{N}) \times (1 + \frac{SR_H}{N}). \end{aligned} \tag{7.7}$$

However, because the reference data are only input once, the on-chip memory size is increased to $(SR_H + N - 1) \times (N - 1)$ to buffer the reference pixels for data re-use.

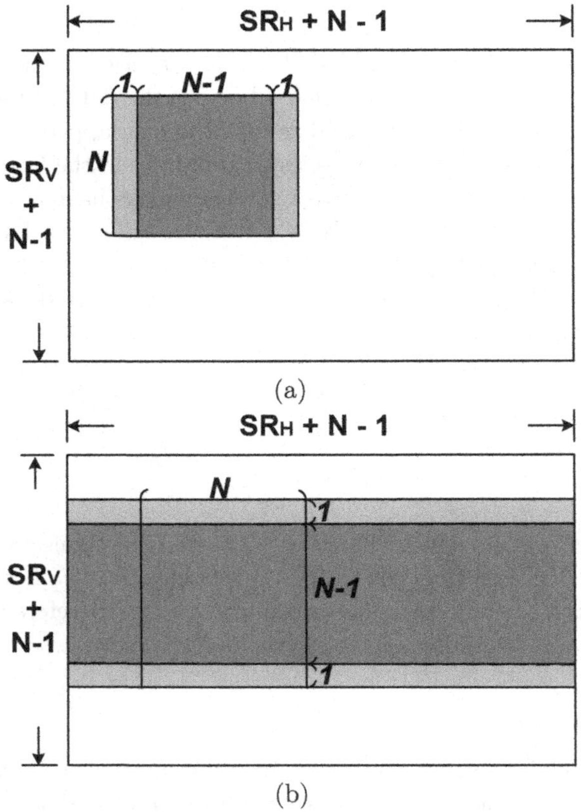

Fig. 7.17 Block-level Data re-use schemes. (a) Level A scheme; (b) Level B scheme; where the heavy gray region is the overlapped and re-used region.

7.3.3.4 *Level C scheme*

Level A and Level B schemes re-use the overlapped region between the reference blocks of the successive search candidates in the *SR-level loop*. However, this kind of data re-use schemes still requires a lot of memory bandwidth, and then they are not enough for a practical system. Hence Level C scheme is developed to re-use the overlapped searching region between two successive current MBs. That is to say, Level C scheme is the data re-use of *MB-level loop*. Level C scheme is similar to Level A scheme and is the data re-use of the *MB-level loop* in the horizontal direction, as shown in Fig. 7.18(a). There is a large overlapped region between two searching regions of successive current blocks in the horizontal direction. For two horizontal successive current blocks, only $N \times (SR_V + N - 1)$ reference pixels are different and required to be loaded. Then, the redundancy access factor of Level C scheme is formulated as

$$Ra_{ME,\ Level\ C} \approx \frac{N \times (SR_V + N - 1)}{N \times N} \approx 1 + \frac{SR_V}{N}. \quad (7.8)$$

The redundancy access factor of Level C scheme is much less than Level A scheme or Level B scheme, but the required on-chip memory size is significantly increased. The whole searching range is required to be stored, so the on-chip memory size is $(SR_H + N - 1) \times (SR_V + N - 1)$ pixels.

7.3.3.5 *Level D scheme*

Compared to the relationship between Level C and Level A schemes, Level D scheme is also similar to Level B scheme but in the *MB-level loop*. Level D scheme can fully re-use the overlapped searching region not only in the horizontal direction but also in the vertical direction and becomes the ultimate block-level data re-use scheme of searching region for one reference frame.

Figure. 7.18(b) shows the concept of Level D data re-use scheme, where W is the width of one frame. Because Level D scheme re-uses the overlapped searching region in both directions, the reference frame is only input once for one current frame, and the redundancy access factor ($Ra_{ME,\ Level\ D}$) is only 1. However, the price is the significant increase of the required on-chip memory size. In order to provide the data re-use in the vertical direction, the searching range of a current MB row is required to be stored, so the on-chip memory size becomes $(SR_V - 1) \times (SR_H + W - 1)$ pixels, where W is the frame width.

7.3.3.6 *Level C+ scheme*

In [165], a new block-level data re-use scheme, Level C+ scheme, is proposed. Level C+ scheme partially re-uses the searching range data in the vertical direction by rescheduling the two loops of *MB-level loop*. Therefore, Level C+ scheme not only can improve the performance of Level C scheme but also requires a much less on-chip memory size than that of Level D scheme.

Figure 7.19 shows the data re-use of Level C+ scheme. In the Level C scheme, the coding order is the raster scan. In the Level C+ scheme,

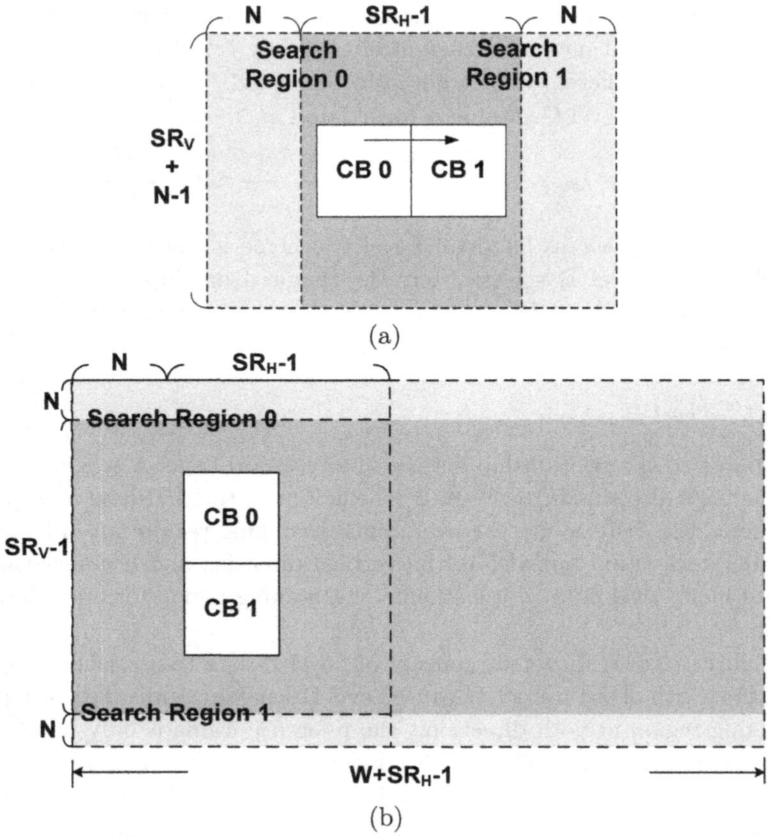

Fig. 7.18 Block-level Data re-use schemes. (a) Level C scheme; (b) Level D scheme; where the heavy gray region is the overlapped and re-used region.

the stripe-based scan is applied, in which several MB rows are stitched and processed at the same time. That is, several successive current MBs in the vertical direction are stitched, and the searching region of these current MBs is loaded, simultaneously. If n successive vertical current MBs are stitched together, which is called n-stitched MBs, only $N \times (SR_V + nN - 1)$ are required to be loaded for these n stitched MBs. Therefore, the redundancy access factor of Level C+ scheme with n-stitched MBs is

$$Ra_{ME,\ Level\ C+} \approx \frac{N \times (SR_V + nN - 1)}{N \times nN} \approx 1 + \frac{SR_V}{nN}. \tag{7.9}$$

The on-chip memory size is also increased. However, because the vertical data re-use only exists in the n-stitched MB rows, not in the whole current frame, the on-chip memory size is only $(SR_V + nN - 1)\times(SR_H + N - 1)$, which is much less than that of Level D scheme.

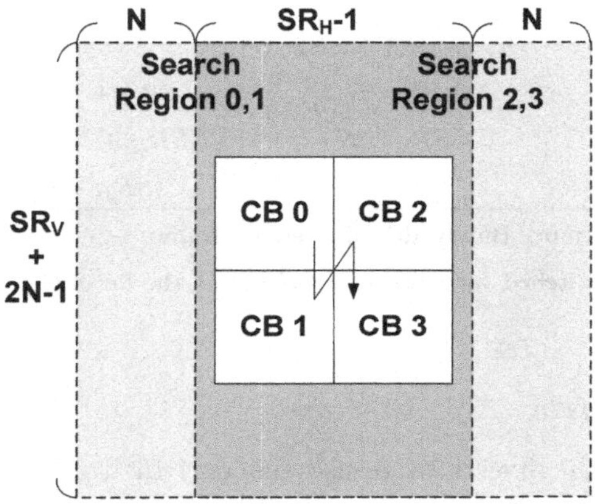

Fig. 7.19 Level C+ scheme with $n = 2$, where the heavy gray region is the overlapped and re-used region.

In the Level C+ scheme, by use of stripe-based scan, not only the overlapped searching region in the horizontal direction can be fully re-used, but also the overlapped searching region in the vertical direction can be partially re-used. Compared to Level C scheme, the reduction ratio of the required memory bandwidth is

$$\frac{1 + {SR_V}/{nN}}{1 + {SR_V}/{N}} \approx \frac{nN + SR_V}{nN + nSR_V}. \tag{7.10}$$

The increase ratio of on-chip memory size is only

$$\frac{(SR_H + N - 1)(SR_V + nN - 1)}{(SR_H + N - 1)(SR_V + N - 1)} \approx \frac{SR_V + nN}{SR_V + N}. \tag{7.11}$$

When SR_V is much larger than nN, Level C+ scheme only requires $1/n$ memory bandwidth and increases nN/SR_V on-chip memory size of Level C scheme. Moreover, Level C+ scheme can provide various tradeoffs between the required memory bandwidth and on-chip memory size by adjusting n. A large n requires much less memory bandwidth, but a large on-chip memory size is needed.

Table 7.1 The comparison of different data re-use schemes for ME.

Re-use Scheme	EMB (Pixels/Pixel)	On-chip Memory Size (Pixels)
Level A	$SR_V \times (1 + SR_H/N)$	$N \times (N-1)$
Level B	$(1 + SR_V/N) \times (1 + SR_H/N)$	$(SR_H + N - 1) \times (N-1)$
Level C	$1 + SR_V/N$	$(SR_H + N - 1) \times (SR_V + N - 1)$
Level C+	$1 + SR_V/nN$	$(SR_H + N - 1) \times (SR_V + nN - 1)$
Level D	1	$(SR_H + W - 1) \times (SR_V - 1)$

EMB: External Memory Bandwidth of reference frame.

n: the number of stitched vertical current blocks in the Level C+ scheme.

7.3.3.7 *Comparison*

We summarize the five data re-use schemes in Table 7.1 from weak to strong. The tradeoff between the required memory access and the on-chip memory size of each data re-use scheme is shown apparently. The smaller the required memory access is, the larger the required on-chip memory size is. We take an example to give a practical comparison. Assume that the block size is 16×16 ($N = 16$), the searching range is $[-64, 64)$ in both directions ($SR_H = SR_V = 128$), and the frame format is D1 size with 30fps. The required memory bandwidth and on-chip memory size of different data re-use schemes are listed in Table 7.2. From Table 7.1 and 7.2, the required memory bandwidth and on-chip memory size are very different among these five data re-use schemes. Level A scheme needs a very huge memory bandwidth but with a very small on-chip memory. Contrarily, Level D scheme requires the smallest memory bandwidth but with a huge on-chip memory size. Moreover, Level A, B, C and D provide the fixed memory bandwidth and on-chip memory size, but Level C+ can provide many different tradeoffs between the required memory bandwidth and on-chip memory size by applying different n. A large n requires much less memory bandwidth but a large on-chip memory size is its price.

7.4 Summary

ME plays an important role not only in the traditional video coding but also in the prediction stage of MCTF. In the last two decades, many al-

Table 7.2 The real-life comparison of different data re-use schemes for ME.

Re-use Scheme	EMB (Pixels/Pixel)	EMB MB/sec.	On-chip Memory Size (Pixels)
Level A	1,152.00	11,943.9	240
Level B	81.00	839.8	2,145
Level C	9.00	93.3	20,499
Level C+ ($n = 2$)	5.00	51.8	22,737
Level C+ ($n = 3$)	3.67	38.1	25,025
Level D	1.00	10.4	107,569

EMB: External Memory Bandwidth of reference frame.

gorithms and architectures are proposed to speed up the computation of ME or improve the coding performance. In this section, the concept of ME algorithm and architectures are introduced as the basic knowledge for the prediction stage of MCTF. The ME algorithms are classified into three categories, full search, fast full search, and fast search algorithms which are further divided into simplification of matching criterion, reduction of search candidates, predictive and hierarchical search. The ME architectures are separated two parts, processing element array and on-chip memory, for discussion. In the processing element array, inter-level, intra-level, and tree-based architectures are three basic ME architectures and are adopted in many ME architectures and video coding systems. On-chip memory is used to significantly save the required memory bandwidth of reference frames in ME, and the five block-level data re-use schemes are discussed to reveal the tradeoffs between the required memory bandwidth and on-chip memory size. In the next section, based on these analysis, we will introduce the analysis of VLSI architecture for MCTF.

Chapter 8

Analysis and Architecture of MCTF

Since motion-compensated temporal filtering (MCTF) is the critical module in the inter-frame wavelet video coding and the coming video coding standard, scalable video coding (SVC) [19], the VLSI design of MCTF becomes important. In this chapter, the VLSI design of MCTF is introduced by analyzing system and memory issues [165, 166]. In the beginning, we introduce the memory access factors of ME and MC, and we use these factors to evaluate the memory issues for one-level MCTF. Moreover, because of the characteristics of open-loop video codings, we also consider the issues of frame-level data re-use in our discussion. Next, based on the analysis of one-level MCTF, the discussion is extended to the system issues of multi-level MCTF. In the analysis of multi-level MCTF, some important factors of multi-level MCTF are introduced first and followed by the system analysis including computation complexity, external memory bandwidth, external memory storage, and coding delay. Based on these analysis, the concept of rate-distortion-computation scalability for a hardware accelerator is developed. That is, we can design a flexible hardware which not only can support various coding schemes of MCTF and traditional motion-compensated prediction (MCP) scheme but also can fit variant system constraints by performing a suitable coding scheme. Finally, we also explore the related system issues of pyramid MCTF after the analysis of multi-level MCTF.

8.1 Memory Access in MCTF

Before the analysis of one-level MCTF, we introduce the memory bandwidth of motion estimation (ME) and motion compensation (MC). The required memory bandwidth of ME and MC depends on the adopted architectures and data re-use schemes. In order to generalize our analysis and easily apply the analyzed results to various architectures and data re-use schemes, we use the redundancy access factors to represent the memory bandwidth of ME and MC. By redundancy access factors, the required memory bandwidth of ME and MC can be easily compared and calculated, even if different ME algorithms, architectures, or data re-use schemes are adopted.

8.1.1 *Redundancy access factor for ME*

In the prediction stage, ME is the most computation-costing part and requires huge memory access. Thus, the block-level data re-use scheme of ME is still very important for MCTF, and in the following analysis, for the sake of simplicity, we adopt the redundancy access factor, Ra_{ME} (pixels/pixel), which is introduced in Section 7.3.3 and defined as

$$Ra_{ME} = \frac{Total\ memory\ bandwidth\ for\ reference\ frame}{Minimum\ memory\ bandwidth\ (pixel\ count\ in\ total)}, \quad (8.1)$$

to represent the required memory access of ME. The redundancy access factor (Ra_{ME}) means that the required memory bandwidth is Ra_{ME} times of the minimum memory bandwidth. In general, if we want to have a small Ra_{ME}, the required on-chip memory size becomes large. By this representation, we can unify the representation of the required external memory access of reference frames in ME with different block-level data re-use schemes and architectures. Therefore, even if the different block-level data re-use schemes of ME are applied, only the real value of redundancy access factor in the analysis results should be changed and the others remain the same.

For example, in Section 7.3.3, there are many block-level data re-use schemes of searching range from Level A to Level D. Among them, Level C scheme provides a better tradeoff between on-chip memory size and external memory bandwidth because of the advancement of manufacturing process, and it is usually used in many previous works. As introduced in Section 7.3.3, Level C scheme re-uses the overlapped searching region between two successive current blocks in the horizontal direction. Figure 8.1 shows Level C scheme, where SR_H and SR_V are the width and height of the searching range, and B_H and B_V are the width and height of the current block, respectively. Therefore, the Ra_{ME} of Level C scheme is

$$Ra_{ME,\ Level\ C} \approx \frac{B_H \times (SR_V + B_V - 1)}{B_H \times B_V} \approx 1 + \frac{SR_V}{B_V}. \tag{8.2}$$

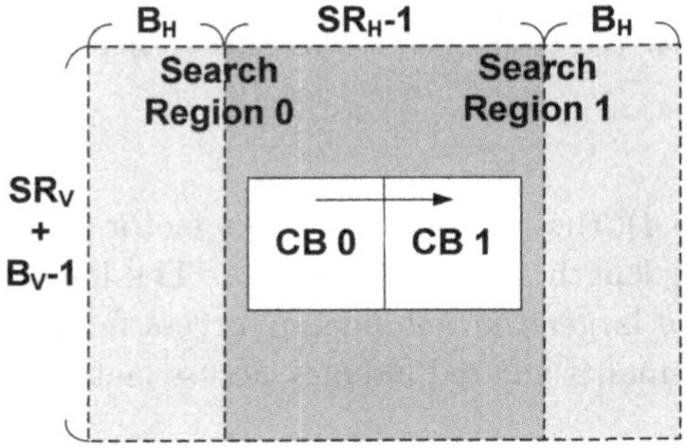

Fig. 8.1 The required data for ME with Level C scheme, where the heavy gray region is the overlapped and re-used region.

8.1.2 *Redundancy access factor for MC*

MC is required in both prediction and update stages of MCTF, and it may require redundant memory access for fractional-pixel MC. MC can be categorized into internal MC (intMC) and external MC (extMC). The intMC performs MC internally without external memory access, because the searching region buffer has sufficient data for fractional-pixel MC. Contrarily, the extMC performs MC by loading data from external memory. If the motion vector is fractional-pixel, more data than one block are required to be input from external memory for the interpolation of fractional-pixel MC, as shown in Fig. 8.2.

For extMC, the total amount of data, A_{extMC}, required from external memory can be formulated as

$$A_{extMC} = (B_{MC,H} + F - 1)(B_{MC,V} + F - 1), \tag{8.3}$$

where $B_{MC,H}$ and $B_{MC,V}$ are the width and height of the block to be performed MC, and F is the interpolation filter length. The corresponding redundancy access factor, Ra_{extMC} (pixels/pixel), can be defined by

$$Ra_{extMC} = \frac{A_{extMC} - B_{MC,H} \times B_{MC,V}}{B_{MC,H} \times B_{MC,V}}. \tag{8.4}$$

Table 8.1 Typical Values of Ra_{extMC} for SVC WD1.0.

MC Block Type	4×4 Block	8×8 Block	16×16 Block
	$B_H = B_v = 4$	$B_H = B_v = 8$	$B_H = B_v = 16$
Ra_{extMC}	4.0625	1.6406	0.7227

Note: H.264/AVC 6-tap interpolation filter is adopted

From (8.3) and (8.4), the redundancy access factor of MC depends on the interpolation filter length and the block size. The longer the interpolation filter length is, the larger the redundancy access factor is. The larger the block size is, the smaller the redundancy access factor is.

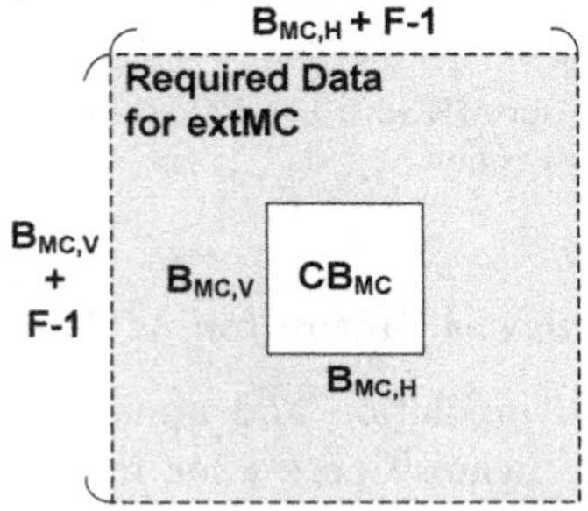

Fig. 8.2 The required data for extMC.

We take SVC WD1.0 as example. In SVC WD1.0, because variable block size motion estimation is supported, there are several kinds of block sizes, such as 4×4, 4×8, 8×8, 16×8, 16×16, and so on. We list several typical values of Ra_{extMC} for different block sizes in Table 8.1 to show the memory access overhead of extMC. For a 4×4 block, the redundancy access factor is 4.0625, which means that the required memory access is $4 \times 4 \times (4.0625 + 1) = 81$ (pixels). Hence the required memory bandwidth of MC is very large. Moreover, the memory access of MC is irregular, which usually induces a low efficiency of memory access.

Finally, in the following analysis, we use these redundancy access factors to represent the required memory bandwidth of ME and MC, so the required memory bandwidth can be easily compared in different data reuse scheme and architectures. Moreover, we summarize the abbreviations

Table 8.2 The List of Abbreviations.

Abbreviation	The Original Representation
Ra	Redundancy access factor of ME
Ra_{extMC}	Redundancy access factor of external MC
DRF	The double reference frames scheme
DCF	The double current frames scheme
m-DCF	The modified double current frames scheme
P-DRF	DRF is adopted in the prediction stage
P-DCF	DCF is adopted in the prediction stage
U-DRF	DRF is adopted in the update stage
EMB	External memory bandwidth
EMS	External memory size
SRB	Searching range buffer

in the following sections in Table 8.2.

8.2 One-Level Motion Compensated Temporal Filtering

In this section, the memory issues of one-level MCTF are introduced based on the redundancy access factors for ME and MC and the assumed architecture of MCTF. MCTF is partitioned into two stages, prediction and update stages, for the discussion. For the prediction stage, several frame-level data re-use schemes are discussed, and for the update stage, its impact is considered. Finally, we will summarize the required external memory bandwidth and external memory size of one-level MCTF with various frame-level data re-use schemes.

8.2.1 *The architecture for MCTF*

Because the operations of MCTF are ME and MC, we assume a general architecture of MCTF would be like that of ME. Figure 8.3 shows the assumed architecture, in which *Processing Engine* is responsible for computing all operations of MCTF, including prediction and update stages, *On-Chip Memory* is used to store the required searching range data for block-level data re-use, and the required reference or current data are stored and loaded from *External Memory* through *External Bus*. In the next subsection, because MCTF is an open-loop video coding, a family of new data re-use schemes, which are called frame-level data re-use schemes, is developed, and its tradeoff between the required external memory bandwidth, on-chip memory size, and external memory storage is also analyzed.

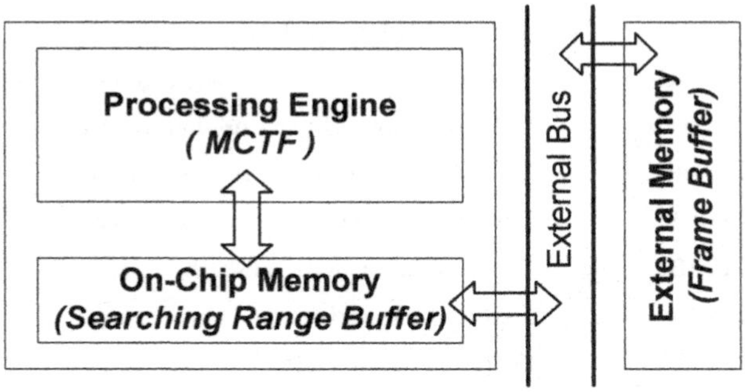

Fig. 8.3 The assumed architecture of MCTF.

8.2.2 *Memory analysis for prediction stage*

The main difference between open-loop MCTF and close-loop MCP is that the reference frames in open-loop MCTF are the original frames or filtered frames, but those in close-loop MCP are the reconstructed or coded frames. Hence ME in close-loop MCP needs to be performed in a frame-by-frame fashion (the close-loop property), but in open-loop MCTF, ME of different frames can be performed simultaneously. This difference is very important, which not only lets the frame-level date re-use scheme be possible but also enlarges the solution space of VLSI architecture design for MCTF. In the following subsections, several frame-level data re-use schemes are introduced, and a summary is given in the last subsection.

8.2.2.1 *Direct implementation*

The direct implementation is introduced, first. There are two ME in the prediction stage, so the direct implementation is to perform the left and right ME separately, as shown the left and right parts in Fig. 8.4(a). Therefore, the external memory access (pixels/pixel) of the direct implementation is

$$\underbrace{[(1 + Ra_{ME})}_{Left\ ME} + \underbrace{1 + Ra_{extMC}}_{Left\ MC} + \underbrace{1}_{H\ output} + \underbrace{(1 + Ra_{ME})}_{Right\ ME\&MC}] \quad /\, 2,$$

where the memory bandwidth of *Left ME* $(1 + Ra_{ME})$ is composed of that of the current and reference frames, the memory bandwidth of *Left MC* is extMC $(1 + Ra_{extMC})$, and the divisor (2) exists because the prediction stage is performed for every two frames. As for the on-chip memory size, the required on-chip memory of the direct implementation is one searching region buffer (SRB) that depends on which block-level data re-use scheme is used.

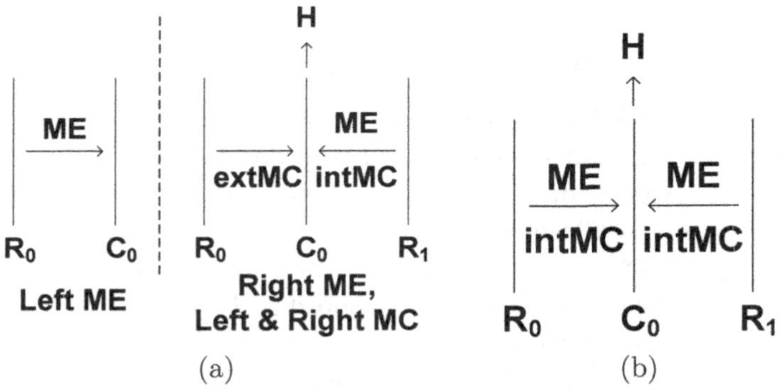

Fig. 8.4 Data re-use schemes for the prediction stage. (C: Current frame; R: Reference frame.) (a) The direct implementation (separate left and right ME). (b) The proposed Double Reference Frames (DRF) scheme.

8.2.2.2 *Double Reference Frames (DRF)*

Instead of the direct implementation which separates two ME into two steps, the left and right ME for one current frame can be performed at the same time, which is called the double reference frames (DRF) scheme and shown in Fig. 8.4(b). In the DRF scheme, because two ME are processed at the same time, not only the Left MC in the direct implementation becomes intMC, but also the memory access of the current frame in the Left ME is eliminated. However, the on-chip memory size is increased to 2 SRB, because two searching ranges are required at the same time. The external memory bandwidth of the DRF scheme is

$$\Big[\underbrace{2Ra_{ME}}_{Left\&Right\ Ref.} + \underbrace{1}_{Cur.\ input} + \underbrace{1}_{H\ output}\Big]\ /\ 2.$$

Compared to the direct implementation, the DRF scheme can save the memory access of the left extMC and current frame, but the penalty is that the required on-chip memory size is double.

In the viewpoint of data processing, the concept of the DRF scheme is to minimize the data lifetime of current frames. That is to say, for one current block, we load all related reference data for the computation and process all computations of one current block simultaneously. Therefore, the current frame is only input once, and the required memory bandwidth of current frames is minimum in the DRF scheme.

8.2.2.3 *Double Current Frames (DCF)*

Because of the open-loop prediction, the frame-level data re-use for the searching region becomes possible, which means that the ME of different current frames can be processed simultaneously. Hence one loaded searching range of reference frames can be shared between several current frames to save the memory bandwidth of reference frames. The double current frames (DCF) scheme is an example, as shown in Fig. 8.5(a). In Fig. 8.5(a), the loaded searching region of the reference frame R_1 can be used for the ME of current frame C_0 and C_1, at the same time. However, the penalties of the DCF scheme are that each current frame is input twice for different reference frames and the MC from frame R_0 to C_0 becomes extMC. Therefore, the required external memory access of the DCF scheme is

$$\Big[\underbrace{Ra_{ME}}_{Ref.\ R_1\ input} + \underbrace{1 + Ra_{extMC}}_{R_0\ MC} + \underbrace{1}_{H\ output} + \underbrace{2}_{Left\&Right\ Cur.}\Big]\ /\ 2.$$

Besides, the required on-chip memory size is $1SRB$, because only one searching region needs to be stored.

Compared to the DRF scheme, the DCF scheme not only reduces half memory access but also saves half on-chip memory size by sharing the reference frame between two current frames. But a large penalty is that extMC is required. From the viewpoint of data processing, the concept of the DCF scheme is to minimize the data lifetime of reference frames. That is to say, when we load one searching range data into on-chip memory, we process all related current blocks, simultaneously. Therefore, the searching range data are only input once, and then the memory bandwidth of reference frames is minimum in the DCF scheme. But the extra memory bandwidth of current frames and extMC may be required.

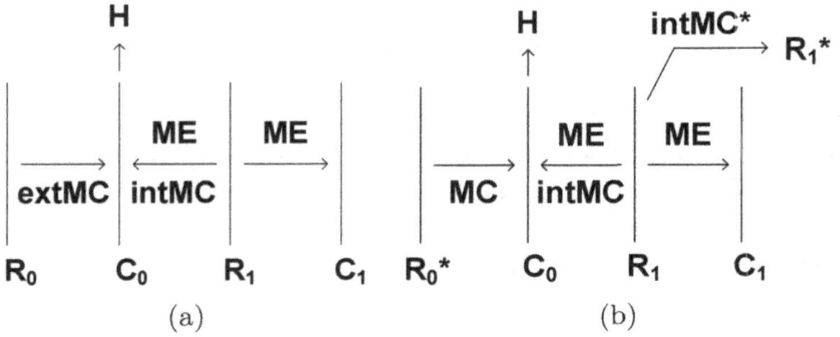

Fig. 8.5 Data re-use schemes for the prediction stage. (C: Current frame; R: Reference frame.) (a) The proposed Double Current Frames (DCF) scheme. (b) The proposed modified Double Current Frames (m-DCF) scheme.

8.2.2.4 *Modified Double Current Frames (m-DCF)*

Although the DCF scheme can reduce the required memory bandwidth of ME by sharing the searching range data between two current frames, it suffers the memory bandwidth overhead of extMC, which depends on the average $\overline{Ra_{extMC}}$ of all blocks. Hence the performance of the DCF scheme depends on $\overline{Ra_{extMC}}$. Compared to the DRF scheme, if $\overline{Ra_{extMC}}$ is larger than $(Ra - 2)$, the overhead of extMC makes the DCF scheme less efficient than the DRF scheme. For example, we assume the average $\overline{Ra_{extMC}}$ of all blocks is equal to 4.0625. If the searching range is $[-64, 64)$ with Level C scheme ($Ra_{ME} = 9$), the DCF scheme has a better performance than the DRF scheme does. But if the searching range is only $[-16, 16)$ ($Ra_{ME} = 3$), the performance of the DRF scheme becomes better than that of the DCF scheme. Moreover, the memory access of extMC is irregular, which may lead to a lower efficiency of external memory access.

Therefore, another kind of the frame-level data re-use scheme, the modified double current frames (m-DCF) scheme, is proposed to improve the DCF scheme. Figure 8.5(b) shows the concept of the m-DCF scheme, which interpolates the best matched blocks of the reference frame R_1 to the MC frame R_1^* for the current frame C_1 in advance and stores R_1^* into the external memory. By this way, the MC from the reference frame R_1 to current frame C_1 becomes intMC, and the penalty is that only the MC frame R_1^* is required to be outputted and input once. Therefore, the required memory access of the m-DCF scheme is

$$[\underbrace{Ra_{ME}}_{Ref.\ R_1\ input} + \underbrace{2}_{R_0^*\ \&R_1^*} + \underbrace{1}_{H\ output} + \underbrace{2}_{Left\&Right\ Cur.}]\ /\ 2,$$

and the on-chip memory size is the same as that of the proposed DCF scheme. Note that besides the reduction of the required memory access, the memory access of R_0^* in the m-DCF scheme becomes regular instead of the irregular memory access of R_0 in the DCF scheme. However, the overhead of the m-DCF scheme is one extra MC frame R_1^* stored in the external memory.

8.2.2.5 *Comparison*

The four mentioned data re-use schemes are summarized in Table 8.3. In terms of external memory bandwidth, the direct implementation is the worst one among the four schemes. As for the three proposed schemes, the performances depend on the values of Ra_{ME} and $\overline{Ra_{extMC}}$. $\overline{Ra_{extMC}}$ is the average Ra_{extMC} of all MC blocks, which is related to motion vector precision (integer-pixel or fractional-pixel) and the MC block size. That is, at different specifications, these three frame-level data re-use schemes have different performances.

We take two examples to illustrate this feature, as shown in Table 8.4. In these two cases, we assume that Level C scheme is used to be the block-level data re-use scheme. The case 1 is that the searching range is $[-16, 16)$ (Ra_{ME}=3) and the average bandwidth of extMC ($\overline{Ra_{extMC}}$) is assumed 2. Then, by use of the above formulas, the ratio of the required memory bandwidth in direct implementation, DRF, DCF and m-DCF schemes is 6 : 4 : 4.5 : 4. The m-DCF scheme has the same performance as the DRF scheme, but the DCF scheme has a worse performance than the DRF scheme due to the overhead of extMC. When the searching range is enlarged to $[-64, 64)$ (Ra_{ME}=9) and the worst case of extMC occurs ($\overline{Ra_{extMC}}$=4) in the case 2, the ratio becomes 13 : 10 : 8.5 : 7. The reduction ratios of the m-DCF scheme are 46% and 30% of the direct implementation and DRF, respectively. Even if the worst case of extMC occurs, the memory bandwidth of the m-DCF scheme is still less than that of the DRF scheme. This is because the required memory bandwidth of reference frames is much larger than that of current frames and the memory bandwidth overhead

Table 8.3 Comparisons of frame-level data re-use schemes for the prediction stage of 5/3 MCTF.

Re-use Scheme	Direct	DRF	DCF	m-DCF
EMB (Pixels/Pixel)	$Ra_{ME} + 2 + \overline{Ra_{extMC}}/2$	$Ra_{ME} + 1$	$Ra_{ME}/2 + 2 + \overline{Ra_{extMC}}/2$	$Ra_{ME}/2 + 2.5$
On-chip Memory Size (Pixels)	1SRB	2SRB	1SRB	1SRB
Regularity of Memory Access	Irregular	Regular	Irregular	Regular

Note: EMB = External Memory Bandwidth.

Table 8.4 Two examples of various frame-level data re-use schemes for the prediction stage of one-level 5/3 MCTF.

	Case1				Case2			
Re-use Scheme	Direct	DRF	DCF	m-DCF	Direct	DRF	DCF	m-DCF
External Memory Bandwidth (Pixels/Pixel)	6	4	4.5	4	13	10	8.5	7
On-chip Memory Size (Pixels)	2,209	4,418	2,209	2,209	20,449	40,898	20,449	20,449

Case1: $[-16, 16)$ with Level C scheme ($Ra_{ME} = 3$), $\overline{Ra_{extMC}} = 2.0$

Case2: $[-64, 64)$ with Level C scheme ($Ra_{ME} = 9$), $\overline{Ra_{extMC}} = 4.0625$

of re-using the reference frames is near a constant. That is, when the required memory bandwidth of reference frames is larger and larger, the performances of the DCF and m-DCF schemes which can share the searching range data become better and better. Besides, the performance of the DCF scheme is seriously degraded if $\overline{Ra_{extMC}}$ is increased from 2 to 4.

In a word, the DCF scheme requires less external memory bandwidth than the DRF scheme does, if $Ra_{ME} \geq \overline{Ra_{extMC}} + 2$. On the other hand, the m-DCF scheme requires less external memory bandwidth than the DRF scheme does, when $Ra_{ME} \geq 3$. As for on-chip memory size, the DCF and m-DCF schemes only require half of on-chip memory size in the DRF scheme. Moreover, because of no extMC in the DRF and m-DCF schemes, the memory access of them is always regular. Contrarily, the memory access of direct implementation and the DCF scheme is irregular. Then, the efficiency of external memory access in the DCF scheme could be lower than that in the DRF or m-DCF scheme. Finally, because the direct implementation is worse than the three proposed schemes, it is excluded from the discussion below.

8.2.2.6 *Extension*

Because of the open-loop video coding scheme, we can extend the DRF and DCF schemes to be the generalized frame-level data re-use schemes. For example, we can further cascade several DRF schemes to reduce more memory bandwidth, which is called the extended DRF (EDRF) scheme. Figure 8.6(a) shows the EDRF scheme. From Fig. 8.6(a), the EDRF scheme is to combine two DRF schemes and process them as the same time. The top part of Figure 8.7 shows the detailed schedules of the DRF and EDRF schemes. In EDRF scheme, the number of reference frames is always one more frame than that of current frames. Therefore, if there are K searching range buffers, we can process $K-1$ current frames simultaneously. And then the required memory bandwidth for each frame is equal to

$$[\underbrace{K \times Ra_{ME}}_{K\ Ref.\ input} + \underbrace{(K-1)}_{K-1\ Cur.\ input} + \underbrace{(K-1)}_{K-1\ H\ output}] \ / \ 2(K-1).$$

In the EDRF scheme with K searching range buffers, $K-2$ reference frames between $K-1$ current frames can be shared, so the required memory bandwidth of reference frames can be reduced but with the increase of on-chip memory size.

Similar to the EDRF scheme, we can develop the extended DCF (EDCF)

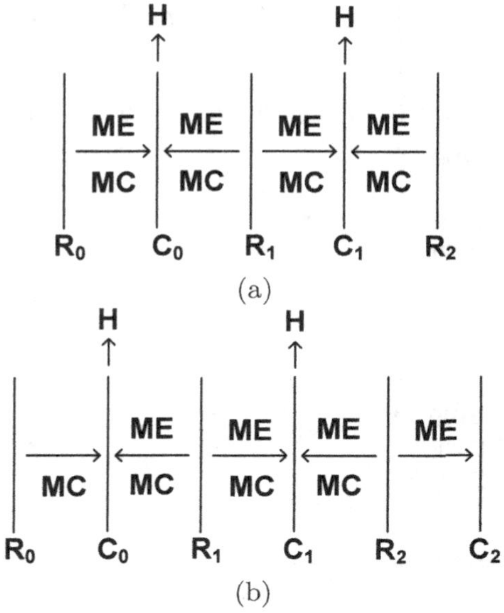

Fig. 8.6 The extended frame-level data re-use schemes (C: Current frame; R: Reference frame): (a) Extended double reference frames with $K = 3$; (b) Extended double current frames with $K = 2$.

scheme, based on the DCF scheme. Figure 8.6(b) shows the EDCF scheme, which cascades two DCF scheme. The detailed schedules of the DCF and EDCF schemes are shown in the bottom part of Fig. 8.7. For the EDCF scheme, the number of reference frames is one less frame than that of current frames. Hence the required memory bandwidth is

$$[\underbrace{K \times Ra_{ME}}_{K\ Ref.\ input} + \underbrace{(1 + Ra_{extMC})}_{Left\ MC} + \underbrace{(K+1)}_{K+1\ Cur.\ input} + \underbrace{(K)}_{K\ H\ output}] \ / \ 2K,$$

if there are K searching range buffers. In the EDCF scheme with K searching range buffers, $K - 1$ current frames between K reference frames can be input once, and only one extMC is required among 2K frames. Therefore, the required memory bandwidth of current frames and extMC can be reduced in the EDCF scheme.

In brief, the DRF and DCF schemes are the basic frame-level data re-use schemes. The EDRF and EDCF schemes are the generalized frame-level data re-use schemes, and they provide various tradeoffs between the required memory bandwidth and the number of searching range buffers. In

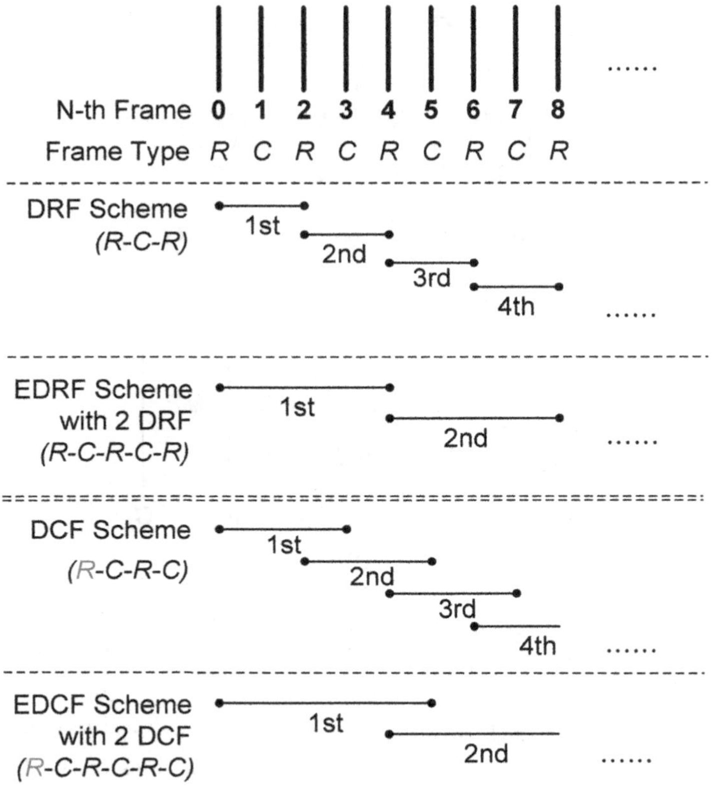

Fig. 8.7 The scheduling of various frame-level data re-use schemes.

the EDRF scheme, because several DRF schemes are cascaded, the reference frames between current frames can be shared. Hence the EDRF scheme not only can minimize the memory bandwidth of current frames but also can further re-use the searching range when the number of searching range buffers is larger than two. As for the EDCF scheme, when the number of searching range buffers is increased, the number of current frames and extMC inputs can be reduced so the memory bandwidth can be saved. Finally, for simplicity, we only discuss the basic frame-level data re-use schemes in the following, and the generalized frame-level data re-use schemes can be easily derived.

8.2.3 Memory analysis for update stage

In the update stage, the motion vectors are derived from those in the prediction stage, so only MC is performed. Since in MC, the motion vectors of two current blocks with the same position in different current frames may be different, the data re-use is hard to be performed. Then, the DCF and m-DCF schemes which re-use the searching region between two current frames cannot provide advantages. Moreover, because only MC is required in the update stage, the MC of the update stage becomes extMC.

The top part of Figure 8.8(a) shows that the DRF scheme is used to implement the update stage. The total external memory access of the update stage is

$$\left[\ \underbrace{2(1+Ra_{extMC})}_{Left\&Right\ Ref.} + \underbrace{1}_{Cur.\ input} + \underbrace{1}_{L\ output}\ \right] / 2,$$

where $2(1 + Ra_{extMC})$ is the memory bandwidth of left and right extMC, and the divisor, 2, exists because the update stage is performed for every two frames. Note that in SVC WD1.0, the computation unit of the update stage is a 4×4 block to perform the MC, which makes the extMC bandwidth overhead very heavy, as shown in Table 8.1.

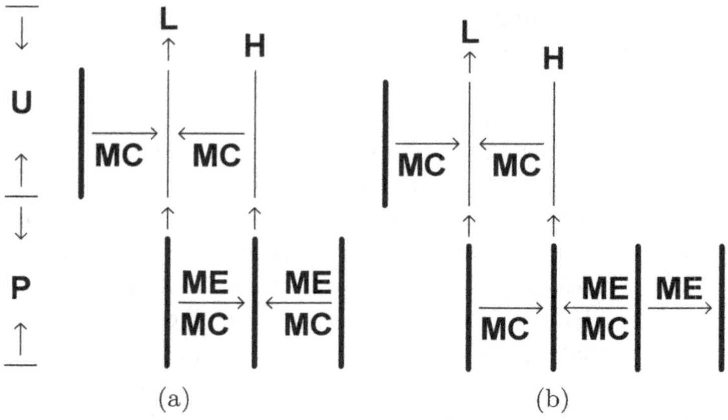

Fig. 8.8 Frame-level data re-use schemes of 5/3 MCTF. (P: Prediction stage; U: Update stage.) (a) P-DRF/U-DRF. (b) P-DCF/U-DRF.

8.2.4 *Memory analysis of one-level MCTF*

The different frame-level data re-use schemes for 5/3 MCTF are shown in Fig. 8.8, where the abbreviation of P-DCF/U-DRF is that the DCF and DRF schemes are applied in the prediction and update stages, respectively. The frames expressed by bold lines represent those need to be stored in the external memory for performing 5/3 MCTF. As shown in Fig. 8.8, because of the frame-level data re-use scheme, the required external memory size (EMS) of the DCF scheme is one more frame than that of the DRF scheme. And if the m-DCF scheme is used in Fig. 8.8(b), one more frame, R_1^*, is required to be stored in the external memory, compared to the DCF scheme.

The analyzed result of one-level MCTF is listed in Table 8.5, in which the average bandwidth ($\overline{Ra_{extMC}}$) is used for extMC in the prediction and update stages. In a word, the update stage has large overheads of external memory bandwidth and memory size, which means that 5/3 MCTF requires more computation resources than 1/3 MCTF does.

In the prediction stage, compared to the DRF scheme, the DCF scheme can save half memory bandwidth and half on-chip memory size by sharing the searching range data between two current frames, but it requires more external memory size for frame-level data re-use. Moreover, the performance of the DCF scheme is degraded due to extMC (Ra_{extMC}), and this can be improved by use of the m-DCF scheme, in which the overhead is the increase of external memory size. Finally, based on our analysis, for different hardware systems and specifications (Ra_{ME} and Ra_{extMC}), a suitable frame-level data re-use scheme can be easily selected to meet the system constraints.

After the theoretical analysis, we show a real case of one-level MCTF with different frame-level data re-use schemes in Table 8.6. The specification is D1 format with 30 fps, and the searching range is $[-64, 64)$ in the both directions with Level C data re-use scheme. As for the external memory bandwidth of extMC ($\overline{Ra_{extMC}}$), we assume it is equal to 2 or 4 in the case1 (EMB^1) or case2 (EMB^2), respectively. From Table 8.6, we can see that the memory bandwidth of 5/3 MCTF is much larger than 1/3 MCTF. This is because that the update stage requires a large memory bandwidth for extMC. When $\overline{Ra_{extMC}}$ is increased from 2 to 4, the memory bandwidth of the update stage is increased from 41 MB/s to 62 MB/s. Therefore, the required memory bandwidth of the update stage becomes a large overhead for the hardware design of 5/3 MCTF.

Moreover, due to $\overline{Ra_{extMC}}$, the performance of the DCF scheme is vari-

Table 8.5 Summary of External Memory Bandwidth (EMB) and External Memory Size (EMS) for one-level MCTF.

	5/3 MCTF			1/3 MCTF		
Prediction	DRF	DCF	m-DCF	DRF	DCF	m-DCF
Update	DRF	DRF	DRF	-	-	-
EMB (Pixels/Pixel)	$Ra_{ME}+3$	$Ra/2+4$	$Ra_{ME}/2+4.5$	$Ra_{ME}+1$	$Ra_{ME}/2+2$	$Ra_{ME}/2+2.5$
	$+\overline{Ra_{extMC}}$	$+3\overline{Ra_{extMC}}/2$	$+\overline{Ra_{extMC}}$		$+\overline{Ra_{extMC}}/2$	
EMS (Frames)	4	5	6	3	4	5
SRB	2	1	1	2	1	1

SRB: searching range buffer.

Table 8.6 The comparison of one-level MCTF with different data re-use schemes.

	5/3 MCTF			1/3 MCTF		
Prediction	DRF	DCF	m-DCF	DRF	DCF	m-DCF
Update	DRF	DRF	DRF	-	-	-
EMB^1 (MB/s)	145.15	122.82	114.05	103.68	77.76	72.58
EMB^2 (MB/s)	165.89	150.34	134.78	103.68	88.13	72.58
EMS (MB)	1.38	1.73	2.07	1.04	1.38	1.73
SRB (KB)	12.48	6.24	6.24	12.48	6.24	6.24

The specification is D1 Format with $Ra_{ME} = 9$.

The EMB of extMC ($\overline{Ra_{extMC}}$) is 2 or 4 in EMB^1 or EMB^2, respectively.

ant. When $\overline{Ra_{extMC}}$ is increased from 2 to 4, the reduction ratio of memory bandwidth in the DCF scheme is deceased from 25% to 15%, compared to the DRF scheme. The m-DCF scheme can improve the DCF scheme by eliminating extMC, and then its performance is better than that of the DCF scheme. But its overhead is the increase of external memory size (EMS). Compared with the DRF scheme, the m-DCF scheme can reduce 30% memory bandwidth and half on-chip memory size but with 66% increase of EMS.

8.3 Multi-Level Motion-Compensated Temporal Filtering

When extending the analysis from one-level MCTF to multi-level MCTF, three preconditions should be discussed and given first: the number of decomposition levels, whether inter-coding L-frames is necessary, and whether update stage is necessary. In the following, three preconditions are introduced, and the system issues of multi-level MCTF are discussed.

8.3.1 *The preconditions of multi-level MCTF*

8.3.1.1 *Decomposition level*

Based on the coding results using SVM3.0, four-level decomposition has the best compression efficiency for CIF sequence *Mobile&Calendar* when 5/3 MCTF is performed, as shown in Fig. 8.9(a). However, two-level or three-level MCTF is the best selection for the sequence *Stefan*, as shown in Fig. 8.9(b). In Fig. 8.9, the coding performance is saturated as the decomposition level increases. When the coding performance is saturated, more decomposition levels cannot bring more quality but it wastes more computation resources.

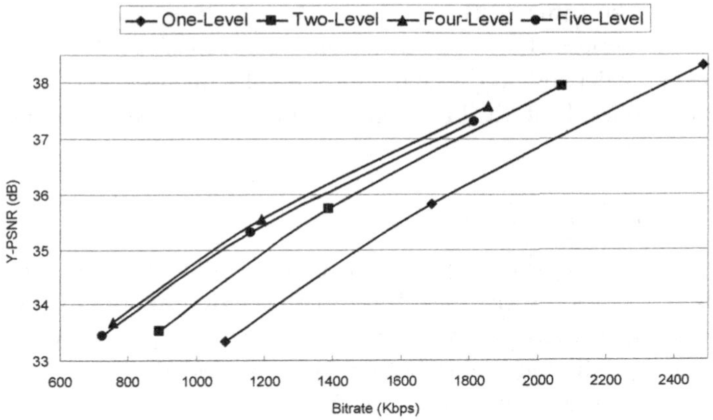

(a)

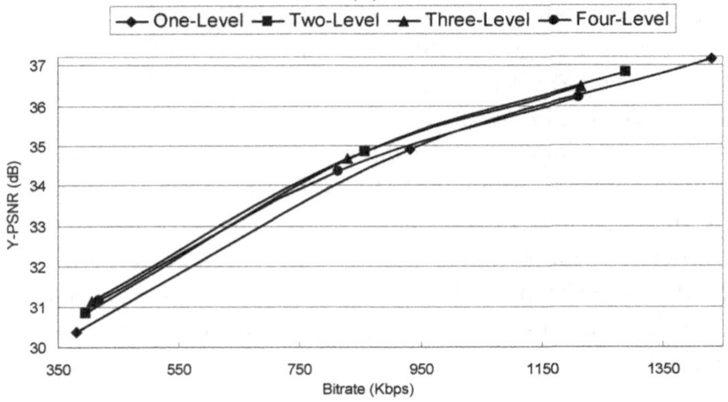

(b)

Fig. 8.9 Rate-Distortion (R-D) curves derived from SVM3.0 for different level decompositions of 5/3 MCTF. (a) *Mobile&Calendar* CIF 30fps, SR:[-16,16]. (b) *Stefan* CIF 30fps, SR:[-32,32].

A high level decomposition does not always bring more quality because of two reasons. The first one is that when the more the number of decomposition level is, the longer the temporal distance in the top decomposition level is. Hence the correlation between two operating frames is lower and the temporal prediction in the top decomposition level is not as good as that in the bottom decomposition level. The second is that the searching range is fixed and limited for all decomposition levels. Even if the temporal distance becomes longer in the higher decomposition level, the searching range is still the same as the original, which reduces the performance of temporal prediction. Therefore, how many decomposition levels should be performed may depend on the characteristics of sequences, and the different decomposition levels of MCTF should be supported in the same multi-level MCTF system.

8.3.1.2 *Inter-coding for L-frames*

The second precondition is to perform inter-coding for the L-frames or not. The L-frames are the base layer in the temporal axis for multi-level MCTF coding systems. They can be inter-coded using close-loop motion-compensated prediction (MCP) schemes or intra-coded without MC in SVC WD1.0. Inter-coding with close-loop MCP schemes can provide a better compression ratio but have a worse error resilience capability. On the other hand, intra-coding can provide a better scalability and error resilience capability but with a large bitrate. The differences of R-D curves between inter- and intra-coded L-frames are shown in Fig. 8.10. Figure 8.10(a) is the result of *Mobile&Calendar* with four-level 5/3 MCTF, where one L-frame exists for every 16 frames, and the difference between inter- and intra-coded L-frames is about 1 dB. Figure 8.10(b) shows the result of *Stefan* with two-level 5/3 MCTF, where one L-frame exists for every four frames, and the difference between inter- and intra-coded L-frames becomes 2–4 dB. That is, as the decomposition level increases, the difference between inter- and intra-coded L-frames decreases. But the intra-coded L-frames still has a large bitrate penalty.

8.3.1.3 *Update stage*

To perform the update stage or not is the third precondition. If the update stage is not performed, it can be decided to perform 1/3 MCTF or Hierarchical B-frame (HB) in SVM3.0. Figure 8.11 gives an example for these different configurations by use of SVM3.0 for *Mobile&Calendar*, where the searching range is $[-16, 16)$, four-level decomposition is adopted in 5/3 MCTF, 1/3 MCTF, and HB. In Figure 8.11, we also add the coding result of H.264/AVC for comparison, where H.264 Main Profile is adopted, the

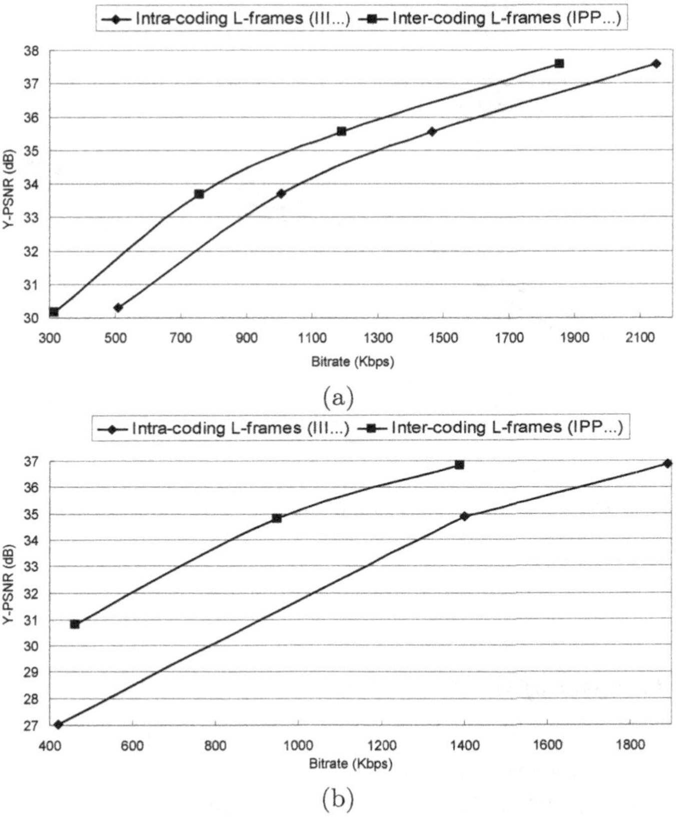

Fig. 8.10 R-D Curves derived from SVM3.0 for inter- and intra-coded L-frames. (a) *Mobile&Calendar* CIF 30fps, SR:[-16,16], Four-level 5/3 MCTF. (b) *Stefan* CIF 30fps, SR:[-16,16], Two-level 5/3 MCTF.

coding scheme is IBBPBBP with five reference frames and the reference software is JM9.0 [167].

Among different coding schemes, 5/3 MCTF can provide the best R-D performance. The coding efficiencies of 1/3 MCTF and HB are nearly the same under the open-loop prediction scheme. Compared 5/3 MCTF and 1/3 MCTF, the update stage can provide 0.5–0.3 dB coding gain. Moreover, from this figure, MCTF is shown to be capable of boosting the coding performance of H.264/AVC. Especially, the H.264 Main Profile configuration uses five reference frames, but SVM3.0 only uses two reference frames for the bi-directional motion estimation of MCTF and one reference frame for the inter-coded L-frames.

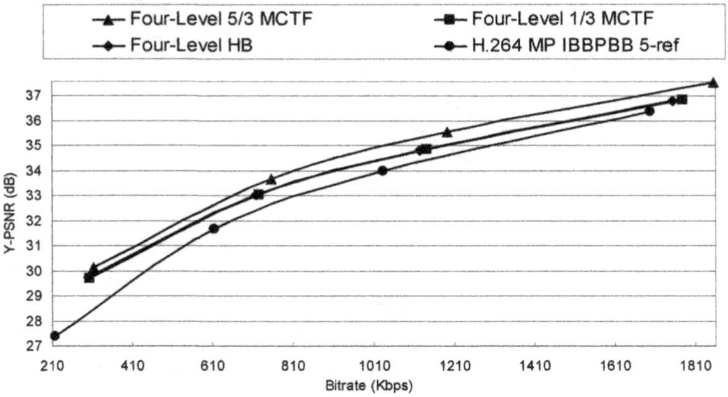

Fig. 8.11 R-D Curve derived from SVM3.0 and JM9.0 for sequence *Mobile&Calendar* CIF 30fps (SR:[-16,16]).

8.3.2 *Analysis of multi-level MCTF*

In the following analysis, MCTF is assumed to use the closest frame as the reference frame of each direction for the prediction stage, and the L-frames are inter-coded as IPPPP.. structure using M previous frames as reference frames. Since the hardware requirements of open-loop 1/3 MCTF and HB are all exactly the same, HB is not discussed in the following.

8.3.2.1 *Computational complexity*

Different MCTF levels have different computation complexity and external memory access. Moreover, the redundancy access factors for extMC (Ra_{extMC}) in different MCTF levels are also variant. In the following, the redundancy access factors are assumed to be the same for every MCTF level. Then the computation complexity and external memory access are exponentially decreased for higher MCTF levels. As shown in Fig. 8.12, the number of input frames in the second level MCTF is only half of that in the first level MCTF. Therefore, the workload (WL) of the second level MCTF is also half of that of the first level MCTF. If the workloads are assumed to be dominated by ME and MC, WL can be formulated as follows:

$$WL_{1^{st}\ level} = \begin{cases} 1ME + 2MC\ for\ 5/3MCTF \\ 1ME + 1MC\ for\ 1/3MCTF \end{cases},$$

$$WL_L = \frac{M \times ME + 1MC}{2^J},$$

$$WL_{J-level} = (1 + \frac{1}{2} + ... + \frac{1}{2^{J-1}})WL_{1^{st}\ level} + WL_L, \quad (8.5)$$

where $WL_{1^{st}\ level}$, WL_L, and $WL_{J-level}$ are average workloads per frame for the first level MCTF, inter-coded L-frames, and J-level MCTF, respectively. It can be found that the computation complexity of J-level MCTF is very close to traditional close-loop MC prediction with two reference frames if $M \leq 2$.

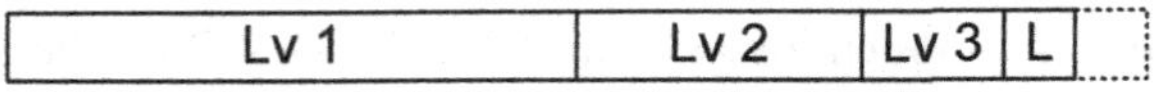

Fig. 8.12 Scaling effect of workload for three-level MCTF and inter-coded L-frames with one reference frame.

8.3.2.2 *External memory access*

The external memory bandwidth (EMB)(pixels/pixel) of multi-level MCTF has a similar scaling effect as the computation complexity, and it can be written as

$$EMB_{J-level} = (1 + \frac{1}{2} + ... + \frac{1}{2^{J-1}})EMB_{1^{st}\ level} + \frac{1 + M \cdot Ra}{2^J}, \quad (8.6)$$

where $EMB_{1^{st}\ level}$ is as shown in Table 8.5 for different frame-level data re-use schemes. From (8.6), $EMB_{J-level}$ is also close to the double of $EMB_{1^{st}\ level}$, when $M \leq 2$.

8.3.2.3 *External memory size*

Compared to the scaling effect in the external memory bandwidth, the required external memory size (EMS) of multi-level MCTF is linearly proportional to the decomposition level J. This is because the number of required stored frames are the same for every decomposition level. For 5/3 MCTF, the external memory size is

$$EMS_{J-level,5/3} = J \cdot EMS_{1^{st}\ level,5/3} + M\ \ (frames), \quad (8.7)$$

where $EMS_{1^{st}\ level,5/3}$ is shown in Table 8.5 and depends on the adopted frame-level data re-use scheme.

For 1/3 MCTF, the frame R_0 in Fig. 8.4 and 8.5 can be shared among all MCTF levels, because no update stages are performed. Thus, for 1/3 MCTF, the external memory size is

$$EMS_{J-level,1/3} = J(EMS_{1^{st}\ level,1/3} - 1) + M \quad (frames), \tag{8.8}$$

where $EMS_{1^{st}\ level,1/3}$ is also shown in Table 8.5 for different frame-level data re-use schemes. The EMS of multi-level MCTF is much larger than the traditional close-loop MCP scheme, when J is large.

8.3.2.4 *Coding delay*

The coding delay is another important issue for the open-loop MCTF prediction, because it is much longer than traditional MC prediction. In [109], only the encoding delay is discussed. In the following, the coding delay is considered, which is defined as the maximum distance between the decoded frame, say X, and the farthest frame that is required to encode frame X. In the other words, the coding delay is the minimum timing delay between the real-time captured video and the decoded video. Figure 8.13(a) and (b) are examples of two-level 5/3 and 1/3 MCTF systems, respectively. For two-level 5/3 MCTF, the coding delay of the P-DRF/U-DRF scheme is nine frames, and that of the P-DCF/U-DRF scheme is twelve frames. For two-level 1/3 MCTF, the coding delay of the DRF scheme is three frames, and that of the DCF scheme is five frames. In the following discussion, the m-DCF scheme has the same property as that of the DCF scheme, so we only discuss the DCF scheme whose results are the same as that of the m-DCF scheme.

The coding delays of 5/3 MCTF and 1/3 MCTF with different frame-level data re-use schemes can be derived by using multi-rate filter bank equations . Figure 8.14(a) shows the original recursive filter-bank representations of J-level MCTF and inverse MCTF (IMCTF). We can change the positions of upsample and downsample, as shown in Fig. 8.14(b), and then all filters of different decomposition levels which are directly cascaded can be synthesized to be one filter. Therefore, the coding delay of 5/3 MCTF with the P-DRF/U-DRF scheme can be formulated as

$$2(2^0 + 2^1 + ... + 2^{J-1}) + (2^0 + ... + 2^{J-1}) = 3(2^J - 1) \quad (frames). \tag{8.9}$$

Similarly, the coding delay of 5/3 MCTF with the P-DCF/U-DRF scheme

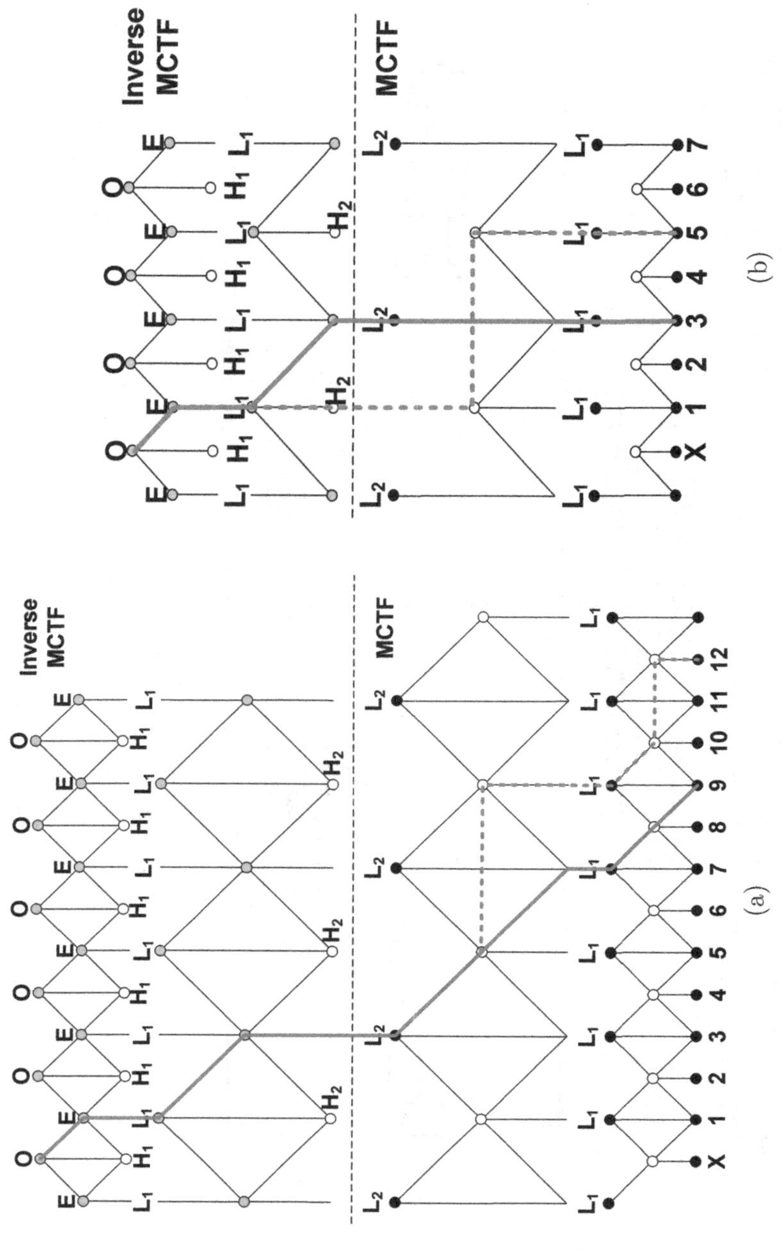

Fig. 8.13 Signal flow graph of two-level MCTF system. (a) 5/3 MCTF, and (b) 1/3 MCTF, where the solid line is P-DRF/U-DRF and the dotted line is P-DCF/U-DRF.

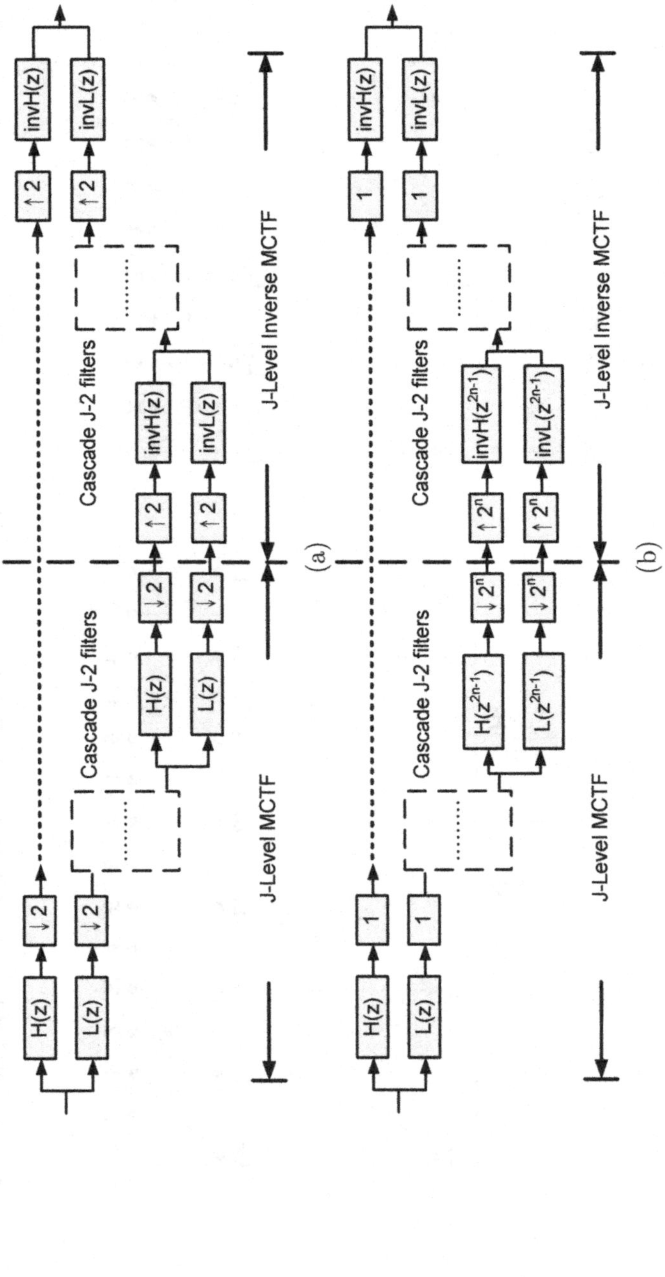

Fig. 8.14 The filter-bank representation of J-level MCTF and inverse MCTF. (a) The original filter-bank representation. (b) The modified filter-bank representations.

Table 8.7 Coding Delays of J-Level 5/3 or 1/3 MCTF with Different Data re-use Schemes.

MCTF	5/3 MCTF		1/3 MCTF	
Scheme	P-DRF/U-DRF	P-DCF/U-DRF	P-DRF	P-DCF
Delay	$3(2^J - 1)$	$4(2^J - 1)$	$2^J - 1$	$2^J + 2^{(J-1)} - 1$

is

$$3(2^0 + 2^1 + ... + 2^{J-1}) + (2^0 + ... + 2^{J-1}) = 4(2^J - 1) \ (frames). \quad (8.10)$$

Note that in [109], the encoding delay of P-DRF/U-DRF scheme is shown to be $2(2^J - 1)$ frames. By the same method, the decoding delay of 5/3 IMCTF can also be derived as $(2^J - 1)$ frames. In the P-DRF/U-DRF or P-DCF/U-DRF scheme, the coding delay is equal to the sum of encoding and decoding delays, because it happens that the coding delay path is the sum of longest delay paths in 5/3 MCTF and 5/3 IMCTF. However, the coincidence does not happen to 1/3 MCTF, which can be found in Fig. 8.13(b). In 1/3 MCTF, the coding delay of the P-DRF or P-DCF scheme can be derived as $(2^J - 1)$ or $(2^J + 2^{(J-1)} - 1)$ frames from the signal data flow, as shown in Fig. 8.13(b), or the filter-bank representation.

The coding delays for different data re-use schemes are summarized in Table 8.7. In a word, the coding delays of multi-level MCTF are exponentially increased with J, and the update stage increases a long delay for coding systems. The ratio of coding delays for 5/3 MCTF with P-DRF/U-DRF, 5/3 MCTF with P-DCF/U-DRF, 1/3 MCTF with P-DRF, and 1/3 MCTF with P-DCF is about 3 : 4 : 1 : 1.5.

8.4 Case Study

To show a real-life system requirement, a case study is given which performs four-level MCTF for D1 sequences with 30fps. The searching range of ME is $[-64, 64)$, and Level C data re-use scheme is adopted such that $Ra_{ME} = 9$. Because of supporting variable block size ME, we assume the extMC is all performed on a 4×4 block such that $Ra_{extMC} = 4.0625$. The L-frames are inter-coded as IPPP... structure with one reference frame. Two configurations of H.264/AVC, IBBPBBP and IBPBP with two reference frames, are also compared (only the MC prediction). For IBPBP configuration, the external memory bandwidth is $2Ra + 1$ because of two reference frames. As for IBBPBBP configuration, the external memory bandwidth (pixels/pixel) is calculated as

$$\frac{\overbrace{2Ra+1}^{P-frames}+\overbrace{2Ra+2}^{B-frames}}{3}=\frac{4}{3}Ra+1,$$

because the searching region of two B-frames can be shared.

The comparisons are listed in Table 8.8. Compared to different frame-level data re-use schemes, the m-DCF scheme reduces the external memory access but requires the largest external storage. The DRF scheme has the smallest external memory size but requires the largest on-chip memory size and external memory bandwidth. Among various coding schemes, the required external memory bandwidth (EMB) of 1/3 MCTF is close to those of H.264/AVC configurations. But due to update stage, 5/3 MCTF requires nearly double of EMB of H.264/AVC. The external storage requirement of MCTF is several times of that of H.264/AVC, but the on-chip memory of MCTF is equal to or less than that of H.264/AVC and depends on which frame-level data re-use scheme is applied.

8.5 Rate-Distortion-Computation Scalability

We summarize the required computation resources of multi-level MCTF. The computation complexity is very similar for all kinds of configurations for multi-level MCTF, which is bounded by the computation complexity of ME with two reference frames per frame if M is equal to one. The external memory bandwidth of multi-level MCTF depends on the frame-level data re-use schemes and update stage, but it is quite similar for different MCTF decomposition levels with the same data re-use scheme. However, the external memory storage requirement is linearly proportional to the MCTF decomposition level, and the coding delay is exponentially increased as the MCTF decomposition level increases.

From the analysis, the required computational ability is similar for different configurations of multi-level MCTF, but the requirements of external memory bandwidth and size are variant. Hence it is very suitable to design one flexible hardware which not only can support all different configurations of multi-level MCTF but also can adapt itself to fit variant external requirements by performing a suitable coding scheme among the supported configurations. That is, the rate-distortion-computation scalability can be

Table 8.8 System requirement comparisons of four-level MCTF and H.264/AVC with two reference frames.

Data re-use Scheme	5/3 MCTF			1/3 MCTF			H.264 IBBP	H.264 IBPBP
Prediction Stage	DRF	DCF	m-DCF	DRF	DCF	m-DCF	-	-
Update Stage	DRF	DRF	DRF	-	-	-	-	-
EMB (MBytes/s)	318.74	290.18	260.42	200.88	172.33	142.56	134.78	196.99
EMS (MBytes)	5.875	7.258	8.640	3.110	4.493	5.875	1.382	1.037
On-chip Memory (KBytes)	12.48	6.24	6.24	12.48	6.24	6.24	12.48	12.48

Note: The specification is D1 Format with 30 fps, and the searching range is $[-64, 64)$

achieved in this flexible architecture.

This system architecture can perform any-level 5/3 MCTF, 1/3 MCTF, HB, and the close-loop MCP with two reference frames. Different coding schemes require various system requirements and provide various coding performances. For example, 5/3 MCTF has the best coding efficiency, but it also requires the largest external memory bandwidth and external memory size. 1/3 MCTF can use the less external memory bandwidth and external memory size with a little degradation of video compression. HB is compatible to H.264, and its performance is similar to 1/3 MCTF. Although the performance of the close-loop MCP scheme is not good, its coding delay is much shorter than that of MCTF or HB. Therefore, it is much suitable for low end-to-end delay applications. Under different system constraints or application requirements, such as available external memory size, external memory bandwidth, delay constraints, or the required compression ratio, this flexible hardware can execute a suitable coding schemes to meet different system or application constraints.

We take an example to illustrate this more clearly. This system architecture can be applied in a hand-held device with various multimedia applications, including Video Conference, Video Camera, and so on. When the user uses this device to attend the video conference, a low coding delay is required and this system architecture can perform the close-loop MCP scheme to meet the low delay requirement. When the device is used to record some event in user's life, the compression ratio becomes much more important. Hence 5/3 MCTF is performed in this system architecture, and based on the video content, the different decomposition levels can be performed to achieve the highest compression ratio. Moreover, when the energy of this device is not enough or the available external memory bandwidth and external memory size are limited, the system architecture can execute different frame-level data re-use schemes, decrease the number of decomposition levels, or use 1/3 MCTF instead of 5/3 MCTF to reduce the usages of external memory resources and battery power. By this way, the rate-distortion-computation scalability is provided.

8.6 Analysis of Pyramid MCTF

After the analysis of multi-level MCTF, we focus on the analysis to pyramid MCTF. Before starting the analysis of pyramid MCTF, *Inter-layer Prediction* should be introduced first. Due to the pyramid MCTF in SVM3.0, the extra redundancy between spatial layers are generated and *Inter-layer Prediction* is developed to remove this redundancy. *Inter-layer Prediction* means that we can use the information of one sequence with a small frame size to predict one sequence with a large frame size. In SVM3.0, when the inter-layer prediction modes are considered, ME is processed twice. One is the original and the other is with the information of previous spatial layer. That is, if *Inter-layer Prediction* is performed in SVM3.0, the required computation complexity is doubled. In the following analysis, we assume the downsample ratio between two spatial layers is δ, and there are P spatial layers, in which the largest frame size is 1, the smallest frame size is δ^{P-1}, and the frame rates in different spatial layers are the same.

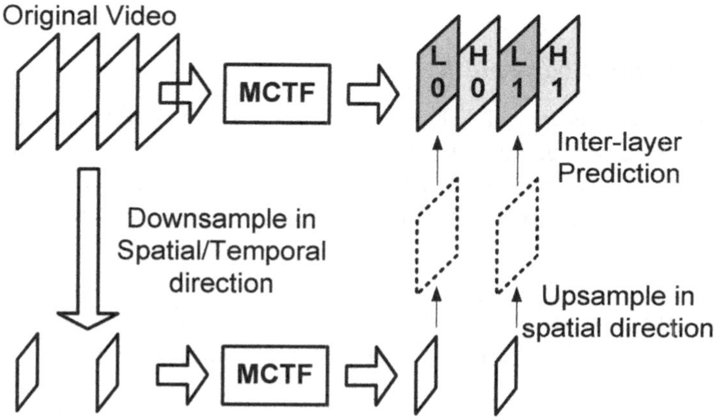

Fig. 8.15 The pyramid MCTF scheme with two spatial layers.

8.6.1 *Computation complexity*

For the computation complexity, motion estimation is still a major part in pyramid MCTF, so we also assume that it dominates the workload of pyramid MCTF. In each spatial layer, the searching range and searching strategy of ME can be different. But for simplicity, we assume all parameters of ME are the same for each spatial layer. Hence the computation complexity of each current macroblock is the same, and the computation complexity of each spatial layer is direct proportional to its frame size. The computation complexity of pyramid MCTF with *Inter-layer Prediction* can be written as

$$\begin{aligned} WL_{P-layer} =&(1+\delta+\delta^2+...+\delta^{J-1}) \times WL_{1-layer} \\ &+(1+\delta+...+\delta^{J-2}) \times WL_{1-layer}, \end{aligned} \tag{8.11}$$

where $WL_{P-layer}$ and $WL_{1-layer}$ are the workload of pyramid MCTF with P spatial layers and MCTF with the largest frame size, respectively. The $WL_{1-layer}$ is equal to (8.5) in the analysis of multi-level MCTF. In (8.11), the first part is the sum of the computation complexity of MCTF in each spatial layer, and the second part is that of *Inter-layer Prediction*. Therefore, if *Inter-layer Prediction* is not adopted or the ME of *Inter-layer Prediction* can be skipped, the computation complexity is only the first part.

8.6.2 *Memory bandwidth*

Because all parameters of ME are the same, the external memory bandwidth of each spatial layer is also direct proportional to the frame size. The required memory bandwidth also can be partitioned into two parts, the memory bandwidth of MCTF and that of *Inter-layer Prediction*, and it can be written as

$$\begin{aligned} EMB_{P-layer} =&(1+\delta+\delta^2+...+\delta^{J-1}) \times EMB_{1-layer} \\ &+(\delta+...+\delta^{J-1}) \times FrameSize \times 30, \end{aligned} \tag{8.12}$$

where $EMB_{P-layer}$ are the memory bandwidth of pyramid MCTF with J spatial layers and $EMB_{1-layer}$ is that of MCTF with the largest frame size, as shown in (8.6). The first part is the summation of the memory bandwidth for MCTF, and the second part is that of *Inter-layer Prediction*, in which the information of sequences with the small frame sizes has to be loaded from external memory. In the second part of (8.12), the series of δ is the amount of data per frame for *Inter-layer Prediction*, $FrameSize$ is the memory bandwidth of one frame, and 30 is the number of frames per second.

8.6.3 *External memory storage*

Due to the inter-layer prediction scheme, P spatial layers cannot be processed in parallel. Therefore, the coding order is from the sequence with the smallest frame size to that with the largest frame size. Then, the external memory storage is

$$EMS_{P-layer} = EMS_{1-layer} + \delta \times FrameSize \times GOPSize \\ + (\delta + ... + \delta^{J-1}) \times M \times FrameSize, \quad (8.13)$$

where $EMS_{P-layer}$ is the external memory storage of pyramid MCTF with P spatial layers, $EMS_{1-layer}$ is that of MCTF with the largest frame size, and $GOPSize$ is the number of frames in one GOP. The first part is the original for one sequence with the largest frame size, as shown in (8.7) or (8.8). The second part is used to store a GOP of the previous spatial layer for the inter-layer prediction scheme, and the third part is used to store the M reference frames of the L frame in each spatial layer.

8.6.4 *Summary*

In pyramid MCTF, the computation complexity and memory bandwidth are direct proportional to the frame size of each spatial layer, when all parameters of ME are the same for each spatial layer. Hence the required computation complexity and memory bandwidth are exponential decreased for these downsampled sequences, but the external memory storage can be re-used, except reference frames of the L frame in each spatial layer. As for *Inter-layer Prediction*, the computation complexity becomes double, the increase of the external memory storage depends on the size of one GOP, and its required memory bandwidth is dependent on the frame size.

Finally, we give an example, in which the downsample ratio is 2 in both directions (δ=1/4), the GOP size is 16, and only one reference frame is used for L-frames ($M = 1$). The computation complexity and memory bandwidth of pyramid MCTF without *Inter-layer Prediction* is close to 4/3 times of the originals, and the external memory storage increases $1/3Frames$. As for *Inter-layer Prediction* in SVM3.0, the computation complexity is 8/3 times of the original, and the extra increase of the memory bandwidth and external memory storage are close to $10Frames/s$ and $13/3Frames$, respectively.

8.7 Conclusion

In this chapter, the system issues of MCTF for VLSI architecture design are introduced. By using the redundant access factors of ME and MC, the external memory bandwidth of ME with block-level searching range data re-use schemes and MC with fractional-pixel resolution is evaluated. Based on these factors, the memory issues of one-level MCTF, including external memory bandwidth, external memory size and on-chip memory size, are discussed. Because of the open-loop prediction scheme, the frame-level data re-use schemes for the prediction stage in MCTF become possible and are discussed. Compared to the direct implementation of MCTF, the DRF scheme can save the external memory bandwidth of extMC, and the DCF scheme can re-use the searching range and reduce on-chip memory size by processing two current frames at the same time. However, the penalty of the DCF scheme is the increase of external memory bandwidth for extMC, and the m-DCF scheme can eliminate it with the increase of external memory size.

After analyzing one-level MCTF, we extend the analysis from one-level MCTF to multi-level MCTF. Three predictions of multi-level MCTF, decomposition level, whether inter-coding L-frames is preformed, and whether update stage is performed, are discussed, first. Next, many important system parameters are formulated, including computation complexity, memory bandwidth, external storage, and coding delay. By the case study, external memory bandwidth, external memory size, and coding delay of multi-level MCTF are much more than traditional MC prediction schemes, but the computation complexity of multi-level MCTF is only equal to that of traditional MC prediction with two reference frames. Based on the analysis of multi-level MCTF, a hardware accelerator with the rate-distortion-computation scalability is possible to be realized. The flexible architecture not only can perform any-level 5/3 MCTF, 1/3 MCTF, HB, and the close-loop MCP with two reference frames but also can fit different system constraints or application requirements by adopting different coding schemes.

Finally, we analyze the related system issues of pyramid MCTF. In pyramid MCTF, the required computation complexity and memory bandwidth are exponential decreased for those downsampled sequences, but the external memory storage can be re-used, except reference frames of the L frame in each spatial layer. As for *Inter-layer Prediction* in SVM3.0, the computation complexity is double, the increase of the external memory storage depends on the size of one GOP, and its required memory bandwidth is dependent on the frame size.

Bibliography

[1] *Information Technology - Digital Compression and Coding of continuous-Tone Still Images.* ISO/IEC 10918-1 and ITU Rec. T.81 Std., 1994.

[2] V. Bhaskaran and K. Konstantinides, *Image and Video Compression Standards: Algorithms and Architectures.* Kluwer Academic Publishers, 2nd edition, 1997.

[3] K. Varma and A. Bell, "JPEG2000 - choices and tradeoffs for encoders," *IEEE Signal Processing Magazine*, pp. 70–75, Nov. 2004.

[4] J. M. Shapiro, "Embedded image coding using zerotrees of wavelet coefficients," *IEEE Transactions on Signal Processing*, vol. 41, no. 12, pp. 3445–3463, Dec. 1993.

[5] A. Said and W. A. Pearlman, "A new, fast, and efficient image codec based on set partitioning in hierarchical trees," *IEEE Transactions on Circuits and Systems for Video Technology*, vol. 6, no. 3, pp. 243–250, June 1996.

[6] D. Taubman, "High performance scalable image compression with EBCOT," *IEEE Transactions on Image Processing*, vol. 9, no. 7, pp. 1158–1170, July 2000.

[7] *JPEG 2000 Image Coding System.* ISO/IEC FDIS15444-1, 2000.

[8] S.-T. Hsiang, "Embedded image coding using zeroblocks of sub-band/wavelet coefficients and context modeling," *IEEE Data Compression Conference*, pp. 83–92, Mar. 2001.

[9] *Information Technology - Coding of Moving Pictures and Associated Audio for Digital Storage Media at up to about 1.5Mbit/s - Part 2: Video.* ISO/IEC 11172-2, 1993.

[10] *Information Technology - Generic Coding of Moving Pictures and Associated Audio Information: Video.* ISO/IEC 13818-2 and ITU-T Recommendation H.262, 1996.

[11] *Information Technology - Coding of Audio-Visual Objects - Part 2: Visual.* ISO/IEC 14496-2, 1999.

[12] J. V. Team, *Draft ITU-T Recommendation and Final Draft International Standard of Joint Video Specification.* ITU-T Recommendation H.264 and ISO/IEC 14496-10 AVC, 2003.

[13] J.-R. Ohm, "Advanced packet-video coding based on layered VQ and SBC

techniques," *IEEE Transactions on Circuits and Systems for Video Technology*, vol. 3, no. 3, pp. 208–221, June 2002.

[14] A. Secker and D. Taubman, "Motion-compensated highly scalable video compression using an adaptive 3D wavelet transform based on lifting," *Proc. IEEE International Conference on Image Processing*, pp. 1029–1032, 2001.

[15] B. Pesquet-Popescu and V. Bottreau, "Three-dimensional lifting schemes for motion compensated video compression," *Proc. IEEE International Conference on Acoustics, Speech, and Signal Processing*, pp. 1793–1796, 2001.

[16] D. Taubman, "Successive refinement of video: fundamental issues, past efforts and new directions," *International Symposium on Visual Communications and Image Processing*, pp. 791–805, 2003.

[17] I. JTC1, "Call for proposals on scalable video coding technology," Oct. 2003.

[18] "Scalable Video Coding and IPMP make big strides," Mar. 2004.

[19] J. Reichel, H. Schwarz, and M. Wien, "Working Draft 1.0 of 14496-10:200x/AMD1 Scalable Video Coding," Jan. 2005.

[20] H. Schwarz, D. Marpe, and T. Wiegand, "Scalable extension of H.264/AVC," Mar. 2004.

[21] T. Wiegand and et al., "MCTF and scalability extension of H.264/AVC," *Proceedings of Picture Coding Symposium*, 2004.

[22] D. Keitel-Schulz and N. Wehn, "Embedded DRAM development: Technology, physical design, and application issues," *IEEE Design and Test of Computers*, vol. 18, no. 3, pp. 7–15, 2001.

[23] F. Catthoor, S. Wuytack, E. D. Greef, F. Balasa, L. Nachtergaele, and A. Vandecappele, *Custom Memory Management Methodology: Exploration of Memory Organization for Embedded Multimedia System Design.* Kluwer Academic Publishers, 1998.

[24] P. de With, P. Frencken, and M. Schaar-Mitrea, "An MPEG decoder with embedded compression for memory reduction," *IEEE Transactions on Consumer Electronics*, vol. 44, no. 3, pp. 545–555, Aug. 1998.

[25] S. Peng and M. Balakrishnan, "DTV and low-cost video decoder," *Proceedings of the IEEE Industrial Electronics Society*, vol. 2, pp. 744–749, 1999.

[26] M. van der Schaar and P. de With, "Near-lossless complexity-scalable embedded compression algorithm for cost reduction in DTV receivers," *IEEE Transactions on Consumer Electronics*, vol. 46, no. 4, pp. 923–933, Nov. 2000.

[27] R. P. Llopis, R. Sethuraman, C. A. Pinto, S. Peters, S. Maul, and M. Oosterhuis, "A low-cost and low-power multi-standard video encoder," *First IEEE/ACM/IFIP International Conference on Hardware/Software Codesign and System Synthesis*, pp. 97–102, 2003.

[28] K. K. Parhi, *VLSI Digital Signal Processing Systems: Design and Implementation.* Wiley, 1999.

[29] M.-Y. Hsu, "Scalable module-based architecture for MPEG-4 BMA motion estimation," Master's thesis, National Taiwan Univ., June 2000.

[30] J.-C. Tuan, T.-S. Chang, and C.-W. Jen, "On the data reuse and memory bandwidth analysis for full-search block-matching VLSI architecture," *IEEE Trans. CSVT*, vol. 12, no. 1, pp. 61–72, Jan. 2002.

[31] I. Daubechies, "Orthonormal bases of compactly support wavelets," *Communications on Pure and Applied Mathematics*, vol. 41, pp. 909–996, Nov. 1988.

[32] S. G. Mallat, "A theory for multiresolution signal decomposition: The wavelet representation," *IEEE Transactions on Pattern Analysis and Machine Intelligence*, vol. 11, no. 7, pp. 674–693, July 1989.

[33] M. Antonini, M. Barlaud, P. Mathieu, and I. Daubechies, "Image coding using wavelet transform," *IEEE Transactions on Image Processing*, vol. 1, no. 2, pp. 205–220, Apr. 1992.

[34] *JPEG 2000 Image Coding System: Motion JPEG 2000.* ISO/IEC FDIS15444-3, 2002.

[35] S. Mallat, *A Wavelet Tour of Signal Processing.* Academic Press, 1998.

[36] P. P. Vaidyanathan, *Multirate Systems and Filter Banks.* Prentice Hall, 1993.

[37] W. Sweldens, "The lifting scheme: a custom-design construction of biorthogonal wavelets," *Applied and Computaional Harmonic Analysis*, vol. 3, no. 15, pp. 186–200, 1996.

[38] I. Daubechies and W. Sweldens, "Factoring wavelet transforms into lifting steps," *The Journal of Fourier Analysis and Applications*, vol. 4, pp. 247–269, 1998.

[39] J. Reichel, "On the arithmetic and bandwidth complexity of the lifting scheme," *Proc. IEEE International Conference on Image Processing*, pp. 198–201, 2001.

[40] M. Unser and T. Blu, "Wavelet theory demystified," *IEEE Transactions on Signal Processing*, vol. 51, no. 2, pp. 470–483, Feb. 2003.

[41] K. K. Parhi and T. Nishitani, "VLSI architectures for discrete wavelet transforms," *IEEE Transactions on Very Large Scale Integration Systems*, vol. 1, no. 2, pp. 191–202, June 1993.

[42] C. Chakrabarti and M. Vishwanath, "Efficient realizations of the discrete and continuous wavelet transforms: From single chip implementations to mappings on SIMD array computers," *IEEE Transactions on Signal Processing*, vol. 43, no. 3, pp. 759–771, Mar. 1995.

[43] M. Vishwanath, R. M. Owens, and M. J. Irwin, "VLSI architectures for the discrete wavelet transform," *IEEE Transactions on Circuis and Systems-II: Analog and digital signal processing*, vol. 42, no. 5, pp. 305–316, May 1995.

[44] C. Chakrabarti, M. Vishwanath, and R. M. Owens, "Architectures for wavelet transforms: A survey," *Journal of VLSI Signal Processing*, vol. 14, pp. 171–192, 1996.

[45] J.-M. Jou, Y.-H. Shiau, and C.-C. Liu, "Efficient VLSI architectures for the biorthogonal wavelet transform by filter bank and lifting scheme," *IEEE International Symposium on Circuits and Systems*, vol. 2, pp. 529–532, 2001.

[46] Y.-H. Shiau, J. M. Jou, and C.-C. Liu, "Efficient architectures for the biorthogonal wavelet transform by filter bank and lifting scheme," *IEICE*

Transactions on Information and Systems, vol. E87-D, no. 7, pp. 1867–1877, July 2004.

[47] W. Jiang and A. Ortega, "Lifting factorization-based discrete wavelet transform architecture design," *IEEE Transactions on Circuits and Systems for Video Technology*, vol. 11, no. 5, pp. 651–657, May 2001.

[48] K. Andra, C. Chakrabarti, and T. Acharya, "A VLSI architecture for lifting-based forward and inverse wavelet transform," *IEEE Transactions on Signal Processing*, vol. 50, no. 4, pp. 966–977, Apr. 2002.

[49] C.-T. Huang, P.-C. Tseng, and L.-G. Chen, "Flipping structure: An efficient VLSI architecture for lifting-based discrete wavelet transform," *IEEE Transactions on Signal Processing*, vol. 52, no. 4, pp. 1080–1089, Apr. 2004.

[50] D. B. H. Tay, "A class of lifting based integer wavelet transform," *Proc. IEEE International Conference on Image Processing*, vol. 1, pp. 602–605, 2001.

[51] Z. Guangjun, C. Lizhi, and C. Huowang, "A simple 9/7-tap wavelet filter based on lifting scheme," *Proc. IEEE International Conference on Image Processing*, vol. 2, pp. 249–252, 2001.

[52] C.-T. Huang, P.-C. Tseng, and L.-G. Chen, "VLSI architecture for forward discrete wavelet transform based on B-spline factorization," *Journal of VLSI Signal Processing Systems*, vol. 40, pp. 343–353, 2005.

[53] ——, "Analysis and VLSI architecture for 1-D and 2-D discrete wavelet transform," *IEEE Transactions on Signal Processing*, vol. 53, no. 4, pp. 1575–1586, Apr. 2005.

[54] M. J. Tsai, J. D. Villasenor, and F. Chen, "Stack-run image coding," *IEEE Transactions on Circuits and Systems for Video Technology*, vol. 6, no. 5, pp. 519–521, Oct. 1996.

[55] N. Polyak and W. A. Pearlman, "A new flexible bi-orthogonal filter design for multiresolution filterbanks with application to image compression," *IEEE Transactions on Signal Processing*, vol. 48, no. 8, pp. 2279–2288, Aug. 2000.

[56] T. Q. Nguyen and P. P. Vaidyanathan, "Two-channel perfect-reconstruction FIR QMF structures which yield linear-phase analysis and synthesis filters," *IEEE Transactions on Acoustics, Speech, and Signal Processing*, vol. 37, no. 5, pp. 676–690, May 1989.

[57] C.-C. Cheng, C.-T. Huang, J.-Y. Chang, and L.-G. Chen, "Line buffer wordlength analysis for line-based 2-D DWT," *IEEE International Conference on Acoustics, Speech, and Signal Processing*, 2006.

[58] H. Choi, W. P. Burleson, and D. S. Phatak, "Optimal wordlength assignment for the discrete wavelet transform in VLSI," *Proceedings of IEEE Workshop on VLSI Signal Processing*, pp. 325 – 333, 1993.

[59] P.-C. Wu and L.-G. Chen, "An efficient architecture for two-dimensional discrete wavelet transform," *IEEE Transactions on Circuits and Systems for Video Technology*, vol. 11, no. 4, pp. 536–545, Apr. 2001.

[60] M. Weeks and M. Bayoumi, "Discrete wavelet transform: Architectures, design and performance issues," *Journal of VLSI Signal Processing Systems*, vol. 35, no. 2, pp. 155–178, Sept. 2003.

[61] N. D. Zervas, G. P. Anagnostopoulos, V. Spiliotopoulos, Y. Andreopoulos, and C. E. Goutis, "Evaluation of design alternatives for the 2-D-discrete wavelet transform," *IEEE Transactions on Circuits and Systems for Video Technology*, vol. 11, no. 12, pp. 1246–1262, Dec. 2001.

[62] P. E. Landman and J. M. Rabaey, "Architectural power analysis: The dual bit type method," *IEEE Transactions on Very Large Scale Integration (VLSI) Systems*, vol. 3, no. 2, pp. 173–187, June 1995.

[63] P.-C. Tseng, C.-T. Huang, and L.-G. Chen, "Generic RAM-based architecture for two-dimensional discrete wavelet transform with line-based method," *Asia-Pacific Conference on Circuits and Systems*, pp. 363–366, 2002.

[64] ——, "VLSI implementation of shape-adaptive discrete wavelet transform," *Proc. of SPIE International Conference on Visual Communications and Image Processing*, pp. 655–666, 2002.

[65] M. Vishwanath, "The recursive pyramid algorithm for the discrete wavelet transform," *IEEE Transactions on Signal Processing*, vol. 42, no. 3, pp. 673–677, Mar. 1994.

[66] C. Chrysafis and A. Ortega, "Line-based, reduced memory, wavelet image compression," *IEEE Transactions on Image Processing*, vol. 9, no. 3, pp. 378–389, Mar. 2000.

[67] C.-T. Huang, P.-C. Tseng, and L.-G. Chen, "Generic RAM-based architectures for two-dimensional discrete wavelet transform with line-based method," *IEEE Transactions on Circuits and Systems for Video Technology*, July 2005.

[68] C. Diou, L. Torres, and M. Robert, "A wavelet core for video processing," *Proc. of International Conference on Image Processing*, pp. 395–398, 2000.

[69] C. Chrysafis and A. Ortega, "Line-based, reduced memory, wavelet image compression," *IEEE Transactions on Image processing*, vol. 9, no. 3, pp. 378–389, Mar. 2000.

[70] Y.-H. Shiau and J. M. Jou, "A high-performance tree-block pipelining architecture for separate 2-D inverse discrete wavelet transform," *IEICE Transactions on Information and Systems*, vol. E86-D, no. 10, pp. 1966–1975, Oct. 2003.

[71] H. Y. et al., "Image processor capable of block-noise-free JPEG2000 compression with 30frames/s for digital camera applications," *IEEE International Solid-State Circuits Conference*, pp. 46–47, 2003.

[72] M.-Y. Chiu, K.-B. Lee, and C.-W. Jen, "Optimal data transfer and buffering schemes for JPEG 2000 encoder," *IEEE Workshop on Signal Processing Systems*, pp. 177–182, 2003.

[73] ——, "Optimal data transfer and buffering schemes for JPEG2000 encoder," *IEEE Workshop on Signal Processing Systems*, pp. 177–182, 2003.

[74] C.-C. Cheng, C.-T. Huang, P.-C. Tseng, C.-H. Pan, and L.-G. Chen, "Multiple-lifting scheme: Memory-efficient VLSI implementation for line-based 2-D DWT," *IEEE International Symposium on Circuits and Systems*, pp. 0–1, 2005.

[75] M. Weeks, "Precision for 2-D discrete wavelet transform processors," *IEEE*

Workshop on Signal Processing Systems, pp. 80–89, 2000.
[76] C.-T. Huang, P.-C. Tseng, and L.-G. Chen, "Memory analysis and architecture for two-dimentional discrete wavelet transform," *IEEE International Conference on Acoustics, Speech, and Signal Processing*, vol. 5, pp. 13–16, 2004.
[77] H.-C. Fang, C.-T. Huang, Y.-W. Chang, T.-C. Wang, P.-C. Tseng, C.-J. Lian, and L.-G. Chen, "81 MS/s JPEG 2000 single-chip encoder with rate-distortion optimization," *IEEE International Conference of Solid-State Circuits*, pp. 328–329, Feb. 2004.
[78] H.-C. Fang, Y.-W. Chang, C.-C. Cheng, C.-C. Chen, and L.-G. Chen, "Memory efficient JPEG 2000 architecture with stripe pipeline scheme," *IEEE International Conference on Acoustics, Speech, and Signal Processing*, vol. 5, pp. 1–4, Mar. 2005.
[79] *JPEG 2000 Verification Model 7.0 (Technical Description).* ISO/IEC JTC1/SC29/WG1 N1684, Apr. 2000.
[80] D. Taubman and M. Marchellin, *JPEG2000: Image Compression Fundamentals, Standards and Practice.* Kluwer Academic Publishers, 2002.
[81] L. Gall and A. Tabatabai, "Sub-band coding of digital images using symmetric short kernel filters and arithmetic coding techniques," *IEEE International Conference on Acoustics, Speech, and Signal Processing*, vol. 2, pp. 761–764, Apr. 1988.
[82] M. Antonini, M. Barlaud, P. Mathieu, and I. Daubechies, "Image coding using wavelet transform," *IEEE Transactions on Image Processing*, vol. 1, no. 2, pp. 205–220, Apr. 1992.
[83] D. Taubman, "High performance scalable image compression with EBCOT," *IEEE Transactions on Image Processing*, vol. 9, no. 7, pp. 1158–1170, July 2000.
[84] D. Taubman, E. Ordentlich, M. Weinberger, and G. Serourssi, "Embedded block coding in JPEG 2000," *IEEE International Conference of Image Processing*, vol. 2, pp. 33–36, Sept. 2000.
[85] (1998, Mar.) The independent JPEG group's JPEG software. [Online]. Available: ftp://ftp.uu.net/graphics/jpeg/jpegsrc.v6b.tar.gz
[86] J. Ribas-Corbera and S. Lei, "Rate control in DCT video coding for low-delay communications," *IEEE Transactions on Circuits and Systems for Video Technology*, vol. 9, no. 1, pp. 172–185, Feb. 1999.
[87] A. Nicoulin, M. Mattavelli, W. Li, A. Basso, A. Popat, and M. Kunt, "Image sequence coding using motion-compensated subband decomposition," M. I. Sezan and R. L. Lagendijk, Eds. Norwell, MA: Kluwer Academic Publisher, 1993, pp. 225–256.
[88] (2004, Nov.) H.264/AVC reference software jm90. [Online]. Available: http://iphome.hhi.de/suehring/tml/download/
[89] *Draft ITU-T Recommendation and Final Draft International Standard of Joint Video Specification.* ITU-T Rec. H.264 and ISO/IEC 14496-10 AVC, May 2003.
[90] Alma Technologies. (2002, Oct.) JPEG2K_E. [Online]. Available: http://www.alma-tech.com/

[91] Analog Devices. (2004, Mar.) ADV202. [Online]. Available: http://www.analog.com/

[92] DSPworx. (2002, Mar.) Cheetah. [Online]. Available: http://www.dspworx.com/cheetah.htm

[93] AMPHION. (2002, Oct.) CS6510. [Online]. Available: http://www.amphion.com/cs6510.html

[94] H. Yamauchi, S. Okada, K. Taketa, T. Ohyama, Y. Matsuda, T. Mori, S. Okada, T. Watanabe, Y. Matsuo, Y. Yamada, T. Ichikawa, and Y. Matsushita, "Image processor capable of block-noise-free JPEG2000 compression with 30 frames/s for digital camera applications," *IEEE International Conference of Solid-State Circuits*, pp. 46–47, Feb. 2003.

[95] P.-C. Tseng, C.-T. Huang, and L.-G. Chen, "Generic RAM-based architecture for two-dimensional discrete wavelet transform with line-based method," *IEEE Asia-Pacific Conference on Circuits and Systems*, vol. 1, pp. 363–366, Dec. 2002.

[96] H. Yamauchi, K. Mochizuki, K. Taketa, T. Watanabe, T. Mori, Y. Matsuda, Y. Matsushita, A. Kobayashi, and S. Okada, "A 1440×1080 pixels 30frames/s motion-JPEG2000 codec for hd movie transmission," *IEEE International Conference of Solid-State Circuits*, pp. 326–327, Feb. 2004.

[97] K. Andra, C. Chakrabarti, and T. Acharya, "A high-performance JPEG 2000 architecture," *IEEE Transactions on Circuits and Systems for Video Technology*, vol. 13, no. 3, pp. 209–218, Mar. 2003.

[98] B.-F. Wu and C.-F. Lin, "Analysis and architecture design for high performance JPEG2000 coprocessor," *IEEE International Conference on Circuits and Systems*, vol. 2, pp. 225–228, May 2004.

[99] C. Chrysafis and A. Ortega, "Line-based, reduced memory, wavelet image compression," *IEEE Transactions on Image Processing*, vol. 9, no. 3, pp. 378–389, Mar. 2000.

[100] C.-T. Huang, P.-C. Tseng, and L.-G. Chen, "Memory analysis and architecture for two-dimentional discrete wavelet transform," *IEEE International Conference on Acoustics, Speech, and Signal Processing*, vol. 5, pp. 13–16, May 2004.

[101] W. Sweldens, "The lifting scheme: a custom-design construction of biorthogonal wavelets," *Appl. Comput. Harmon. Anal.*, vol. 3, no. 15, pp. 186–200, 1996.

[102] C.-T. Huang, P.-C. Tseng, and L.-G. Chen, "Flipping structure: An efficient VLSI architecture for lifting-based discrete wavelet transform," *IEEE Transactions on Signal Processing*, vol. 52, no. 4, pp. 1080–1089, Apr. 2004.

[103] Y.-W. Chang, H.-C. Fang, C.-C. Cheng, C.-C. Chen, C.-J. Lian, and L.-G. Chen, "124 msmples/s pixel-pipelined motion-jpeg 2000 codec without tile memory," *IEEE International Conference of Solid-State Circuits*, 2006.

[104] D. Taubman and A. Zakhor, "Multi-rate 3-D subband coding of video," *IEEE Transactions on Image Processing*, pp. 572–588, 1994.

[105] J.-R. Ohm, "Three dimensional subband coding with motion compensation," *IEEE Transactions on Image Processing*, vol. 3, pp. 559–571, Sept. 1994.

[106] F. Dufaux and J. Konrad, "Efficient, robust, and fast global motion estimation for video coding," *IEEE Transactions on Image Processing*, vol. 9, pp. 497–501, Mar. 2000.

[107] *Video Codec for Audiovisual Services at p × 64 Kbit/s.* ITU-T Recommendation H.261, Mar. 1993.

[108] D. Secker and D. Taubman, "Highly scalable video compression using a lifting-based 3D wavelet transform with deformable mesh motion compensation," *Proc. IEEE International Conference on Image Processing*, pp. 749–752, 2002.

[109] G. Pau, B. P.-Popescu, M. Schaar, and J. Vieron, "Delay-performance trade-offs in motion-compensated scalable subband video compression," *Advanced Concepts for Intelligent Vision Systems*, 2004.

[110] I. JTC1, "Scalable Video Model 3.0," Oct. 2004.

[111] N. Bozinovic, J. Konrad, W. Zhao, and C. Vazquez, "On the importance of motion invertibility in MCTF/DWT video coding," *IEEE International Conference on Acoustics, Speech, and Signal Processing*, vol. 2, pp. 49–52, 2005.

[112] N. Bozinovic, J. Konrad, T. Andre, M. Antonini, and M. Barlaud, "Motion-compensated lifted wavelet video coding: toward optimal motion/transform configuration," *Proceeding Twelfth European Signal Processing Conference*, Sept. 2004.

[113] V. Valentin, M. Cagnazzo, M. Antonini, , and M. Barlaud, "Scalable context-based motion vector coding for video compression," *IEEE EURASIP Picture Coding Symposium*, Apr. 2003.

[114] C. Vazquez, E. Dubois, and J. Konrad, "Reconstruction of irregularly-sampled images in spline spaces," *IEEE Transaction on Image Processing to appear*, June 2004.

[115] J. R. Ohm, "Advanced in scalable video coding," *IEEE Proceeding*, vol. 93, no. 1, pp. 42–56, June 2005.

[116] S.-J. Choi and J. W. Woods, "Motion-compensated 3-D subband coding of video," *IEEE Trans. Image Processing*, vol. 8, no. 2, pp. 155–167, Feb. 1999.

[117] T. Rusert, K.Hanke, and J. R. Ohm, "Transition filtering and optimized quantization in interframe wavelet video coding," *Proc. of SPIE Visual Commun. Image Processing (VCIP'03)*, pp. 682–694, 2003.

[118] A. Golwelkar and J. W. Woods, "Scalable video compression using longer motion compensated temporal filters," *Proc. of SPIE Visual Commun. Image Processing (VCIP'03)*, pp. 1406–1417, 2003.

[119] M. Flierl and B. Girod, "Investigation of motion compensated lifted wavelet transforms," *Proc. of Picture Coding Symp.*, pp. 59–62, 2003.

[120] Y. Andreopoulos, M. van der Schaar, A. Munteanu, J. Barbarien, P. Schelkens, and J. Cornelis, "Full-scalable wavelet video coding using in-band motion compensated temporal filtering," *Proc. of IEEE Conf. Acoustics, Speech and Signal Processing*, pp. III417–III420, 2003.

[121] A. Secker and D. Taubman, "Lifting-based invertible motion adaptive transform (LIMAT) framework for highly scalable video compression," *IEEE*

Trans. Image Processing, vol. 12, no. 12, pp. 1530–1542, Dec. 2003.

[122] H. W. Park and H. S. Kim, "Motion estimation using low-band-shift method for wavelet-based moving picture coding," *IEEE Trans. Image Processing*, vol. 9, no. 4, pp. 577–587, Apr. 2000.

[123] G. V. der Auwera, A. Munteanu, J. Barbarien, P. Schelkens, and J. Cornelis, "Scalable wavelet video coding with in-band prediction - the bottom-up overcomplete discrete wavelet transform," *Proc. of IEEE Conf. Image Processing*, pp. 729–732, 2002.

[124] *Video Coding for Low Bit Rate Communication.* ITU-T Recommendation H.263, May 1996.

[125] I. JTC1, "Scalable Video Model 2.0," July 2004.

[126] D. V. C. Group, *ITU-T recommendation H.263 software implementation.* Telenor R&D, 1995.

[127] W. Li and E. Salari, "Successive elimination algorithm for motion estimation," *IEEE Trans. Image Processing*, vol. 4, no. 1, pp. 105–107, Jan. 1995.

[128] J. N. Kim and T. S. Choi, "A fast full-search motion-estimation algorithm using representative pixels and adaptive matching scan," *IEEE Trans. Circuits Syst. Video Technol.*, vol. 10, no. 7, pp. 1040–1048, Oct. 2000.

[129] C. K. Cheung and L. M. Po, "Normalized partial distortion search algorithm for block motion estimation," *IEEE Trans. Circuits Syst. Video Technol.*, vol. 10, no. 3, pp. 417–422, Apr. 2000.

[130] X. Q. Gao, C. J. Duanmu, and C. R. Zou, "A multilevel successive elimination algorithm for block matching motion estimation," *IEEE Trans. Image Processing*, vol. 9, no. 3, pp. 501–504, Mar. 2000.

[131] M. Brünig and W. Niehsen, "Fast full-search block matching," *IEEE Trans. Circuits Syst. Video Technol.*, vol. 11, no. 2, pp. 241–247, Feb. 2001.

[132] C. Zhu, W. S. Qi, and W. Ser, "A new successive elimination algorithm for fast block matching in motion estimation," *Proc. of IEEE Int. Symp. Circuits Syst. (ISCAS'04)*, pp. 733–736, 2004.

[133] M. Bierling, "Displacement estimation by hierarchical block matching," *Proc. of SPIE Visual Commun. Image Processing (VCIP'88)*, pp. 942–951, 1988.

[134] B. Liu and A. Zaccarin, "New fast algorithms for the estimation of block motion vectors," *IEEE Trans. Circuits Syst. Video Technol.*, vol. 3, no. 2, pp. 148–157, Apr. 1993.

[135] Z. L. He, C. Y. Tsui, K. K. Chan, and M. L. Liou, "Low-power VLSI design for motion estimation using adaptive pixel truncation," *IEEE Trans. Circuits Syst. Video Technol.*, vol. 10, no. 5, pp. 669–678, Aug. 2000.

[136] J. Y. Tham, S. Ranganath, M. Ranganath, and A. A. Kassim, "A novel unrestricted center-biased diamond search algorithm for block motion estimation," *IEEE Trans. Circuits Syst. Video Technol.*, vol. 8, no. 4, pp. 369–377, Aug. 1998.

[137] S. Zhu and K. K. Ma, "A new diamond search algorithm for fast block-matching motion estimation," *IEEE Trans. Image Processing*, vol. 9, no. 2, pp. 287–290, Feb. 2000.

[138] A. M. Tourapis, O. C. Au, M. L. Liou, G. Shen, and I. Ahmad, "Optimizing

the mpeg-4 encoder - advanced diamond zonal search," *Proc. of IEEE Int. Symp. Circuits Syst. (ISCAS'00)*, pp. 674–677, 2000.

[139] A. M. Tourapis, O. C. Au, and M. L. Liu, "Highly efficient predictive zonal algorithms for fast block-matching motion estimation," *IEEE Trans. Circuits Syst. Video Technol.*, vol. 12, no. 10, pp. 934–947, Oct. 2002.

[140] T. Koga, K. Iinuma, A. Hirano, Y. Iijima, and T. Ishiguro, "Motion compensated interframe coding for video conferencing," *Proc. Nat. Telecommun. Conf.*, pp. C9.6.1–C9.6.5, 1981.

[141] J. Jain and A. Jain, "Displacement measurement and its application in internal image coding," *IEEE Trans. Commun.*, vol. COM-29, no. 12, pp. 1799–1808, Dec. 1981.

[142] M. J. Chen, L. G. Chen, and T. D. Chiueh, "One-dimensional full search motion estimation algorithm for video coding," *IEEE Trans. Circuits Syst. Video Technol.*, vol. 4, no. 5, pp. 504–509, June 1994.

[143] R. Li, B. Zeng, and M. L. Liou, "A new three-step search algorithm for block motion estimation," *IEEE Trans. Circuits Syst. Video Technol.*, vol. 4, no. 4, pp. 438–442, Aug. 1994.

[144] L. M. Po and W. C. Ma, "A novel four-step search algorithm for fast block motion estimation," *IEEE Trans. Circuits Syst. Video Technol.*, vol. 6, no. 3, pp. 313–317, June 1996.

[145] L. K. Liu and E. Feig, "A block-based gradient descent search algorithm for block motion estimation in video coding," *IEEE Trans. Circuits Syst. Video Technol.*, vol. 6, no. 4, pp. 419–422, Aug. 1996.

[146] Y. W. Huang, S. Y. Ma, C. F. Shen, and L. G. Chen, "Predictive line search: an efficient motion estimation algorithm for mpeg-4 encoding systems on multimedia processors," *IEEE Trans. Circuits and Syst. Video Technol.*, vol. 13, no. 1, pp. 111–117, Jan. 2003.

[147] C. W. Lam, L. M. Po, and C. H. Cheung, "A novel kite-cross-diamond search algorithm for fast video coding and videoconferencing applications," *Proc. of IEEE Int. Conf. Acoust., Speech, and Signal Processing (ICASSP'04)*, pp. 365–368, 2004.

[148] D. Tzovaras, M. G. Strintzis, and H. Sahinolou, "Evaluation of multiresolution block matching techniques for motion and disparity estimation," *Signal Processing: Image Commun.*, vol. 6, pp. 56–67, 1994.

[149] J. H. Lee, K. W. Lim, B. C. Song, and J. B. Ra, "A fast multi-resolution block matching algorithm and its VLSI architecture for low bit-rate video coding," *IEEE Trans. Circuits Syst. Video Technol.*, vol. 11, no. 12, pp. 1289–1301, Dec. 2001.

[150] J. H. Lee and N. S. Lee, "Variable block size motion estimation algorithm and its hardware architecture for H.264," *Proc. of IEEE Int. Symp. Circuits Syst. (ISCAS'04)*, pp. 740–743, 2004.

[151] A. Joch, F. Kossentini, H. Schwarz, T. Wiegand, and G. J. Sullivan, "Performance comparison of video coding standards using lagragian coder control," *Proc. of IEEE International Conference on Image Processing*, 2002.

[152] K. M. Yang, M. T. Sun, and L. Wu, "A family of VLSI designs for the motion compensation block-matching algorithm," *IEEE Trans. Circuits Syst.*,

vol. 36, no. 2, pp. 1317–1325, Oct. 1989.

[153] T. Komarek and P. Pirsch, "Array architectures for block matching algorithms," *IEEE Trans. Circuits Syst.*, vol. 36, no. 2, pp. 1301–1308, Oct. 1989.

[154] J. F. Shen, T. C. Wang, and L. G. Chen, "A novel low-power full search block-matching motion estimation design for H.263+," *IEEE Trans. Circuits Syst. Video Technol.*, vol. 11, no. 7, pp. 890–897, July 2001.

[155] H. Yeo and Y. H. Hu, "A novel modular systolic array architecture for full-search block matching motion estimation," *IEEE Trans. Circuits Syst. Video Technol.*, vol. 5, no. 5, pp. 407–416, Oct. 1995.

[156] Y. K. Lai and L. G. Chen, "A data-interlacing architecture with two-dimensional data-reuse for full-search block-matching algorithm," *IEEE Trans. Circuits Syst. Video Technol.*, vol. 8, no. 2, pp. 124–127, Apr. 1998.

[157] S. F. Chang, J. H. Hwang, and C. W. Jen, "Scalable array architecture design for full search block matching," *IEEE Trans. Circuits Syst. Video Technol.*, vol. 5, no. 4, pp. 332–343, Aug. 1995.

[158] L. D. Vos and M. Stegherr, "Parameterizable VLSI architectures for the full-search block-matching algorithm," *IEEE Trans. Circuits Syst.*, vol. 36, no. 2, pp. 1309–1316, Oct. 1989.

[159] N. Roma and L. Sousa, "Efficient and configurable full-search block-matching processors," *IEEE Trans. Circuits Syst. Video Technol.*, vol. 12, no. 12, pp. 1160–1167, Dec. 2002.

[160] Y. S. Jehng, L. G. Chen, and T. D. Chiueh, "An efficient and simple VLSI tree architecture for motion estimation algorithms," *IEEE Trans. Signal Processing*, vol. 41, no. 2, pp. 889–900, Feb. 1993.

[161] W. M. Chao, C. W. Hsu, Y. C. Chang, and L. G. Chen, "A novel motion estimator supporting diamond search and fast full search," *Proc. of IEEE Int. Symp. Circuits Syst. (ISCAS'02)*, pp. 492–495, 2002.

[162] S. Dutta and W. Wolf, "A flexible parallel architecture adopted to block-matching motion estimation algorithms," *IEEE Trans. Circuits Syst. Video Technol.*, vol. 6, no. 1, pp. 74–86, Feb. 1996.

[163] H. D. Lin, A. Anesko, and B. Petryna, "A 14-GOPS programmable motion estimator for H.26X video coding," *IEEE J. Solid-State Circuits*, vol. 31, no. 11, pp. 1742–1750, Nov. 1996.

[164] S. C. Cheng and H. M. Hang, "A comparison of block-matching algorithms mapped to systolic-array implementation," *IEEE Trans. Circuits Syst. Video Technol.*, vol. 7, no. 5, pp. 741–757, Aug. 1997.

[165] C.-T. Huang, C.-Y. Chen, Y.-H. Chen, and L.-G. Chen, "Memory analysis of VLSI architecture for 5/3 and 1/3 motion-compensated temporal filtering," *Proc. IEEE International Conference on Acoustics, Speech, and Signal Processing*, 2005.

[166] C.-Y. Chen, C.-T. Huang, Y.-H. Chen, and L.-G. Chen, "System analysis of VLSI architecture for motion-compensated temporal filtering," *Proc. of International Conference on Image Processing*, 2005.

[167] J. V. T. of ISO/IEC MPEG and I.-T. VCEG, *H.264/AVC Reference Software JM9.0*, 2004.

Index